D0380200

BIOETHICS

Fourth Edition

BIOETHICS

*basic writings on the
key ethical questions that surround
the major, modern biological
possibilities and problems*

edited by
THOMAS A. SHANNON

Cover Design: Tim McKeen

Library of Congress Cataloging-in-Publication Data

Bioethics : basic writings on the key ethical questions that surround the major, modern
     biological possibilities and problems / edited by Thomas A. Shannon. — 4th ed.
          p.   cm.
     Includes bibliographical references.
     ISBN 0-8091-3444-6
     1. Medical ethics.   2. Bioethics.   I. Shannon, Thomas A. (Thomas Anthony), 1940–.
R724.B47   1994
174'.2—dc20   93-23504
                                                                                    CIP

Published by Paulist Press
997 Macarthur Blvd.
Mahwah, New Jersey 07430

Printed and bound in the
United States of America

Contents

PART THREE
CONSENT, THERAPY, AND RESEARCH

PART FOUR
PUBLIC POLICY ISSUES

ACKNOWLEDGEMENTS

The following articles have been used with permission of the proper copyright holders. All rights reserved.

1. Daniel Callahan, "An Ethical Challenge to Prochoice Advocates," *Commonweal* 117 (23 November 1990): 681–687. Copyright Commonweal Foundation © 1990.

2. Thomas A. Shannon and Allan B. Wolter, "Reflections on the Moral Status of the Pre-embryo," *Theological Studies* 51 (December 1990): 603–626.

3. Scott Aaron, "The Choice in 'Choose Life'," *Commonweal* 119 (28 February 1992), 15–18. Copyright Commonweal Foundation © 1992.

4. Brenda Almond and Carole Ulanowsky, "HIV and Pregnancy," *Hastings Center Report* 20 (March/April 1990): 16–21.

5. Maura A. Ryan, "The Argument for Unlimited Procreative Liberty: A Feminist Critique," *Hastings Center Report* 20 (July/August 1990): 6–12.

6. Richard A. McCormick, "Therapy or Tampering: The Ethics of Reproductive Technology and the Development of Doctrine," in *The Critical Calling: Reflections on Moral Dilemmas Since Vatican II* (Washington, D.C.: Georgetown University Press, 1989): 329–352.

7. Marc Lappé, "Ethical Issues in Manipulating the Human Germ Line," *The Journal of Medicine and Philosophy* 16 (December 1991): 621–639.

8. W. French Anderson, "Human Gene Therapy: Why Draw A Line?" *The Journal of Medicine and Philosophy* 14 (December 1989): 681–693.

9. Hans Jonas, "The Burden and Blessing of Mortality," *Hastings Center Report* 22 (January/February 1992): 34–40.

10. Timothy E. Quill, "Death and Dignity: A Case of Individualized Decision Making," *The New England Journal of Medicine* 324 (7 March 1991): 691–694.

11. Thomas A. Shannon and James J. Walter, "The PVS Patient and the Forgoing/Withdrawing of Medical Nutrition and Hydration," *Theological Studies* 49 (December 1988): 623–647.

12. William A. Gray, Robert J. Capone, Albert S. Most, "Unsuccessful Emergency Medical Resuscitation: Are Continued Efforts in the Emergency Department Justified?" *The New England Journal of Medicine* 325 (14 November 1991): 1393–1398.

13. The Atlanta Archdiocese, "Friend-of-the-Court Brief for Larry James McAfee," *Origins* 19 (28 September 1989): 273, 275–279.

14. Ezekiel J. Emanuel and Linda L. Emanuel, "Living Wills: Past, Present, and Future," *The Journal of Clinical Ethics* 1 (Spring 1990): 9–19.

15. Albert R. Jonsen, "Initiative 119: What Is at Stake?" *Commonweal* 118 (9 August 1991): 466–468. Copyright Commonweal Foundation © 1991.

16. Andrew W. McThenia, "Deciding for Others: Issues of Consent," *Second Opinion* 5 (1987): 76–99.

17. Steven H. Miles, "Informed Demand for 'Non-beneficial' Medical Treatment," *The New England Journal of Medicine* 325 (15 August 1991): 512–515.

18. Terrence F. Ackerman, "Balancing Moral Principles in Federal Regulations on Human Research," *IRB: A Review of Human Subjects Research* 14 (January/February 1992): 1–6.

19. Carol Levine, Nancy Neveloff Dubler, and Robert J. Levine, "Building a New Consensus: Ethical Principles and Policies for Clinical Research on HIV/AIDS," *IRB: A Review of Human Subjects Research* 13 (January/April 1991): 1–17.

20. Giles R. Scofield, "Is Consent Useful When Resuscitation Isn't?" *Hastings Center Report* 21 (November/December 1991): 28–36.

21. Dorothy C. Wertz and John C. Fletcher, "Privacy and Disclosure in Medical Genetics Examined in an Ethics of Care," *Bioethics* 5 (July 1991): 212–232.

22. Susan Wendell, "Toward a Feminist Theory of Disability," in Helen Bequaert Holmes and Laura M. Purdy (eds.), *Feminist Perspectives in Medical Ethics* (Bloomington: Indiana University Press, 1992), 63–81. Also appeared in *Hypatia* 2 (Summer 1989): 104–124.

23. John La Puma and Edward F. Lawlor, "Quality-Adjusted Life-Years: Ethical Implications for Physicians and Policymakers," *Journal of the American Medical Association* 263 (6 June 1990): 2917–2921. Copyright © 1990, American Medical Association.

24. David C. Hadorn, "The Oregon Priority-Setting Exercise: Quality of Life and Public Policy," *Hastings Center Report* 20 (May/June 1991): 11–16.

25. James F. Childress, "Ethics, Public Policy, and Human Fetal Tissue Transplantation Research," *Kennedy Institute of Ethics Journal* 1 (June 1991): 93–121.

26. Robert M. Veatch, "Routine Inquiry About Organ Donation: An Alternative to Presumed Consent," *The New England Journal of Medicine* 325 (24 October 1991): 1246–1249.

27. Leon R. Kass, "Organs for Sale? Propriety, Property, and the Price of Progress," *The Public Interest* 107 (Spring 1992): 65–86. With permission of the author.

28. Alexander Morgan Capron, "Which Ills To Bear? Reevaluating the 'Threat' of Modern Genetics," *Emory Law Journal* 39 (Summer 1990): 665–696.

29. Ronald Bayer, "Public Health Policy and the AIDS Epidemic: An End to HIV Exceptionalism?" *The New England Journal of Medicine* 324 (23 May 1991): 1500–1504.

30. Nancy S. Jecker and Robert A. Pearlman, "An Ethical Framework for Rationing Health Care," *The Journal of Medicine and Philosophy* 17 (February 1992): 79–96.

Preface to the Fourth Edition

I am honored by the decision of the editors of Paulist Press to produce the fourth edition of this Reader. I am pleased that faculty and students continue to find this Reader a helpful addition to their classes.

As one would expect, the problems in the field of bioethics have become even more complicated and new ones are added on an almost daily basis. Consequently the selection process for articles continues to present major challenges.

To reflect changing times and needs, this fourth edition will be different in four major ways. First, it will contain fewer articles. My hope is that the brevity will make the Reader more useful in the classroom. Additionally too large a text can be intimidating. One of my colleagues refers—fondly, I trust—to the third edition as the "telephone book." The desire to be too inclusive in content and articles can be dysfunctional conceptually as well as pedagogically. Second, none of the articles in this edition is carried over from previous editions. The third edition retained seven articles from the original 1976 edition. These articles I still regard as classic essays, but times and needs change. Third, I have developed a new method of organizing the traditional topics. I have grouped articles around four general themes—abortion and reproduction; death and dying; consent, therapy, and research; and public policy issues. I hope this will be a format that is easily adapted to the general way courses are organized. Fourth, not all of the standard commentators are represented. The reason for this is simply that newer scholars are making significant contributions and these need to be recognized.

My hope is that these articles, organized in this fashion and with these general criteria, will provide a context for the continuing discussion and debate of these most critical problems.

I am particularly thankful to Russ Conners, Pat McCormick, Steve Lammers, and Jim Walter who took the time to consider my proposal and to suggest other authors and articles. I appreciate their help as well as the continuing conversations I have with them.

I would also like to express my continuing gratitude to Jon Strauss, the President of WPI, and JoAnn Manfra, Department Chair, and my colleagues in the Humanities Department for their continuing support and encouragement of my work. Such collegiality is a rare, but deeply appreciated, gift.

Thomas A. Shannon
Department of Humanities
Worcester Polytechnic Institute
Winter, 1993

introduction | *Thematic Ethical Issues*

Thomas A. Shannon

To prepare you for some of the discussions that will emerge in the various topics and to help give you a basic framework for ethical analysis, this essay will present, first, a discussion of ethical theories or methods and, second, definitions of basic ethical concepts.

1. Ethical Theories

In general, an ethical theory is the process by which we justify a particular ethical decision. It is the basis on which we organize complex information and competing values and interests to formulate an answer to the question "What should I do?" The main purpose of a theory is to provide consistency and coherence in our decision making. That is, an ethical theory or framework gives us a coherent way to approach various problems. If we have a theory, we don't have to figure out where to begin each time we meet a new problem. A theory also allows us to develop some degree of consistency in our decision making. We will begin to see how different values relate to each other. If we are consistent and coherent in our decision making, we will have a greater degree of internal unity and integrity in our decision making. Given the complexity of problems to be addressed, these qualities are extremely worthwhile.

a. *Consequentialism*

The ethical theory of consequentialism answers the question "What should I do?" by giving priority to the consequences of the various answers. That is, what is ethical is that consequence which brings about the greatest number of advantages over disadvantages or which brings about the greatest good for the greatest number of people. Basically, in this method, one looks to outcomes, to consequences, to the situation, and, from that perspective, one decides what is ethical. The ethical theories of situation ethics and utilitarianism are frequently mentioned types of consequentialist ethical theories.

The major benefit of this theory is that it looks to the actual impact of a

3

particular decision and asks how people will be affected by it. Consequentialism is attuned to the nuances of life and seeks to be responsive to them. The major problem of this theory is that the theory itself provides no standard by which one would measure one outcome against another. That is, while being sensitive to the circumstances, consequentialism has no basis for evaluating one outcome against another.

b. *Deontologism*

Deontological ethics, which derives its name from the Greek word for duty, *deon,* looks to one's obligations to determine what is ethical. This theory answers the question "What should I do?" by specifying my obligations or moral duties. The ethical act is one in which I meet my obligations, my responsibilities, or fulfill my duties. For a deontologist, obligation and rules are primary, for only by attending to these dimensions of morality can one be sure that self-interest does not override moral obligations. The Ten Commandments and Kant's Categorical Imperative are probably the most common examples of deontological ethics.

The major benefit of deontological ethics is the clarity and certainty of its starting point. Once the rules are known or the duties determined, then what is ethical is evident. The major problem is the potential insensitivity to consequences. By looking only at duty, one may miss important outcomes of a resolution of a dilemma.

c. *Rights Ethics*

This theory resolves ethical dilemmas by first determining what rights or moral claims are involved. Then dilemmas are resolved in terms of the hierarchy of rights. Paramount for a person of this orientation is that the moral claims of individuals—their rights—are taken seriously. The ethical theory of rights is a popular one in our American culture. Consider, for example, the central role this theory plays in the abortion and euthanasia debates.

The main advantage of a rights theory is that it highlights the moral centrality of the person and his or her moral claims in a situation of ethical conflict. On the other hand, this theory does not tell us how to resolve conflicts of rights between individuals. The theory makes the claims of the individual central without telling us how to resolve potential conflicts of rights between individuals or groups.

d. *Intuitionism*

Intuitionism resolves ethical dilemmas by appealing to one's intuition, a moral faculty of the person which directly apprehends what is right or wrong. Thus an intuitionist knows what is right or wrong, not by appeal to circumstances, duties, or rights, but by appeal to one's moral sense. While one's intuition may confer duties, the duty is not the point of departure; one's moral sense is.

We all know of situations in which all we can say is "I'm doing this because I know it's right," and that is the end of the moral argument. Experientially we know that we frequently rely on this method, and the strength that comes from such a moral intuition is great. Nonetheless, if we cannot externalize or publicize in some fashion our process of decision making, we cannot be totally accountable to others. Thus while intuitionism may give us the necessary courage of our convictions, it does not provide us with a way of convincing others that our way is correct.

2. ETHICAL TERMS

In the course of this book various terms will be frequently used. Philosophers, like physicians, nurses, lawyers, and other professionals, have their own language and jargon. This section will introduce you to some of the basic terms used in bioethical discussions so you can join in on the conversations.

a. *Autonomy*

Autonomy is a form of personal liberty of action in which the individual determines his or her course of action in accordance with a plan of his or her own choosing. Autonomy involves two elements. First is the capacity to deliberate about a plan of action. One must be capable of examining alternatives and distinguishing between them. Second, one must have the resources to put this plan into action. Autonomy includes the ability to actualize or carry out what one has decided.

In many ways, autonomy is the all-American value or virtue. It affirms that we ought to be the master of our own fate or the captain of our ship. Autonomy mandates a strong sense of personal responsibility for our own lives. Autonomy celebrates the hardy individualism for which our country is famous. It emphasizes creativity and productivity while being the enemy of conformity. Autonomy mandates that we choose who we wish to be and take responsibility for that.

But too heavy a reliance on individuality and control of one's self can isolate one from the community, from one's family, from one's friends. While ultimately I am responsible for myself and my actions, the community can also be involved in my learning what my responsibilities are and can also set obligations that I need to respect as I make my decisions. While autonomous, I still live within a social network that can make important contributions to my well-being.

Thus, while autonomy is important, and plays a critical role in bio-ethics, it needs to be understood within the context of the community as well as other moral responsibilities that I may have.[1]

b. *Nonmaleficence*

Nonmaleficence is the technical way of stating that we have an obligation not to harm people. One of the most ancient ethical principles of medical ethics is "First of all, do no harm," derived from the Hippocratic tradition. If we can't benefit someone, then at least we should do him or her no harm.

The harm we are to avoid is typically understood as physical or mental. But harm can also include injuries to one's interests such as having my property unjustly taken or having my access to it restricted. Or I can be harmed by having my liberty of speech or action unfairly restricted. Although there is no necessary physical impact on me from these latter harms, nonetheless these are genuine harms to me.

The duty of nonmaleficence clearly imposes an obligation not to harm someone intentionally or directly. But this duty also prohibits exposing others to a risk of harm. For example, if I am driving too fast, I may not actually harm someone, but I am clearly exposing individuals to the risk of harm. Thus the duty of nonmaleficence would prohibit speeding.[2]

But there are other situations in which individuals are exposed to actual harm or the risk of harm and the duty of nonmaleficence is not violated. An individual receiving chemotherapy is exposed to various risks of harm from the therapy. Can such risks of harm be justified and, if so, how?

The traditional method for examining the legitimation of risks or harmful effects is the principle of double effect. This tradition has its origin in traditional Roman Catholic theology but has gained wide acceptance as a means of judging the moral acceptability of risks and harms.

The principle of double effect[3] has four conditions:

1. What we are going to do must not be evil or wrong.

2. The harm we are considering must not be the means of producing the good effect.

3. The evil or harmful effect may not be intended, but merely permitted or tolerated.

4. There must be a proportionate reason for performing the action in spite of the consequences the act has.

As traditionally stated, this principle makes certain assumptions about actions, namely that there are some actions that are known to be wrong independent of circumstances, e.g. abortion or euthanasia. Thus no amount of consideration of circumstances could ever permit an act of direct euthanasia because such an act would be considered wrong in itself and would never meet the first criterion. Debates over whether acts are wrong in themselves or not have led many to focus on the fourth criterion as the key element in moral decision making. That is, the fourth criterion suggests that one might not know in advance whether or not an action is wrong and that a major element in discerning this is to determine whether or not there is a proportionate reason for performing the act.

Richard McCormick[4] has identified three factors to take into consideration in determining whether a reason is proportionate. First, there is at stake a value at least equal in importance to the one sacrificed. Second, there is no less harmful way, here and now, of protecting the good we are seeking to attain. Third, the way the value is achieved should not undermine that value in the future.

McCormick's point is that establishing a proportionate reason is not like solving an arithmetic problem. Rather we need to exercise prudence and gauge the effect of our acts on other values. The duty of nonmaleficence stands as a strong reminder that we have an obligation not to harm, but that when some harm or risk of harm appears to be necessary, then we need to be morally accountable for determining that decision. The principle of double effect provides that process of justification.

c. Beneficence

Beneficence is the positive dimension of nonmaleficence. The duty of beneficence claims that we have a duty to help others further their interests when we can do this without significant risk to ourselves. Thus the duty of beneficence argues that we have a positive obligation to regard the welfare of others, to be of assistance to others as they attempt to fulfill their plans. The duty of beneficence is based on a sense of fair play, suggesting that because we have received benefits from others or because we have been helped along the way, we have an obligation to return that same favor to others. Beneficence is a way of ensuring reciprocity in our relations and of passing along to others the goods we have received in the past.[5]

But this duty is not without limit. The limit is harm to one's self. Beauchamp and Childress have identified a process which one can use to evaluate the risk of harm to determine our degree of obligation. First, the individual we are to help is at risk of significant loss or danger. Second, I can perform an act directly relevant to preventing this loss or damage. Third, my act is likely to prevent this damage or loss. Fourth, the benefits that the individual receives as a consequence of my actions (a) outweigh harms to self and (b) present minimal risk to self.[6]

Again we have the necessity of making a prudential calculation about risks and benefits. Sometimes this calculation may be clear. If someone is drowning and I cannot swim, I am not obligated to go in the water to help the person, although I would be obligated to assist in other ways. But the calculation may be problematic. Does a health care professional have a duty to care for someone with AIDS? Here the moral calculus is complicated because of unclarity about the efficiency of various modes of transmission, the time of incubation, and the effectiveness of traditional isolation techniques, as well as the as yet incurable nature of the disease.

d. *Justice*

On the one hand, the basic meaning or intent of justice is rather straightforward. Justice deals in various ways with the distribution of benefits and burdens, of goods and services according to a just standard. But determining that just standard has perplexed and puzzled people down through the ages.[7]

There are two basic types of justice. Comparative justice argues that what one person or group receives is determined by balancing the competing claims of other individuals or groups. In comparative justice, what one receives is determined by one's conditions or needs, and how those relate to similar needs of others in society. Thus one person may need a kidney transplant more than another because person A is dying of renal failure while person B has just been diagnosed as having kidney disease. The point of comparative justice is a balancing of the needs of individuals competing for the same resource.

Noncomparative justice determines distribution of goods or resources by a standard independent of the claims of others. Here we have a principle of distribution or treatment, not an evaluation of the specifics of the case or the needs of individuals. Good examples of noncomparative standards are the distribution according to strict numerical equality experience or the attempt by the state of Oregon to provide therapies based on a legislatively determined cost-benefit analysis, not the needs of the patient. In noncomparative justice, allocation, distribution or treatment is determined by principle, not need.

Similarly, there are two basic principles of justice: formal and material. The formal principle of justice specifies a procedure to be followed in allocating goods or distributing burdens. The traditional principle of justice is derivative from the Greek philosopher, Aristotle: equals are to be treated equally and unequals unequally. Or to restate it, to each, his or her own.

The formal principle of justice is noncomparative in that it states a rule by which distributions are to be measured. It proposes a standard independent of needs or individuals. However, the rule does not tell how we determine what qualifies for equality or inequality. That is, with respect to what standard is someone equal or unequal? What is morally relevant in our determining equality and inequality? The strength of the formal principle of justice is that it gives us a clear rule; its major deficit is that it does not specify its moral content.

To cope with the problem of applications, material principles of justice have been devised. Generally speaking, a material principle of justice identifies some relevant property or criterion on the basis of which a distribution can be made. Thus material principles of justice are typically, though not always, comparative in that they examine needs or qualifications and on that basis determine what to do. Let me illustrate this by identifying several of these material principles of justice.

First is the noncomparative material principle of to each an equal share. The standard is strict numerical equality, and one arrives at this by dividing what is to be allocated by the number of actual recipients. Second is distribution according to individual need. Here one looks at specific needs of individuals and judges them, one against the other. This, like the third principle of justice—social worth—is obviously comparative. Social worth criteria go beyond needs and evaluate the status of an individual or his or her actual or potential contributions to society. The final form of material justice, which is also comparative, is distribution according to individual effort. This criterion does not examine accomplishments but looks at what one attempted and the efforts to realize that. The higher the effort, the greater the reward.

Each of these principles has its benefits and problems and because of this a middle way has been suggested. This method of allocation emphasizes formal equality but shifts this by utilizing equality of opportunity rather than one of the comparative forms of justice. This method of distribution is randomization either through a lottery or by distribution to people as they show up.

The obvious benefit of this method is that it protects strongly our intuitive sense of respect for people. That is, randomization provides a formal rule of allocation that does not force us to make invidious and potentially harmful choices between people based on assumptions about social worth. Individuals maintain their dignity because they will be treated fairly by having an equality of opportunity. Finally, such a system will help maintain trust between members of the health care team and the patient. The patient is not at the mercy of biases of an institution or individuals, but rather knows that he or she will be treated fairly.

On the other hand, this standard does not deal with some important questions. First, should there be some medical screen through which one should pass before entering the randomization schema? Second, should one's condition or likelihood of benefit be considered? That is, if a fifteen year old is more likely to benefit from a procedure than an eighty year old, should the eighty year old have an equal opportunity for treatment? Third, the mode of distribution assumes an endless supply of resources in that the only relevant criterion is equality of opportunity, not appropriateness of intervention or resource allocation.

e. *Informed Consent*

Informed consent is, I think, the most critical problem in bioethics. This is the time when health care professionals and patients can discuss value implications of treatments or clarify what is important for each of them. Consent negotiations allow discussions of issues of importance for all involved parties.

Informed consent is the knowledge of and consent to a particular form of treatment before that treatment is administered. There are four major elements in this definition.[8]

1. *Competence.* Competence generally refers to a person's capacity for decision making. A person may experience full competence, in that he or she is in control of one's life. Or competence may be limited. A person may have decision making capacities in one area but not another. An individual may not comprehend the value of money and may be restrained in its use but may be quite capable of making other decisions of daily living concerning nutrition, personal hygiene, or appointment making. Age may also limit competence in that one may be competent for some activities but not others. Finally, and most difficultly, one may be intermittently competent. Consider, for example, a person in the early stages of senility. At times this individual may be competent, but at other times he or she may be unaware of the implications of his or her choices.

To help sort out the difficult issues of evaluating competence, three different standards will be presented in order of increasing complexity. The first standard states that a person is competent when he or she has made a decision. When presented with a choice, the individual chooses an alternative. The fact of a choice is evidence of competence. Second is the capacity to give reasons for one's choice. Competence here requires some process of justification, an articulation of why one made this choice. The third standard argues that not only should one be able to give reasons for one's choice, but also that this choice should be a reasonable one.

Each of these standards is different and raises a variety of value judgments. What is most critical is that individuals be aware of what standard of competence they are using and recognize that it may conflict with the judgments of others.

2. *Disclosure.* Disclosure refers to the content of what a patient is told during the consent negotiation. There are two general standards for disclosure. The more traditional standard is the professional standard: what a person is told is what professionals typically tell patients. The obligation to inform patients is fulfilled by telling a patient what one's colleagues would tell that same patient. The obvious problem with this standard is that one's colleagues may tell a patient little or nothing. That is, the professional standard may be simply to tell a patient as little as possible about one's condition. In this situation, the standard is met, the obligation fulfilled, but the patient remains ignorant.

The more recent standard is that of the reasonable person. Here the health care provider is obligated to disclose what the reasonable person would want to know. One cannot fulfill the obligation by saying nothing; some information must be communicated. And the degree of specificity is centered outside the profession in the hypothetical reasonable person. Such a standard promotes autonomy and is protective of patients' rights. Nonetheless it remains on a general level.

This level of generality is why I think it important to go further and determine what this particular patient wants to know. Such a standard of disclosure recognizes a patient's right to be informed but, more importantly, it qualifies that right with respect to the patient's desires. Some patients may want to know nothing; others may want additional reading they can do. Only by determining what this particular patient wants to know can his or her rights be respected and protected.

3. *Comprehension.* In addition to having information disclosed, one must also comprehend that information. If a patient doesn't understand what he or she has been told, there is no way that individual can use the information.

Comprehension presents many problems and may test the patience of health care professionals. Some may assume that patients simply cannot understand the complexity of the issues. Others may assume that one does not comprehend unless one receives a mini-course in medicine. Or one may assume that there is not sufficient time to fully inform an individual.

Several issues should be noted here. First, from the fact that someone is not "fully" informed, it does not follow that he or she is not "adequately" informed. Second, health care professionals have a professional language. While that language is appropriate for peer communication, it is inappropriate for communication with patients. Thus, professionals need to translate their terms and jargon so it will be intelligible to others. Third, comprehension typically requires time, especially when the diagnosis is poor. Being informed does not necessitate being told everything at once. Fulfilling the condition of comprehension requires a sensitivity to what a patient can take in at one time.

4. *Voluntariness.* Voluntariness refers to one's ability to make a choice without being unduly pressured to make a particular choice by any specific person. Being free in making a decision means that we own the decision, that the decision is ours, that we have chosen the option.

Yet we know that no decision is ever made without some constraints or pressures. No one chooses in a vacuum, in the absence of values or experiences. The moral issue is to remove as much coercion or undue influence as possible so that the decision is the individual's, not someone else's.

Coercion refers to the use of an actual threat of harm or some type of forceful manipulation to influence the person to choose one alternative rather than another. Coercion may take physical, psychological or economic forms. The nature of coercion is perhaps best captured in the widely quoted phrase from the movie "The Godfather": "I made him an offer he couldn't refuse." This connotes the illusion of choice (made an offer) but, in effect, forecloses all options but one (the one that can't be refused).

Undue influence refers to the use of excessive rewards or irrationally persuasive techniques to short-circuit a person's decision making process. Thus one may use behavior modification techniques to get someone to agree with your decision. One may offer large cash payments or the promise of benefits to induce people to participate in research that has a high risk.

But in either case, the appeal is not to a person's interests, rights, or values. The purpose of coercion or undue influence is to do an end run around choice or judgment so the patient will do what he or she might not ordinarily have done.

f. *Paternalism*

Generally speaking, paternalism involves some sort of interference with the individual's liberty of action. Typically this interference is justified with reference to the person's own good. Paternalism may be active in that one acts on behalf of a person but not at his or her request. One may provide a therapy for a person that he or she has not asked for. Or paternalism may be passive in that one refuses to help another achieve some goal he or she may have. For example, a physician may refuse to prescribe a tranquilizer because of fears of its abuse by the patient.

James Childress identified several types of paternalism that refine this general idea and indicate its different aspects.[9]

(1) *Pure and Impure.* Pure paternalism bases its intervention into a person's life on an appeal to the welfare of that person alone. This is the classic model in which parents tell children to eat spinach because it's good for them. Impure paternalism justifies interference with another person because of the welfare of that person and the welfare of another. Thus, some argue that a parent who is also a Jehovah's Witness should have a blood transfusion not only because of the good for that person, but also for the good of his or her children.

(2) *Restricted and Extended.* A restricted paternalistic intervention is one which overrides an individual's act because of some defect in the person. Thus, one may prohibit a child from doing something because of chronological or psychological incompetence. In extended paternalism, an individual is restrained because what he or she wants to do is risky or dangerous. Thus there are laws that mandate wearing helmets while riding motorcycles or prohibit bungee jumping.

(3) *Positive and Negative.* A positive paternalistic act, such as forcing a patient into a rehabilitation program, seeks to promote his or her own good. A negative paternalistic intervention, such as taking cigarettes away from someone, seeks to prevent a harm.

(4) *Soft and Hard.* In a soft paternalistic act, the values used to justify the intervention are the patient's values. For example, unconscious or comatose patients are frequently removed from life support systems because they stated that preference in advance of being in that situation. In hard paternalism, the values used to justify an act are not the patient's. This is the classic case of someone else knowing what is good for you and then having you do it or having it done to you.

(5) *Direct and Indirect.* In direct paternalism, the person who receives the alleged benefit is the one whose values are overridden. The motorcyclist forced to wear the helmet is the one who assumedly will benefit if there is an accident. In indirect paternalism, one person is restrained so that another individual can receive a benefit. A classic instance is child abuse in which parents are restrained in some fashion to benefit the child.

The desire to help or provide a benefit for someone runs deep within the human spirit. Also there are the specific obligations of nonmaleficence and beneficence that we discussed earlier in this chapter. Yet people are autonomous. They know their interests and what is important to them. Respect for persons mandates a presumption against paternalistic interventions. Yet we see harm being done that could be prevented. Can the issues be resolved?

One argument for a paternalistic intervention included these four steps:

(a) The recipient of the paternalistic act actually has some incapacity which prevents or inhibits him or her from making a decision. The person is under undue stress, is a minor, or his or her judgment is impaired in some way.

(b) There is the probability of harm unless there is an intervention. Here one needs to determine if all harms are equal. Are physical, mental, or social harms interchangeable?

(c) Proportionality. The probable benefit of intervention outweighs the probable risk of harm from nonintervention. Here one needs to be careful of uncritical interventions of extended paternalism.

(d) The paternalistic intervention is the least restrictive, least humiliating and least insulting alternative. This criterion argues that one remain as respectful of the individual as possible during the intervention.

This method will not resolve all issues connected with paternalism, but it will force individuals to recognize and justify such paternalistic interventions.[10]

g. *Rights*

The term "rights" is one of the most frequently used in ethics and bioethics. Yet the term is problematic because of its varied meanings and different connotations. This problem is evident even in the origin of the term "rights." In the medieval ethical tradition, we do not find the term "rights"; rather, we find the term "duty" which referred to the reciprocal obligation members of a community had to each other. Duties were specific ways in which each helped the other realize the common good. In the modern tradition, beginning with the Enlightenment, rights referred to claims of the individual against the state. Rights were a means of carving out a zone of privacy or protection against the ever increasing powers of the state. Thus the term "rights" has two major historical origins and two different connotations.

Current usages of rights language reflect elements of this history. Some think of rights as privileges, as social goods that go beyond routine moral obligations. Others think of rights as a sort of social immunity, a protection from powers of the state. Rights are also seen as powers, capacities to act in society. Entitlements are another way of thinking of rights. These are social responses which are seen as deserved, as derivative from being a member of a society. Finally, rights are seen as claims, a moral demand made upon someone or on society.

Also there are different ways to think of rights. One way is to understand them as moral. Moral rights are based on an ethical argument and exist prior to and independent of the guarantees of any institution. Frequently these moral rights are rooted in the nature of the person and his or her dignity and are, therefore, understood to be universal and inalienable. A second type of right is legal: those rights spelled out by the laws, constitution or political institutions of a particular country or political unit. Legal rights are only those rights granted to citizens by the government. They are specific to particular cultures and are subject to social qualifications.

A positive right is a claim to a positive action on the part of another person. A positive right entails a duty on the part of someone else to do something. For example, the right of informed consent confers an obligation on the part of a health care professional to tell me relevant information about my diagnosis and treatment options. A negative right establishes an obligation for someone to refrain from action. Negative rights establish obligations of noninterference. The legal right to abortion, for example, does not secure an obligation for someone to perform an abortion, rather only that a woman not be interfered with in seeking an abortion.

One of the most difficult problems in rights theory is establishing who is the subject of a right and on what basis. Animal rights activists argue, for example, that to have rights one need only be capable of feeling pain or be sentient. Others would suggest that consciousness is enough to secure rights. Still others argue that only self-consciousness can secure rights. Another suggestion is that one be able to use a language. This of course presents interesting issues with respect to the chimps who have been taught sign language as well as with other animals who appear to have some form of communication. Finally, the argument is made that only persons are bearers of rights. Persons are generally understood to be moral agents with an enduring concept of self and capable of autonomous actions. The question of rights is quite complex on the level of definition and determining the subject of rights. When rights are interjected into the social order and made the basis of entitlements, then the picture becomes much more complex and difficult. We will encounter this difficulty in almost every topic presented in this book.

NOTES

1. Tom L. Beauchamp and James F. Childress, *Principles of Biomedical Ethics*. New York: Oxford University Press, 1977, 56.

2. Ibid., pp. 97ff.

3. For a thorough discussion of the principle of double effect, see the article "The Hermeneutical Function of the Principle of the Double Effect" by Peter Knauer, S.J., in *Readings in Moral Theology No. 1*, eds. Charles Curran and Richard McCormick. New York: Paulist Press, 1979.

4. Richard McCormick, S.J., *Ambiguity and Moral Choice*. Department of Theology, Marquette University, p. 93.

5. Beauchamp and Childress, pp. 135ff.

6. Beauchamp and Childress, p. 140.

7. Beauchamp and Childress, pp. 169ff.

8. Beauchamp and Childress, pp. 66ff.

9. James Childress. *Who Shall Decide? Paternalism in Health Care*. New York: Oxford University Press, 1982.

10. James F. Childress. *Priorities in Biomedical Ethics*. Philadelphia: The Westminster Press, 1981, p. 27.

DISCUSSION QUESTIONS

1. What major ethical theory do you primarily use in decision making?
2. Do you think a health care professional has a moral obligation to care for someone with AIDS?
3. Why is the concept of informed consent so important? What functions does it perform for both patient and health care professional?
4. What method of allocation of resources seems most just to you?
5. Do you think people should have the right to refuse treatment?
6. Can you justify treating someone against his or her will?

BIBLIOGRAPHY

Ashley, Benedict, O.P. and Kevin O'Rourke, O.P., *Health Care Ethics*. St. Louis: The Catholic Hospital Association, 1982.

Bayles, Michael (ed.), *Contemporary Utilitarianism*. New York: Doubleday, 1968.

Curran, Charles, *Issues in Sexual and Medical Ethics*. Notre Dame: University of Notre Dame Press, 1978.

Denise, T. C. and S. P. Paterfreund, *Great Traditions in Ethics*, seventh edition. Belmont: Wadsworth Publishing Co., 1992.

Dworkin, Ronald, *Taking Rights Seriously*. Cambridge: Harvard University Press, 1977.

Emanuel, Ezekiel, *The Ends of Human Life*. Cambridge: Harvard University Press, 1991.

Gula, Richard, *Reason Informed by Faith*. Mahwah: Paulist Press, 1989.

Gustafson, James, *Ethics from a Theocentric Perspective,* Vols. I and II. Chicago: University of Chicago Press, 1981.

Hauerwas, Stanley, *A Community of Character.* Notre Dame: University of Notre Dame Press, 1981.

Lustig, B. Andrew (ed.), *Bioethics Yearbook,* Vol. I. Boston: Klower Academic Publishers, 1991.

MacIntyre, Alasdair, *After Virtue.* Notre Dame: University of Notre Dame Press, 1981.

Maguire, D. C. and A. N. Fargauli, *On Moral Grounds: The Art/Science of Ethics.* New York: Crossroad, 1991.

Munson, Ronald, *Interventions and Reflections: Basic Issues in Medical Ethics.* Belmont: Wadsworth Publishing Co., 1992.

Pense, Gregory E., *Classical Cases in Medical Ethics.* New York: McGraw-Hill Publishing Co., 1990.

Shannon, Thomas A. *An Introduction to Bioethics.* New York: Paulist Press, 1987.

Veatch, Robert M. (ed.), *Medical Ethics.* Boston: Jones and Bartlett Publishers, 1989.

PART ONE

ABORTION AND REPRODUCTION

Daniel Callahan
Thomas A. Shannon
Allan B. Wolter, O.F.M.
Scott Aaron
Brenda Almond
Carole Ulanowsky
Maura A. Ryan, Ph.D.
Richard A. McCormick, S.J.
Marc Lappé, Ph.D.
W. French Anderson

1 *An Ethical Challenge to Prochoice Advocates*

Abortion & The Pluralistic Proposition

DANIEL CALLAHAN

Dr. Daniel Callahan is the director of the Hastings Center. His recent books include Setting Limits *and* What Kind of Life.

A t the heart of much moral debate in America lies a simple and popular conviction: the law should leave to the individual conscience choice about those acts that are private, do not command a moral consensus, and are not harmful to others. I will call this the pluralistic proposition. The abortion debate of the past three decades has, in great part, been about this proposition. Those who call themselves "prochoice" argue that the abortion choice is private and personal to women and should thus be left to them without the interference of the law. The "prolife" side, by contrast, has held that the decisive harm abortion does to the fetus and its right to life removes it from the private realm and makes it a matter of legitimate government regulation.

I do not want here to examine directly the struggle between those two positions, the general structure of which is by now all too familiar, painfully so, from the endless public debate. I want instead to look at the subject of abortion as a case study of the problems and paradoxes of the pluralistic proposition, particularly as it has manifested itself in the logic and politics of the prochoice position. One question, above all, troubles me. Is it possible, simultaneously and with equal seriousness, to hold that abortion should (a) be left to the individual and private choice of women, and (b) that each such decision should be understood as a genuine moral choice, one that can be good or bad, right or wrong?

This question is important for the abortion debate, but no less impor-

This article originally appeared in Commonweal *117 (23 November 1990): 681–687.*

tant for many other ethical debates that come down to deciding between private choice and government intervention. If we opt for private choice, what is this likely to mean to the idea of personal morality and what are its possible social implications? Can we entertain a meaningful and substantive notion of personal morality in a pluralistic society? Or is it the case that the pluralistic proposition—in practice if not necessarily in theoretical formulation—encourages a thin and minimalist, relativistic idea of personal morality? Could it be that a strong notion of pluralism requires a weak notion of personal morality, or that a strong notion of personal morality requires a weak notion of pluralism?

Why am I interested in these questions? Over twenty years ago I published a book on abortion, *Abortion: Law, Choice and Morality* (Macmillan, 1970). Reversing my own earlier convictions, I concluded that the universality of a resort to abortion even if illegal and dangerous, the inherently uncertain moral status of the fetus (at least the relatively early fetus), and the value in a pluralistic society of keeping the law out of controverted and delicate moral issues whenever possible, made the "prochoice" position morally and politically compelling. I have not changed my view on the legal issue in any significant way.

I also argued, no less strongly, that even though the choice should be the woman's, and that it should be a private choice, it was still a serious moral choice. Once women had the choice, it would then become important for them in their private lives to give thought to what could count as a morally justifiable choice; and it would be no less appropriate to have some public discussion about the standards and criteria appropriate for such choices, much as we might about other moral matters not subject to law but of common interest and importance. To be sure, the private moral wrestling would and could be a source of anguish and pain, but that is true of all critical moral choices, hardly unique to abortion. The goal that I proposed seemed, then, perfectly compatible with what I understand the pluralistic proposition to be: leave the choice to women but understand the choice to be a grave one, worthy of public no less than private reflection.

I could not have been more naive, more hopelessly optimistic in thinking that such reflection would be acceptable. The prochoice movement has in fact never known quite what to do with the moral issue. For most of its leaders, it is simply set aside altogether, left to the opaque sphere of personal morality, itself a subject of uncertainty and discomfort. Is it not the nature of personal morality, many seem to think, that it is so unique and idiosyncratic to the individual, so subject to private, self-determined moral standards, that nothing meaningful can be said about it, and certainly not enough for public debate? The tacit answer to this question is clear enough. There is a great deal of sociological literature on why women have abortions, and many interesting journalistic accounts of women's experience in making abortion decisions. Yet there is remarkably little written about how women ought to make such private decisions, that is, thoughtful writing on the appropriate moral uses of free choice for those who have the legal right to do so.

Yet if silence or uneasiness is the predominant response to the moral problem, there are others in the prochoice movement—a small but seemingly growing minority—for whom even the idea of discussion of the moral choice is repugnant (see: Jason DeParle, "Beyond the Legal Right: Why Liberals and Feminists Don't Like to Talk About the Morality of Abortion," the *Washington Monthly*, April 1989, pp. 28–44). They either want to declare that abortion is not, in its substance, a moral question at all (only the woman's *right* to choose an abortion is taken to be a moral issue); or that women should not have to struggle and suffer over the choice even if it is; or that, in any case, to concede that it is a *serious* moral choice and to have a public discussion about that choice is politically hazardous, the opening wedge of a discussion that could easily lead once again to a restriction of a woman's right to an abortion. Better to declare the whole topic of the morality of abortion off limits.

One way or another, then, the prochoice movement has not been able to tolerate the fullness of the pluralistic proposition. It can support the choice side more readily than the morality side. At best it is uneasy about the moral issue, at worst dismissive and hostile toward it.

That stance has an important practical implication for the future of the prochoice movement: its inability or unwillingness to come to grips with the moral issue threatens its political credibility. The majority of Americans, the public opinion polls indicate, are greatly troubled about the moral reasons for abortion in different circumstances (see: E.J. Dionne, Jr., "Polls Find Ambivalence on Abortion Persists in U.S.," the *New York Times*, August 3, 1989, p. A18). Not all private reasons are accepted as equally valid, and a large proportion of people report themselves uncertain about their own views, not just those of others. The prolife movement has effectively capitalized on this uncertainty, appealing to the moral uneasiness of many and bringing to the surface qualms and doubts shunted aside by the prochoice movement.

If, for some people, to have choice is itself the beginning and end of morality, for most people it is just the beginning. It does not end until a supportable, justifiable choice has been made, one that can be judged right or wrong by the individual herself based on some reasonably serious, not patently self-interested way of thinking about ethics. That standard—central to every major ethical system and tradition—applies to the moral life generally, whether it be a matter of abortion or any other grave matter. An unwillingness to come to grips with that standard not only puts the prochoice movement in jeopardy as a political force. It has a still more deleterious effect: it is a basic threat to moral honesty and integrity. The cost of failing to take seriously the personal moral issues is to court self-deception, and to be drawn to employ arguments of expediency and evasion. I want to show how that has happened in at least some strands of the prochoice movement and why it reduces the moral strength of that position.

Before I develop that thesis, however, a caution is in order. Despite the harsh things I have to say about elements of the prochoice position, I think in the end it is the only one that is viable in our society. For all of its faults, it is the position I embrace. Though there is room for change and compromise, it would be a great loss to have the substance of *Roe* v. *Wade* overturned, that of leaving early abortions in the private hands of women and their physicians. I am searching for two things simultaneously: a *permanent* and *secure* place in American law for the right of women to make their own choice, and a far richer, more sensitive notion of the nature of that choice than is now commonly the case.

Let me begin that task by looking, first, at the history of arguments used by the prochoice movement, that movement which achieved its greatest victory in the 1973 *Roe* v. *Wade* decision, which is now in jeopardy; and then, secondly, at the developments in the arguments since that time.

During the 1950s and into the late 1960s, the movement to legalize abortion rested on a number of contentions: that a vast number of illegal abortions was doing great harm to the health of women, killing and maiming them; that women should have available a backup to ineffective contraception, though the latter should always remain the primary method of birth control; that the number of unwanted pregnancies, thought to be large, should be reduced and only wanted children should be born—the welfare of children was as much at stake as that of women; that, while an abortion decision is and must be difficult morally and psychologically, a woman should have a right to make such a decision; and that, while abortion should be legally available and financially affordable, everything possible should be done to change those economic and domestic circumstances that force women into unwanted pregnancies.

While this set of arguments looked strongly to the freedom and welfare of women, it was not exclusively a feminist argument by any means. It stressed the common benefits of abortion reform, particularly to children and the society, and it drew heavily on the pluralistic proposition, which bears on a wide range of personal choices for men and women, not simply the abortion choice for women.

Many of those arguments are still, of course, part of the movement. But there have been a number of developments since the early 1970s, some political, some scientific, and some ideological. The most obvious political change has been the emergence of a strong, well-organized, and well-financed prolife movement. It has been able to press its case effectively in legislatures and with the general public (even though public opinion has remained remarkably stable and stationary on abortion for nearly two decades). While this movement has often been stereotyped by its opponents as nothing but religious conservatism, that is hardly accurate. It has grassroots support among many who are otherwise politically liberal. It has also of late gained the support of many women who are feminists. They see in abortion a resort to violence similar to that used for centuries by men against women: the use of power by the strong against the weak, both the physical power of violence and the cultural power to define the unwanted out of the human community altogether (see: Sidney Callahan, "Abortion and the Sexual Agenda," *Commonweal*, April 25, 1986, pp. 232–238). More generally, the prolife movement has found its greatest strength in its focus on precisely that issue that the prochoice movement has found most discomforting and awkward: the moral status of the fetus.

The most important scientific developments have been threefold. There is the growing medical interest in fetal health and development, a trend that has nothing directly to do with the abortion issue, but reflecting research and public health concerns. There is the lowering age of fetal viability, now down to twenty-four weeks, a result of the great improvements in neonatology (though perhaps, for the time being, stalled at that level). There is the widespread use of the sonogram, allowing a woman to see her fetus *in utero* (see: Daniel Callahan, "How Technology is Reframing the Abortion Debate," *Hastings Center Report*, February 1986, pp. 35–42). Taken together, these scientific developments have brought the fetus more squarely before the public eye. The prolife movement did not create that trend, but has effectively capitalized upon it by tying it into its moral focus on the fetus.

The most striking ideological development has been the emergence into leadership positions in the prochoice movement of some feminists who have scanted many of the original arguments for abortion reform. They have shifted the emphasis almost entirely to a woman's right to an abortion, whatever her reasons and whatever the consequences. Much less is heard about the social harm of unwanted pregnancies, much less about the terrible or tragic choice posed by an abortion, much less about the moral nature of the choice, and practically nothing about the need to reduce the number of abortions, now running at a rate of 1.6 million a year. No number of abortions seems to be too many.

It is as if, in face of the prolife movement, some feminist leaders have decided to be as single-minded and unmeasured as their opponents; and they have become in many respects a mirror-image of them. If the prolife movement exclusively stresses the rights of the fetus, then the prochoice movement must exclusively stress the rights of women. If the prolife movement says that abortion is oppressive and murderous, the prochoice movement must then say it is liberating and morally unimportant. If the prolife movement says that every abortion choice is wrong, whatever the reason, then the prochoice leadership implies that every choice is right, whatever the choice. From a movement that in the 1950s and 1960s was measured, careful, open to larger concerns, it now runs the risk of becoming narrow and ideologically rigid. I do not claim that this characterization is true of all prochoice leaders, far from it, only that it is strongly present, and growing, and in a way that was not the case two decades ago. It has come to overshadow the writings and work of other feminists, no less intent on preserving women's freedom of choice, but also on setting that freedom in a context of the common good of men and women, children, and families.

Why has this shift taken place? The most obvious reasons are the growing pressures and successes of the prolife movement, forcing a more defensive, intransigent position; the prospect of a Supreme Court gutting or reversal of *Roe* v. *Wade;* and the impact of the media, with its predilection for polarized positions, encouraging one-dimensionality on both sides of the debate. Yet we might speculate on a more subtle additional possibility: that of the actual difficulty of managing the pluralistic proposition in the face of insistent moral issues that cannot be successfully denatured by exclusive reduction to choice.

Public opinion polls over the years have persistently displayed two distinctive features. When asked a *general* question about the right of women to have an abortion, a majority favors such a right; it has been steadily supportive of *Roe* v. *Wade.* At the same time, when questioned more precisely, a majority also wants morally to distinguish among abortion choices. In that respect, the public has never been unambiguously prochoice or prolife; some 60 percent of the public falls in a zone of ambivalence and nuance (see: Dionne, ibid., and also *Gallup Poll Monthly,* April 1, 1990, p. 41).

The prochoice movement is unable effectively to respond to these findings, partly because of its own ideology (which wants no such distinctions) and partly because of deficiencies in the pluralistic proposition on which it relies to make its general case. The consequence of these deficiencies is that, when pressed on the personal moral issues, the pro-choice leadership usually reacts with anger, confusion, or denial. It does not know what else to do with them.

Why has this happened? I offer a hypothesis. To make its advocacy case, the prochoice movement has partially relied on a set of beliefs and assertions that are either false or highly misleading. It has had to do that because, if looked at too closely, the actual complexity of the abortion situation raises disturbing questions about both the political realities and issues of personal morality. To admit that complexity would be to admit the importance of some portions of the prolife argument, a highly distressing prospect. I offer a partial list of those assertions, counterpoised against what I take to be the more complex truth of the matter.

1. *Abortion restrictions represent a war of men against women, with men intent upon keeping women in reproductive thralldom.* Yet every survey for nearly twenty years shows women themselves divided on the issue, marginally but consistently more opposed to fully permissive abortion than men. The strongest supporters of legal abortion over the years have been young males. Should we be surprised at that? Molly Yard, president of NOW, said after the *Webster* decision that the Court has begun "a war against women." The polls would suggest that abortion is as much a war among women as against women (with class and education a significant element of that war). Faye D. Ginsburg's important recent book, *Contested Lives* (University of California Press, 1989), underscores that point.

2. *Abortion should not be promoted as a primary means of birth control, but as a back-up to a contraceptive failure.* Yet some 40 percent of all abortions are now repeat abortions, a figure that has steadily grown over the years. There are, moreover, some 1.6 million abortions a year, with no diminution in sight. Those figures suggest, though do not prove, a primary and growing dependence for many upon abortion as the first line of defense against unwanted pregnancy, not a back-up method (and reminiscent of the pattern that developed in Eastern Europe in the aftermath of abortion liberalization in the 1960s and 1970s).

3. *Abortion will diminish the dependence of women upon men, giving them full control over their reproduction.* If legal abortion has given women more choice, it has also given men more choice as well. They now have a potent new weapon in the old business of manipulating and abandoning women. For if women can have abortions, then there is no compelling leverage for women to use in demanding that men take responsibility for the children they procreate. That men have long coerced women into abortion when it suits their purposes is well-known but rarely mentioned. Data reported by the Alan Guttmacher Institute indicate that

some 30 percent of women have an abortion because someone else, not the woman, wants it (see: Rachel Benson Gold, *Abortion and Women's Health*, The Alan Guttmacher Institute, 1990, p. 20). The same data indicate that that is not necessarily the exclusive reason, but it is remarkably difficult to find much prochoice probing into the reality of coerced abortions. It is as if there is an embarrassed, sheepish silence on what would seem a matter of obvious concern for those committed to choice.

4. *Given freedom of choice, women will make free choices.* Why is it, then, that many women feel coerced economically into having an abortion? (Poor black women, mainly young, are proportionately the largest group to choose abortion.) Why is it, then, that there is now a whole genre of literature and reports of women who regret their abortions, who felt coerced by others or their social circumstances into having an abortion they would not otherwise have chosen? (See: David C. Reardon, *Aborted Women: Silent No More*, Loyola University Press, 1987.) While it may be an accident that resources for the poor have diminished in parallel with the increased access to abortion, exactly that has happened. But is it wholly an accident that our country combines the world's most liberal abortion laws with the poorest social support and systems for women, mothers and children? (See: Mary Ann Glendon, *Abortion and Divorce in American Law: American Failures, European Challenges*, Harvard University Press, 1987.)

5. *It does not matter what choice women make as long as they have the freedom to make their own choice.* But that is a hard position to sustain, even for the single-minded, when the choice is to abort a female fetus simply because it is female; or to have an abortion to please (or spite) a husband or boy friend; or to have repeat abortions because of a casual attitude toward the use of contraceptives; or to conceive fetuses for experimental purposes or commercial profit.

I cite that list of arguments to show that "choice" covers a multitude of realities, not all of them quite so tidy as some mainline prochoice ideology would have it. Those realities reveal a disturbingly obvious point: not all opponents of abortion are men, not all arguments against abortion are antiwoman, and not each and every abortion choice is equally justifiable, either because of the social circumstances or setting of the choice, or because of the actual content of the choice.

Of course to concede even the moral possibility that some abortion choices could be reprehensible, to admit that some choices can be morally wrong, would be to agree that choice itself is not the end of the moral matter. As a theoretical issue, the pluralistic proposition surely encompasses that possibility. To admit that much in the case of particular abortion choices, however, would be to show the hazards of the pluralistic proposition in its actual political usage. At the least it would be to concede implicitly that the fetus has enough moral status to force a judgment that not all reasons for its destruction are morally defensible. There are good choices, and there are bad choices.

Even contemplating this possibility poses a hard dilemma for the prochoice leadership. Consider two possible alternatives here. One of them is to reject altogether the contention that abortion represents a moral choice of any consequence, and some take that route. But that view is hardly likely to be persuasive to most prochoice supporters, who know better. The other alternative is to concede the validity of the moral worries, the importance of the moral substance of choice, and thereby open the door to a public moral discussion of abortion itself. That would require seriously considering at least some prolife arguments and perspectives, and would of course lay the basis for a moral rejection of some abortions, perhaps many.

Note an interesting parallel. A number of prominent feminists—including Betty Friedan and Gloria Steinem, it might be recalled—came to reject a pure choice ideology in the case of surrogate motherhood (during the debate over the Baby M case). The choice of becoming a surrogate mother, they argued, is not necessarily a good choice or beneficial to women, however much it may have the virtue of being a choice that a woman can legally make. That was a little-noted revolution in feminist thinking, though it was foreshadowed by those feminists who have condemned pornography and prostitution even in cases where women freely choose to take part. The same kind of thinking applied to the abortion debate would represent a genuine upheaval—asking not just whether it is good for women to have choice, but to ask also what constitutes a good choice. How can it make sense to favor the right to choice, but to be morally indifferent about the use of that right? We all favor the right to free speech, but we are not unconcerned—nor do we withhold our public condemnation—when that right is used to insult or demean those of other races. Those are not thought to be, nor are they, contradictory positions.

I conclude that only the second alternative noted above is tenable, to admit the moral seriousness of the abortion choice. I have already suggested one set of reasons for moving in that direction: the high price paid in credibility for evasion of problems of real moral concern to probably a majority of prochoice supporters (and surely of great concern to those who are not certain just where they stand). Such a move will surely be risky. Once they start taking the moral choice seriously, some people are likely to change their position on abortion in general. Yet in the long run, if the prochoice position is to prevail, it will have to run such risks. It has not so far planted solid roots and it has out of anxiety and muddle put to one side moral questions that are as urgent as they are real. More generally, the pluralism proposition can not itself well endure unless it finds a stronger place for a consideration of private moral choices. A strong commitment to legal freedom and choice combined with a weak commitment to substantive moral examination and ethical choice is an unsatisfactory combination. The latter simply goes underground, eating away corrosively at the commitment to legal freedom.

Is it possible in the case of abortion to combine legal freedom and seriousness about the moral questions? That would require the meeting of at least four conditions: (1) recognizing that the prochoice position represents only one important moral tradition in our culture, and must exist in tension with and appreciation of the no less important tradition embodied in the prolife movement, that of a respect for life; (2) accepting the need for active public debate about individual moral choices and the likelihood that some will be judged more negatively than others; (3) accepting the necessity for some compromise in the law as a way of taking seriously the objections of the prolife position; (4) agreeing on the need to make every effort to change those economic and social circumstances that lead women to make coerced abortion choices, and on the need for meaningful counseling of women who are considering abortion.

1. *Abortion and the traditions of morality.* One reason for the intensity and intractability of the abortion debate is that it pits two important moral traditions against each other, that of respect for choice, and that of respect for life. The prolife position speaks eloquently and meaningfully about the value of nascent, defenseless life. It is a morally serious position, one compatible with a wide range of other values that seek to protect and preserve life.

Where it fails in the eyes of many of us, however, is in moving from its premise of respect for life to its conclusion that embryonic or fetal life merits the same protection as life after birth. At the least, that is a difficult question, not so perspicuously self-evident as prolife advocates would have us believe.

A prolife position that would resolutely put to one side the value of free choice in grappling with, and acting upon, that question must fail to make a fully persuasive case. It assumes that it has solved a moral problem for everyone that has, in actuality, never found any single and enduring historical solution. It confuses moral fervor and noble intentions with ethical justification. It would impose upon the unwilling a position that does not command their moral agreement and would force them to act against their conscience.

To say all that is not to imply that the prochoice position is free of problems. There are, in fact, varied ways of formulating that position and it makes a difference which one chooses. A prochoice position that would make the value of early human life depend solely upon private choice and the individual exercise of power—the view that a woman confers value on a fetus by her decision to accept it—fails to understand the importance of communal safeguards against capricious power over life and death. It is no less insensitive to the all-too-common tendency to define out of the human community those lives that are threatening or burdensome. It is prone morally to confuse being unwanted with being valueless, a blurring of categories that puts the value of all human life at risk. A viable prochoice stance for the future must come to grips with those hazards in far more effective ways than it has done in the past. The first step is to be willing to talk about them, having the nerve to put aside worries about the political hazards of doing so.

It *is* hazardous. But the importance of running that risk is that by doing so the prochoice movement will put itself in a far more secure long-term position. The state of public opinion provides one reason for thinking about this possibility. Why is there, as public opinion polls suggest, a broad agreement on the general right of women to make an abortion choice, yet considerable disagreement on morally acceptable reasons for abortion? The most plausible reason is that most people are trying to find a suitable balance between the traditions of choice and those of respect for life. While *Roe* v. *Wade* is tolerable for a majority if asked a yes or no question, it does not capture well the shadings of their actual feelings and evaluation; it is too crude. In the long run, a nuanced position that makes some distinctions among and between reasons for abortion is likely to be taken more seriously than one which wants, once and for all, to resolve the tension. A prochoice position that opposes any political compromise fails to understand that for most people their own moral judgment is already a compromise.

2. *Moral choice and moral judgment.* Only a willingness to make room for an ongoing—and no doubt never-ending—debate about the morality of individual abortion choices can preserve the status of abortion as a serious moral issue. A prochoice movement unwilling or unable to do that will be forever in jeopardy, hiding from itself but not from others its underlying moral insecurity. In practice that kind of openness will mean accepting the likelihood that some reasons for abortion will be judged reasonable and acceptable, and others unreasonable and unacceptable. It no less means that women will and should have a difficult and highly troubling debate with themselves about their own abortions and will, if the public discussion has been full and rich, have to struggle with the conflicting moral views. Nothing has so baffled me over the years as the

faintly patronizing, paternalistic way in which, in the name of choice, it has been thought necessary to protect women from serious moral struggle.

I take it to be a good rule of ethical thinking that an important moral choice is one that can give a principled defense of itself and that is not, under most circumstances, simply a self-interested defense of personal preference (called ethical egoism in the philosophical literature). In this case, that would at the least require some sensitive reflection on the values encompassed in that moral tradition that presses for a respect for life. It should not, moreover, be assumed that, just because there is psychological anguish or ambivalence about abortion, there is moral seriousness present; they are not necessarily the same. Anguish and ambivalence can result from trying to decide what one really wants to do, fear of the procedure itself, worry about the reaction of others. Serious ethical reflection goes beyond those matters. It requires thinking carefully about the moral status of the fetus, and about the best way to live a life and to shape a set of moral values and ideals.

3. *Compromise and accommodation.* The Supreme Court, in its 1989 *Webster* decision, gave to the states the right to set some conditions on abortion, and it will probably allow even further restrictions in the future. It may even overturn the *Roe* v. *Wade* decision, but that is thought less likely. An immediate response of the prochoice leadership to *Webster* was hostility to the decision and to any and all compromise. Planned Parenthood, in a series of advertisements after the decision, said that there could be "no middle ground." That kind of stance is a mistake. The *Webster* decision already assures that there will be such ground, like it or not. More importantly, it seems increasingly clear that, *with some compromise,* an accommodation might be developed that would have a good chance of both enduring and allowing for the great majority of present abortions.

What accommodations might be reasonable? A restriction on late abortions, already made more difficult by the *Webster* decision, would meet widespread approval. A large number of hospitals have, for some years, established an informal cut-off point of twenty weeks, so a restriction of this kind would not have a major impact. A parental notification requirement for minors seeking abortion would win widespread support as well (even if, as I believe, it would have some unhappy, damaging results). A continuing limitation on the use of federal facilities, while also troublesome, is doubtless likely in the future. Most abortions are not carried out for strictly medical or health reasons, but for private and personal reasons. It is hard, then, to see how a strong case can be made for the use of federal or federally-supported facilities in the face of widespread public opposition, and in the light of the prochoice definition of abortion as a private matter, outside the scope of government intervention.

I do not claim that such compromises will be without pain. A number of women might in the future be denied abortions, for economic or other reasons, that are now available. I am only saying that compromises of this sort are most likely to find a middle ground that will be acceptable to public opinion, to be sustainable by the legislatures and courts, and yet also to be most likely to insure that women will still be left with a wide range of choice in the future.

4. *Taking choice seriously.* There are three major obstacles to taking choice seriously. The first I have already discussed at length, that of the fear of, and reluctance to, even discuss openly what might count as an unjustifiable moral choice. The morality of the choice is thereby trivialized. The second obstacle is the absence of serious counseling on abortion, particularly in the clinics that do such a large number of abortions. They rarely explore with women their own thinking, the implications for their lives of their choice, or the possibility that they are being influenced or coerced into abortions they would not otherwise want. There can be no serious choice apart from those conditions. If one believes in real choice—in abortion or any other serious matter that requires reflection and psychological freedom—then the proposal in many states that there be a mandatory waiting period of a few days seems a reasonable accommodation for the prochoice movement to make. A flat rejection of that possibility suggests a desire to maximize abortion rather than to increase choice.

I would be considerably less reassured about going in this direction, I should stress, unless good counseling services were in place. There will, it is true, be practical problems here. Good counseling programs are never easy to organize. But then the present situation is hardly adequate either. It allows women little occasion for considered and assisted reflection, and inadequate help in implementing a range of different choices. This is even more true of the poor than the affluent.

Counseling will, however, have little meaning unless there is an enormous improvement in the services and social benefits available to women. The United States lags far behind every other industrialized nation in the provision of protections, choices, and benefits for pregnant women and mothers. If abortion provides for some women a meaningful alternative to the bearing of a child they can not afford and will be unable properly to care for, it also has the ironic effect of taking pressure off the government and society to give them decent help to allow them to choose instead to have a child. Abortion is often a cheap solution to deeply social problems, and all the more seductive if it is dressed up in the language of choice, pretending that poor women really have mean-ingful choices. The only plausible way to resist that outcome is to make clear that abortion should never be an alternative to full and decent social policy, and that the presence of permissive abortion laws provides no excuse not to put into place needed policy reforms.

What might an abortion policy in the future look like with that aim in mind and in light of the accommodations I have suggested? It would encompass two major ingredients. On the one hand, there would be a sharp restriction of late abortions, parental notification for teenagers, federally supported abortions only for medical or clear health reasons, mandatory counseling and waiting periods, and serious efforts to reduce the number of abortions, especially repeat abortions. There would be, on the other hand, a significant improvement in maternal and child benefits, improved counseling, and more effective family planning and contra-ceptive education and services.

The prochoice movement would, in its future work, stress the need for serious choice, the moral character of that choice, and be receptive to public debate about standards for the making of private choice. Even if it comes to a different conclusion about the moral status of the fetus—as it doubtless will—the prochoice side should show itself no less probing about the importance of that question than the prolife side. That kind of probing will probably lead to a loss of some people from its side, perhaps many. But its willingness to engage in such probing, and to run that risk, will itself have a powerful appeal to many prolife adherents who are themselves ambivalent about denying all choice to women. Some of them will come over.

If the prochoice movement presents itself as principally a move-ment about the rights of women, it is likely to lose in the long run. The abortion issue is broader, deeper, and more complex than that. It is surely about those rights, but it is also about the welfare of families and children, about the obligations of males toward women and toward the children they procreate, and about the family and the place of child-bearing within it. The prochoice movement can show itself to be one of nuance and responsibility, of choice and moral seriousness, of women's right to self-determination and their demonstrated and undoubted ca-pacity to put that commitment in the larger context of a common social good.

At stake here as well is the future of the pluralistic proposition. A pluralism that tries to buy social peace at the expense of moral probity, or considers public issues of far greater importance than private moral issues, can not long endure. It will be beset from within by those who give thought to their private choices and who wonder about the meaning and impact of those choices in their lives and the lives of others. It will and should be troubled when it recognizes that many so-called private choices are shaped, even determined, by social circumstances and mores. The idea that we can draw a sharp line between the public and the private sphere, between public and private choices, is a great myth. They constantly influence and reflect each other.

A strong pluralism is one that just as actively debates the nature and content of private choice as it does that of public, legal, and political choice. The only crucial difference is its supporters agree that, however the debate about that content goes, it will and should in the end leave choice to the individual. The great weakness of the prolife movement is that it has not been willing to trust individuals with free and private moral choice. The prochoice movement has fallen into a different trap. It has been unwilling to trust the moral issues to public debate.

I hope that the prochoice movement would now be willing to run that greatest of all risks, but the only one that seems to me credible for the common good: the willingness to entertain a robust, thick, and probing conception of personal morality, one just as strong in its way as the pluralism and toleration at the level of law and politics is in its way. The prochoice movement has tried to make do with a thin, near-to-vanishing idea of personal morality. That serves neither its own long-term interests nor those of the pluralistic proposition.

2 Reflections on the Moral Status of the Pre-Embryo

Thomas A. Shannon and Allan B. Wolter, O.F.M.

Thomas A. Shannon is Paris Fletcher Distinguished Professor of the Humanities at Worcester Polytechnic Institute. Allan B. Wolter, O.F.M. is Professor Emeritus (Catholic University of America) in retirement at Old Mission, Santa Barbara, California.

In this paper we wish to review contemporary biological data about the early human embryo in relation to philosophical and theological claims made of it. We are seeking to discover more precisely what degree of moral weight it can reasonably bear. While other ethical conclusions might well be drawn from the results of such a reflective investigation, we limit ourselves to a few moral considerations based on our current knowledge of how human life originates. As Catholics, we too believe that "from the moment of conception, the life of every human being is to be respected in an absolute way because man is the only creature on earth that God 'wished for himself' and the spiritual soul of each man is 'immediately created' by God."[1] But we are also vitally concerned as to when one might reasonably believe such absolute value could be present in a developing organism. We would also like to defuse some of the polar opposition fanned by the rhetoric of both prolife and prochoice advocates that creates a legislative dilemma for morally and religiously responsible politicians. We even hope that a rational analysis of available scientific data might lead to some broad consensus among concerned citizens that the term "human life" is not necessarily a univocal conception.

All life is a many-splendored creation on the part of God; this is especially true of human life at any stage of its development. But we suggest that appropriate protection of the human organism changes with

This article first appeared in Theological Studies *51 (December 1990): 603–626.*

36

its developmental stages. We wish to present a theory which recognizes the right of every potential mother to a meaningful life and a healthy personality development,[2] but which condemns irresponsible destruction of fetal life.

One of the hallmarks of the Catholic tradition, with certain conspicuous exceptions, has been to be in dialogue with the philosophy and science of its day and to use such insights in articulating the vision of Catholicism. Such efforts have been done better and worse. Many have taken time to evaluate the correctness or usefulness of a particular articulation. But in almost all cases, because of new discoveries in science, changes in scientific theory, and the use of new philosophical frameworks, the insights and articulation of the faith of one generation have differed from those of another. Sometimes such differences have led to severe conflict. One remembers the Copernican revolution, the case of Galileo in the 17th century, and the tensions introduced by the rediscovery of Aristotelian science in the 13th century. Nor can historians of medieval theology forget that certain philosophical views of Aquinas himself were regarded as theologically dangerous by two successive archbishops of Canterbury and condemned by the bishop of Paris in 1277 on the advice of the prestigious university theological faculty, a condemnation that was lifted insofar as it applied to St. Thomas only two years after the saint's canonization in the 14th century.

Anyone who has studied the history of ideas, scientific, philosophical, or theological, knows that there is a usefulness in reviewing the theoretical conceptions of the past, since they have a habit of recurring cyclically in a new and useful scientific garb.[3] The same is true of the theoretic conceptions used by theologians in articulating their faith. We argue that the most recent scientific discoveries fit in more admirably with the epigenetic conception of how a human being originates that was held for centuries by the great theologians and doctors of the Church than does the more recent and now more commonly accepted—though happily not defined—moment of fertilization as coincident with the time of animation. The widespread acceptance of the theory of immediate animation is of post-Tridentine origin,[4] having entered into the tradition only in the early 17th century, and in 1869 the distinction between the formed and unformed fetus was no longer canonically recognized. This assumption about immediate animation still plays a large part in contemporary ecclesiastical documents, as well as do references to the scientific literature purporting to buttress arguments supporting the theory, as we will discuss later.

We would also like to remind our readers, however, that some 40 years ago two learned priests from the University of Louvain,[5] where this theory of immediate animation was originally introduced, repudiated its scientific standing and went to some lengths to explain historically how this mistaken interpretation of empirical data was initially accepted. We claim that the most recent scientific evidence concerning fertilization and the development of the very early human embryo does even more to reinforce their view that any theory of immediate animation seems to have become as untenable today as it was commonly held to be for centuries by Catholic thinkers. We think that since scientific observations, now recognized as erroneous, played such a historical role in the development of the position favoring such a theory, new and respected scientific evidence should be utilized by Catholic theologians when they discuss the process of fertilization and conception to determine its moral implications.

We hope our analysis will be welcomed because of our acceptance and use of the methodology of the tradition and because we take seriously the role of science in helping articulate the context of moral problems, as do current ecclesiastical documents. While our conclusions may differ from those of these documents, we think such differences are to be cherished because they help the community understand its beliefs and values at a much deeper level and allow some of the forgotten riches of our Catholic tradition to be expressed to a new audience.

This rearticulation needs careful examination, however, for the fact that something is new does not *ipso facto* make it good or correct. Thus a careful and prayerful process of discernment should also be an important part of the way we rearticulate our tradition, for the community must genuinely receive the reconceptualization of the tradition before it is authentic. This essay is an attempt at such a process of discernment by setting out an account of the process of individuation in the early human embryo in light of modern biology and reflecting on it in the light of some important theological and philosophical insights that seem to have perennial vitality.

The medievals and post-Renaissance theologians articulated their theory of the person, the body, and ensoulment in light of the biology and philosophy of their day. On the basis of this they appropriately drew moral conclusions. We know now that the biology used at any one time, if not out of date, may well need updating. But the philosophy and history of science also make it clear that there is a significant difference as to how our scientific knowledge of the wonder of God's creation grows. We believe that such a moment of review is necessary today if we are to give a reasonable defense of the respect Catholics have traditionally had for human life. For we know that in the male seed there is no homunculus, but it was not until the 1700s that mammalian sperm was discovered, and not until the 1800s that the mammalian egg was found and its role revealed. Modern diagnostic technologies such as ultrasound and feto-scopy have given us a whole new perspective on the development of the human embryo. Thus, while we can correctly say that the biological data of a past era are inadequate in light of the discoveries of modern science, we cannot dispose as easily of the basic philosophical or theological way our scholastic predecessors interpreted those data. And we certainly cannot fault their use of the most advanced scientific knowledge available to them as a necessary condition for articulating any rational philosophico-theological conception of the person, the body, and en-soulment. It is in that spirit that we present this brief review of what embryology has to tell us today.

CONTEMPORARY PERSPECTIVES ON THE HUMAN EMBRYO

1. The Pre-embryo[6]

In mammalian reproduction an egg and sperm unite to produce a new and almost always genetically unique individual. The process, how this occurs, is undergoing tremendous reconceptualization and remod-eling in the light of new studies and new diagnostic technologies which allow access to this entity.

A critical discovery of the past two decades is that of capacitation, "the process by which sperm become capable of fertilizing eggs."[7] Hu-man sperm need to be in the female reproductive tract for about seven hours before they are ready to fertilize the egg. This process removes or deactivates "a so-called decapacitating factor that binds to sperm as they pass through the male reproductive tract."[8] This permits the acrosome reaction to occur, which is the means by which lytic enzymes in the sperm "are released so that they can facilitate the passage of the sperm through the egg coverings."[9] Then the sperm are able to penetrate the egg so fertilization can begin.

Fertilization usually occurs in the end of the Fallopian tube nearest the ovary. Sperm usually take about ten hours to reach the egg, and if not "fertilized within 24 hours after ovulation, it dies."[10] Fertilization, how-ever, is not just a simple penetration of the surface of the egg. Rather, it is a complex biochemical process in which a sperm gradually penetrates various layers of the egg. Only after this single sperm has fully pene-trated the egg and the haploid female nucleus, one having only one chromosome pair, has developed, do the cytoplasm of the egg and the nuclear contents of the sperm finally merge to give the new entity its diploid set of chromosomes. This process is called syngamy. It takes about 24 hours to complete and the resulting entity is called the zygote. Thus the process of fertilization (and it is important to note that it is a process) generally takes between 12–24 hours to complete,[11] with another 24-hour period required for the two haploid nuclei to fuse.

Fertilization accomplishes four major events: giving the entity the complete set of 46 chromosomes; determination of chromosomal sex; the establishment of genetic variability; and the initiation of cleavage, the cell division of the entity.

Now begins a very complex set of cell divisions as the fertilized egg begins its journey down the Fallopian tube to the uterus. About 30 hours after fertilization, there is a two-cell division; around 40–50 hours there is a division into four cells; and after about 60 hours the eight-stage cell division is reached. "When the embryo approaches the entrance to the uterus, it is in the 12–16 cell stage, the morula. This occurs on the fourth day."[12] Although the cells become compacted here, there is yet no predetermination of any one cell to become a specific entity or part of an entity. On around the sixth or seventh day the organism, now called the blastocyst, reaches the uterine wall and begins the process of its implantation there so that it can continue to develop. Here we have a differentiation into two types of cells: the trophectoderm, which becomes the outer wall of the blastocyst, and the inner cell mass, which becomes the precursor of the embryo proper. This process of implantation is completed by the end of the second week, at which time there is "primitive uteroplacental circulation."[13]

Critical to note is that from the blastocyst state to the completion of implantation the pre-embryo is capable of dividing into multiple entities.[14] In a few documented cases these entities have, after division, recombined into one entity again. Nor must this particular zygote become a human; it can become a hydatidiform mole, a product of an abnormal fertilization which is formed of placental tissue.

Note also that the zygote does not possess sufficient genetic information within its chromosomes to develop into an embryo that will be the precursor of an individual member of the human species. At this stage the zygote is neither self-contained nor self-sufficient for such further development, as was earlier believed. To become a human embryo, further essential and supplementary genetic information to what can be found in the zygote itself is required, namely

> the genetic material from maternal mitochondria, and the maternal or paternal genetic messages in the form of messenger RNA or proteins. In terms of molecular biology, it is incorrect to say that the zygote has all the informing molecules for embryo development; rather, at most, the zygote possesses the molecules that have the potential to acquire informing capacity.[15]

That potential informing capacity is given in time through interaction with other molecules. . . . This new molecule with its
informing capacity was not coded in the genome. Thus, the
determination to be or to have particular characteristics is given
in time through the information resulting from the interaction
between the molecules.[16]

The development of the zygote depends at each moment on several
factors: the progressive actualization of its own genetically coded information, the actualization of pieces of information that originate *de novo*
during the embryonic process, and exogenous information independent
of the control of the zygote.

2. The Embryo

The next major stage of development is that of the embryo. This is
the beginning of the third week of pregnancy and "coincides with the
week that follows the first missed menstrual period."[17] This phase begins
with the full implantation of the pre-embryo into the uterine wall and
the development of a variety of connective tissues between it and the
uterine wall. Eventually the placenta develops and is the medium
through which maternal-embryonic exchanges occur.

Two major events now occur. The first is the completion of gastrulation, "profound but well-ordered rearrangements of the cells in the
embryo."[18] This process results in the development of various layers
which ultimately give rise to the tissues and organs of the entity and is
completed by the third week. At this time all expressions of the genes are
switched off except those that determine what a particular cell will be.
There are now three layers present which are responsible for the development of much of the organism:

The embryonic ectoderm gives rise to the epidermis; the nervous system; the sensory epithelium of the eye, ear, and nose;
and the enamel of the teeth. The embryonic endoderm forms
the linings of the digestive and respiratory tracts. The embryonic mesoderm becomes muscle, connective tissue, bone and
blood vessels.[19]

The second major event, the process of embryogenesis or organogenesis, now begins and is completed by the end of the eighth week.
This process results in the development of all major internal and external structures and organs.

By the end of the third week the primitive cardiovascular system
has begun to form with the development of blood vessels, blood cells,

and a primitive heart. Since the "circulation of blood starts by the end of the third week as the tubular heart begins to beat,"[20] the cardiovascular system reaches a functional state first.

The nervous system progresses from a neural tube to the essential subdivisions of the brain into forebrain, midbrain, and hindbrain.[21] During this time also the upper and lower limb buds begin to appear. The digestive tract begins to form, as do all the external structures such as the head and the eyes and ears. Hands and feet make their appearance, as do, by the end of the eighth week, distinct fingers and toes.

The development of the nervous system is critical because this is the basis for the "generation and coordination of most of the functional activities of the body."[22] The rudimentary brain and spinal cord are present around the third week but are as yet "unspecialized or undifferentiated for neural function."[23] Neuron development begins around the fifth week, and around the sixth week the "first synapses . . . can be recognized."[24] Carlson observes that at about the seventh week "the embryo is capable of making weak twitches in the neck in response to striking the lips or nose with a fine bristle."[25] Grobstein notes "the earliest continuous neuronal circuitry for reflex conduction and behavior could be initiated as early as six weeks."[26] Such a pattern, Carlson says, "signifies that the first functional reflex arcs have been laid down."[27]

In a rather thorough review of the literature Michael Flower describes various embryonic movements and the neural basis necessary for their possibility.[28] Flower notes that the earliest reported elicited reflex response from an embryo occurred at 7.5 weeks. This was a movement away from a stroking stimulus to the mouth. Such movements were typical during this period of the eighth week of development.[29] In the middle of the ninth week the patterns make a transition to whole body responses, and during the 12th week local reflexes dominate. These data indicate a critical level of integration of the nervous system.

This review of embryonic development up to the eighth week shows a dramatic process of development from the initiation of fertilization to the formation of an integrated organism around mid-gestation. The rest of the paper will concentrate on examining what moral implications these data might have. The intent is not to draw a moral ought from a biological is, but to reconsider the compatibility of moral and philosophical claims with what we know of developmental embryology.

MORAL CONSIDERATIONS

1. Conception

A critical finding of modern biology is that conception biologically speaking is a process beginning with the penetration of the outer layer of the egg by a sperm and concluding with the formation of the diploid set of chromosomes. This is a process that takes at least a day. This raises a question as to how one ought to understand the term "moment of conception" frequently used in church documents.

One could understand "moment" metaphorically as referring to the process as a whole, or if it is meant to convey an instant of time, then it would seem to refer to either the end of the process of biological conception when the zygote has become an embryo, or to some prior stage of development that has been reached in which this human life form (fertilized egg, zygote, or pre-embryo) has acquired a distinct set of properties. However, it seems that the theologians who framed these carefully crafted documents wished to convey the idea that at the moment of conception (whatever stage of development of human life obtains) everything is present that is required essentially for this human organism to be a person in the philosophical/theological, if not psychological, sense of the term: a rational or immortal soul has been created and infused into the organic body. At the same time, while they wished to set forth guidelines, they declared it was still a theoretically open question and hence they did not want to specify, or define, the moment when such passive conception (as it was called by Catholic theologians for many centuries) took place. Prayerful reflection on what embryology and our Catholic tradition tell us may not yield any direct positive knowledge of when passive conception takes place, but it does seem to throw considerable light on when it has not occurred.

Biologically understood, conception occurs only after a lengthy process has been completed and is more closely identified with implantation than fertilization.[30] The pastoral letter *Human Life in Our Day* speaks of conception "initiating a process whose purpose is the realization of human personality."[31] Such a phrase is biologically correct if applied to implantation and seems to be a reasonable moral description of the typical outcome of conception.

2. Singleness

Clearly and without any doubt, once biological conception is completed we have a living entity and one which has the genotype of the human species. As Grobstein nicely phrases it, "conception (fertilization) is the beginning of a new generation in the genetic sense. . . ."[32] This zygote is capable of further divisions and is clearly the precursor of all that follows. But can we say with *Donum vitae*, quoting the "Declaration on Procured Abortion," "From the time that the ovum is fertilized, a new life is begun which is neither that of the father nor of the mother; it is rather the life of a new human being with his own growth"[33]?

How are we to understand this phraseology in the light of the biology of development? For, while it is correct to say that the life that is present in the newly fertilized egg is distinct from the father and mother and is in fact usually genetically unique, it is not the case that this particular zygote is fully formed and it is not a single human individual, an "ontological individual," as Ford suggests.[34] Because of the possibility of twinning, recombination, and the potency of any cell up to gastrulation to become a complete entity, this particular zygote cannot necessarily be said to be the beginning of a specific, genetically unique individual human being. While the zygote is the beginning of genetically distinct life, it is neither an ontological individual nor necessarily the immediate precursor of one.

Second, the zygote gives rise to further divisions "resulting in an aggregate of cells, each of which remains equivalent to a zygote in the sense that it can become all or any part of an embryo and its extra-embryonic structure."[35] Such cells at this stage are totipotent:

> Within the fertilized ovum lies the capability to form an entire organism. In many vertebrates the individual cells resulting from the first few divisions after fertilization retain this capability. In the jargon of embryology, such cells are described as totipotent. As development continues, the cells gradually lose the ability to form all the types of cells that are found in the adult body. It is as if they were funneled into progressively narrower channels. The reduction of the developmental options permitted to a cell is called restriction. Very little is known about the mechanisms that bring about restriction, and the sequence and time course of restriction vary considerably from one species to another.[36]

Such a process of restriction is completed when the cells have become "committed to a single developmental fate. . . . Thus determination represents the final step in the process of restriction."[37] Such determination begins during gastrulation, three weeks into embryonic development.

Genetic uniqueness and singleness coincide on one level only after the process of implantation has been completed and on another after the restriction process is completed. Thus, if we take implantation as the marker of both conception and human singleness, this does not occur until about a week after the initiation of fertilization. If we use determination and restriction, because of their signaling of the loss of totipotency of the cells, as the markers of human singleness, then individuality does not occur until about three weeks after fertilization. Of critical importance is Ford's observation: *"The teleological system of the blastocyst should not be identified with the ontological unity of the human individual that will develop from it.*"[38]

There is, then, a partial answer to the very interesting question[39] *Donum vitae* asks: "How could a human individual not be a human person?"[40] A Catholic philosopher might well object or reply that this is certainly a very muddled question, for "traditionally speaking" individuality has been considered a necessary, though not sufficient condition for human personhood. The rational soul has never been considered the formal reason why something human is individual. Obviously, "human individual" can have several meanings. If it refers to a fertilized ovum, this is indeed something both human (qua product) and numerically single. Yet, until the process of individuation is completed, the ovum is not an individual, since a determinate and irreversible individuality is a necessary, if not a sufficient, condition for it to be a human person.

Something human and individual is not a human person until he or she is a human individual, that is, not until after the process of individuation is completed. Neither the zygote nor the blastocyst is an ontological individual, even though it is genetically unique and distinct from the parents. The potential for twinning remains until the beginning of gastrulation, although it is rare for it to occur this late. Additionally, a zygote that divides can reunite and one individual will emerge. Furthermore, each cell can form a total individual. A human individual, to use the language of the document, cannot be a human person until after individuality is established.

Also, as Grobstein noted, genetic uniqueness does not necessarily imply singleness.[41] That is, when fertilization is complete and the haploid state is reached, the organism has its full complement of genetic information. At this point it is genetically unique. But because of the potentiality for twinning, this uniqueness may be shared by more than one organism. Thus, even though unique, the organism is not necessarily single. Singleness or individuality occurs after the genetically unique organism has implanted and its development is restricted to forming one unified organism.

An individual is not an individual, and therefore not a person, until the process of restriction is complete and determination of particular cells has occurred. Then, and only then, is it clear that another individual cannot come from the cells of this embryo. Then, and only then, is it clear that this particular individual embryo will be only this single embryo.

One can reasonably conclude, then, that if there is no single human entity, there is no person. For the one is the presupposition of the other. Thus, when *Donum vitae* approvingly refers to the findings of modern science and argues "that in the zygote . . . resulting from fertilization the biological identity of a new human individual is already constituted,"[42] does not this statement of the Congregation fail to make a critical distinction between genetic uniqueness and singleness? In using "individual" rather than "person" in this meticulously worded statement, the Congregation may have sought to sidestep the controversial question of when personhood begins. But if "individual" be taken in its philosophical or technical meaning, scientific data available today hardly justify the claim that a particular zygote is necessarily both genetically unique and an individual.

This is particularly important in assessing the theological intent of the Congregation, particularly since it argues that the "conclusions of science regarding the human embryo provide a valuable indication for discerning by the use of reason a personal presence at the moment of this first appearance of a human life."[43] As the statement stands, three concepts appear to be conflated here: genetic uniqueness, singleness, and personal presence. The argument for the first presence of human and personal life in the zygote relies heavily on scientific claims about the fertilized egg. However, such claims of singleness and personhood cannot be made, the former scientifically and the latter philosophically. We assume that the Congregation would want to adjust its findings in the light of these distinctions.

3. Ensoulment[44]

In this section and elsewhere, we will be discussing the principle of immaterial individuality or immaterial selfhood. In the Catholic tradition, and clearly in many of the sources we cite, the usual term for this is "soul." Our practice will be to use the term "soul" when speaking within a clear traditional context. But when we develop our own presentation, we will use the term "immaterial individuality" or "immaterial selfhood," because the term "soul" has many connotations and images connected with it and in so far as possible we wish to avoid problematic usages and confusing images.

a. Issues

Although far from being a defined doctrine, there is support in Roman Catholic moral theology for the position that ensoulment is coincident with fertilization or, at least, as early as possible after conception. This position apparently dates from the early-17th-century writings of Thomas Fienus, professor on the faculty of medicine at Louvain.[45] This opinion gradually caught on and became the dominant opinion. This position was complemented by teachings that held that the embryo "possesses all the essential parts of a human body, though very minute in size."[46] This teaching on immediate animation eventually worked its way into the mainstream of Catholic moral theology. If doctors of medicine were Catholics, explains Dorlodot,

> they were told that the theologians of their time held that the soul is created by God immediately after fecundation. The theologians in turn based themselves on the opinion of the doctors, as these did on that of the theologian. In other words, *caecus caeco ducatum praestat*. Finally, the moral theologians, who completely forgot the principles which, according to the great doctors of Catholic morality, render abortion always illicit, invoked the danger of favouring abortive or sterilizing practices.[47]

Additionally, the removal from canon law in 1896 of the distinction between the formed and unformed fetus suggests that there is not a time when the body is unformed.[48] The *Ethical and Religious Directives for Catholic Health Facilities* provide another reason when they include in the definition of an abortion the "interval between conception and implantation."[49] Also, we have the 1981 testimony of Cardinal Cooke and Archbishop Roach in support of the Hatch amendment: "We do claim that each human individual comes into existence at conception, and that all subsequent stages of growth and development in which such abilities are acquired are just that—stages of growth and development in the life cycle of an individual already in existence."[50] Finally, in *Donum vitae* we read: "nevertheless, the conclusions of science regarding the human embryo provide a valuable indication for discerning by the use of reason a personal presence at the moment of this first appearance of a human life."[51]

If this statement is to be accepted as it stands, we suggest that the conclusions of science should be interpreted differently, particularly if we reflect on what we know from science in the light of a centuries-long tradition among Catholic philosophers and theologians. For like them we are struck by both the wonder and sacredness of human life even from its obscure beginnings, as well as to when we could begin to suspect a personal presence might be there. Nor can we forget that for some 17 centuries the Church indeed condemned abortion, but not on the ground that it might by even the most remote possibility be in all cases a question of murder. Certainly some of the greatest minds and doctors of the Church refused to believe, as many today seem to do, that ensoulment is coincident with fertilization or that we must trace the genesis of each human person back to that moment. Obviously, the Sacred Congregation for the Doctrine of Faith had no intention of definitively settling this question, for it stated pointedly, "This declaration expressly leaves aside the question of the moment when the spiritual soul is infused. There is not a unanimous tradition on this point and authors are as yet in disagreement."[52] It did not believe, however, that such theoretical openness should lead to any rash or precipitous practical action, for it goes on to say: "From a moral point of view this is certain: even if a doubt existed concerning whether the fruit of conception is already a human person, it is objectively a grave sin to dare to risk murder."[53]

Several very critical questions arise here, particularly since abortion was traditionally considered a sin against marriage but not homicide. One of them, concerning the moral possibility of acting on probable knowledge, has already been masterfully treated by Carol Tauer.[54] Others concern practical and philosophical issues relating to the development of the pre-embryo and embryo. It is to these issues that we now turn.

The dominant position of the moral tradition on ensoulment was the acceptance of a time during the pregnancy when the fetus was not informed by the rational soul. Two distinctions were used in discussing this. The first distinction is between active and passive conception and is exemplified in *De festis* of Benedict XIV, in which the pope comments on the doctrine of the Immaculate Conception.

> Conception can have a twofold meaning, for it is either active, in which the holy parents of the Blessed Virgin, joining each other in a marital role, have accomplished those things which have to do most of all with the formation, organization, and disposition of the body itself for receiving a rational soul to be infused by God; or it is passive, when the rational soul is coupled with the body. This infusion and union of the soul with a duly organized body is commonly called passive conception, namely, that which occurs at that very instant when the rational soul is united with a body consisting of all its members and its organs.[55]

Thus the pope would seem to understand active conception, in our terminology, as the physical union of egg and sperm that will become the embryo, while passive conception would be the moment the rational soul is infused into a suitably organized body, one that results from (begins with) organogenesis.

The second distinction is between mediate and immediate animation by such a soul. The theory of mediate animation is succinctly stated as follows:

Animation by the intellectual soul is impossible so long as the parts of the brain which are the seat of the imagination and the vis cogitativa (and we might add, the memory) are not suitably organized. But it still is more evident that there cannot be animation by the intellectual soul when the brain is not even outlined, or again, when even the embryo really does not as yet exist. Now that is precisely the case with the ovum, and the morula, and of that which results from its development, so long as there has not appeared, on a particular part of the germ, that which by its ulterior development will become a fetus.[56]

Immediate animation occurs coincidentally with the fusion of egg and sperm, known as the moment of conception. This is the position utilized in the teachings referred to at the beginning of this section. This distinction is also thoroughly discussed by Donceel, as previously noted.[57]

Medieval theologians were particularly interested in clarifying the technical meaning of "conception" in their justification of the celebration of the popular feast of the Bl. Virgin Mary's conception. Henry of Ghent, following common scholastic reasoning, distinguished between the "conception of the seed when fetal life begins" and the conception of the human soul some "35 or 42 days later [when], depending on the sex, a rational soul is created."[58] Such a position echoes St. Anselm's perceptive judgment, "No human intellect accepts the view that an infant has a rational soul from the moment of conception."[59]

Had this saint known of the empirical data on wastage, he would have considered such a claim not only irrational but blasphemous.[60] For only about 45% of eggs that are fertilized actually come to term. The other 55% miscarry for a variety of reasons. Some are related to the biochemistry of the uterus, others are a function of low levels of necessary hormones, while yet other reasons have to do with structural anomalies within the pre-embryo or embryo itself.[61] Such vast embryonic loss intuitively argues against the creation of a principle of immaterial individuality at conception. What meaning is there in the creation of such a principle when there is such a high probability that this entity will not develop to the embryo stage, much less come to term?

Also, given the fact that twinning and recombination is a possibility, what is one to say about the presence of immaterial individuality during that process? If this principle is initiated at fertilization and then a twin is formed, how does one explain the relation of the original principle to the zygote that splits off? And should recombination occur, how does one explain coherently the fate of such a principle of immaterial individuality? Should one freeze the pre-embryo, all organic processes stop for the duration. What is the status of immaterial individuation then? It is genuinely unclear what to think of that in terms of the standard theory of immediate ensoulment. Then there is the issue of whether a soul, in the classic sense of the form of the body, is needed for the fertilized egg to develop into its possible subsequent forms.

b. Commentary

The question of the moral significance of the morula and of embryonic wastage has been noted previously in the moral literature. In 1976, for example, Bernard Häring brought together much of the scientific literature and examined its moral significance. His conclusion concurs with one suggestion in our analysis and opens the door to other issues: "the argument that the morula cannot yet be a person or an individual with all the rights of the members of the human species seems to me to be convincing as long as we follow our traditional concept of personhood."[62] This conclusion opens up several areas for consideration.

First, we concur with Haring and particularly with the analysis of Ford that, given the biological evidence, there is no reasonable way in which the fertilized egg can be considered a physical individual minimally until after implantation. Maximally, one could argue that full individuality is not achieved until the restriction process is completed and cells have lost their totipotency. Thus the range of time for the achievement of physical individuality is between one and three weeks. One simply cannot speak, therefore, of an individual's being present from the moment of fertilization.

Second, given the standard definition of personhood used in Catholic moral theory—an individual substance of a rational nature—questions are raised about the rational nature. When might one consider such a rational nature to be present? Ford suggests the formation of the primitive streak, which coincides with the time of the formation of the neural tube, as an appropriate criterion.[63] Another criterion would be around eight weeks, when the first elicited responses have been recorded. These are the result of a simple three-neuron circuit. Thus, towards the end of the embryonic period some neural activity is present. A third answer would be the formation of a relatively integrated nervous system, which occurs around the 20th week of fetal development. Of critical importance here is the connection of neural pathways through the thalamus to the neocortex. This allows stimuli to be received, as well as activities to be initiated.

One can speak of a rational nature in a philosophically significant sense only when the biological structures necessary to perform rational actions are present, as opposed to only reflex activities. The biological data suggest that the minimal time of the presence of a rational nature would be around the 20th week, when neural integration of the entire organism has been established. The presence of such a structure does not argue that the fetus is positing rational actions, only that the biological presupposition for such actions is present.

Third, the pre-embryonic form as a system is not totally passive, the recipient only of actions from the outside as it were. It has its own activities arising from the released potencies of the novel combination of its constituent materials. Such potencies are released when these elements form a system, e.g. the embryo. This development of new systems gives rise to new activities and possibilities and serves as the foundation or presupposition for other stages of development. Philosophically speaking, we have every reason to believe that the dynamic properties of the organic matter—the elements of the fully formed zygote—owe their existence to their organizational form or the system. Important to note is that "where there are only material powers—that is, the ability to form material systems—, there is only a material nature or substance."[64] Thus the material system or form of the developing body can explain its own activity. We conclude that there is no cogent reason, either from a philosophical or still less from a theological viewpoint, why we should assert, for instance, that the human soul is either necessary or directly responsible for the architectonic chemical behavior of nucleo-proteins in the human body.

Among the scholastic theologians and doctors of the Church, perhaps St. Bonaventure has given the most helpful model for what we have in mind. For in his interesting Aristotelian interpretation of how St. Augustine's theory of seminal reasons might be explained according to the science of his own day, he argued that if the potencies be understood as active rather than passive, then the Aristotelian formula that the new substantial *form is educed from the potency of matter* made sense. For "the philosopher of nature says that matter first receives the elementary form and by its means it comes to the form of the mineral compound and by means of the latter to the organic form, for he looks to that potency of matter according to which it is progressively actualized by the operation of nature."[65]

If we interpret this in more contemporary terms, it means simply that the new substantial form is nothing more than that of the organic system itself, and that its new and unique dynamic properties stem from the complementary interaction of elements that make up the system. All that is needed is some external agent to bring the elements of that system together, for, as Bonaventure puts it, "in matter itself there is something cocreated with it from which the agent acting in matter educes the form. Not that this something from which the form is educed is such that it becomes some part of the form to be produced, but it is rather that which can be and will become the form, even as a rosebud becomes a rose."[66]

These remarks suggest that the principle of immaterial individuality is indeed the ultimate actualization of all the potencies contained within the forms or systems that constitute the organic life of the human being. Thus, finally, we can say that while it is necessary to recognize the distinctions between higher and lower vital functions in the human being, nonetheless there may be "an area where the biochemical theory is the more plausible explanation, and another area where the animistic position seems to be the only tenable view."[67]

The question of when such a principle comes into being is dependent on which level of the system of the human being one is examining and what activities are performed here. The strong implication of these suggestions is that immaterial individuality comes into existence late in the development of the physical individual.

CONCLUSIONS

1. Biological Data

a. Physical Individuality

Two biological data mandate a revision of our understanding of the beginning of individuality: (1) the possibility of twinning, which lasts up to implantation, which occurs about a week after fertilization begins, and (2) the completion of the restriction process, which prevents individual cells from forming another individual, about three weeks into the pregnancy. While one can speak of genetic uniqueness, in that the fertilized egg has its own genetic code distinct from any other entity (except an identical twin, triplet, etc.), we simply cannot speak of an individual until in fact that individual is present, and the earliest that can be is about two or three weeks after fertilization begins.

b. Neural Development

Three markers are significant in neural development: (1) gastrulation, the development of the various layers in the pre-embryo which give rise to the whole organism; (2) organogenesis, the presence of all major systems of the body, occurring around the eighth week, and (3) the development of the thalamus, which permits the full integration of the nervous system, around the 20th week.

Critical here is the necessity of a functioning and probably integrated nervous system for the possibility of rational activity. For if there is no nervous system functioning, it is not clear that the rational part of the definition of a person can be fulfilled, even though the individual part might be. The functioning nervous system is a necessary condition for the possibility of a new stage of development to emerge and is also a sign that the organism is prepared for this. Thus any of the three markers noted immediately above could serve as an indicator of the capacity for rationality, though not necessarily its actuality.

c. Developmental Autonomy

Given the philosophical discussion on nature and substance, it is reasonable to argue that the developing body as an organized system is a new substance or nature and has the capacity to elicit the potencies within its own reality. That is, a fully formed zygote is a new nature because it has its own actuality and potentiality. It is in itself a sufficient explanation of its own development and activities. The same is true on each new level of development as the zygote becomes an embryo and, finally, a fetus. On a genetic level, the clearest marker of the presence of self-directing activity which would manifest such a new nature would appear in the zygote after it developed the capacity to manufacture its own messenger RNA and thus be developmentally, though not physically, independent of the mother.

2. Moral Implications

a. Physical Individuality

We find it impossible to speak of a true individual, an ontological individual, as present from fertilization. There is a time period of about three weeks during which it is biologically unrealistic to speak of a physical individual. This means that the reality of a person, however one might define that term, is not present at least until individualization has occurred. Individuality is an absolute or necessary condition for personhood.

We conclude that there is no individual and therefore no person present until either restriction or gastrulation is completed, about three weeks after fertilization. To abort at this time would end life and terminate genetic uniqueness, to be sure. But in a moral sense one is certainly not murdering, because there is no individual to be the personal referent of such an action.

Since the zygote is living, has the human genetic code, and indeed possesses genetic uniqueness, this entity is valuable, and its value does not depend on the presence or absence of any or a particular quality or characteristic such as intelligence or capacity for relationships.[68] Thus the zygote and the blastomers derived from it, because they are living, possess ontic value and are in themselves valuable. Thus the general argument made here is not a so-called "quality of life" argument.

Nonetheless, until the completion of restriction or gastrulation, the zygote and its sequelae are in a rather fluid process and are not physical individuals and therefore cannot be persons. The pre-embryo at this state, we conclude, cannot claim absolute protection based on claims to personhood grounded in ontological individuality. Yet, since the pre-embryo is living and possesses genetic uniqueness, some claims to protection are possible. But these may not be absolute and, if not, could yield to other moral claims.

b. Immaterial Individuality

If one assumes, as we think correct to do, that the potencies actualized in the formation of the new nature of the fertilized egg have the inherent capacity to ground its growth and development, then there is no need to posit a principle of individual immateriality, understood as the Aristotelian *nous* or as the entelechy of the body, in pre-embryonic development.

Since the evidence for such a principle comes from the internal evidence of those who experience it, it is difficult at best to ground any speculation as to when it comes into existence. We would make this argument. On the one hand, the developing pre-embryo as a new nature has within it the potential for future development. On the other hand, if the will as a rational potency is what genuinely distinguishes the person from a nature, then one needs to look to biological presuppositions which enable such a potency to exist. We would argue that the earliest time is around the eighth week of gestation, because then the nervous system is fully integrated.

3. Summary

We have reviewed some of the salient biological data about the initial stages of the development of human life, with a view to evaluating the philosophical and theological claims made of them. Reflecting on these from a historico-theological perspective, we have tried to discover whether there exists some rational justification for the absolute value that is attributed to the zygote or pre-embryonic state based on claims to personhood, or whether our earlier long-standing Catholic tradition of mediate animation by a rational soul does not provide a more satisfactory philosophical and theological account. For if we consider judiciously what the great scholastic doctors had to say about the "moment of conception," we seem to have good reason to reintroduce, in interpreting the data of present-day science, the theological distinction between active and passive conception made by Pope Benedict XIV in discussing Mary's immaculate conception.

We thus affirm that any abortion is a premoral evil. That is, it is the ending of life. Consequently we do not want to be understood as proposing or supporting an "abortion on demand" position or assuming that early abortions are amoral. Abortion is a serious issue, because life is involved and one needs always to respect life. We have made one major argument, however, in this essay. Given the findings of modern biology, there is no evidence for the presence of a separate ontological individual until the completion of either restriction or gastrulation, which occurs around three weeks after fertilization. Therefore there is no reasonable basis for arguing that the pre-embryo is morally equivalent to a person or is a person as a basis for prohibiting abortion. That is, there is no biological support for the position that the fertilized egg is from the beginning of the process of fertilization a distinct individual needing no outside agency to develop into a person. Neither is there good philosophical evidence that the principle of immaterial individuality need be present from the beginning to explain the physical development of the pre-embryo.

This position obviously does not support the argument that abortion is to be prohibited because a person is present from the beginning of fertilization. The earliest such an argument could reasonably be made is after the completion of gastrulation. We recognize that this argument will dismay many and comfort others. Our intention in proposing the argument of this essay is to gain a greater coherence between moral theology and modern embryology.

In this sense we are complementing the work of the Roman Congregations and bringing it up to date. We also wish to test the strength of our argument, already subjected to review by several colleagues, in review by a wider and more diverse audience. Additionally, our intention is to develop a position that is reasonable and can be reasonably defended in the public sector.[69] Finally, we think our position on the pre-embryo and embryo can stand rigorous scrutiny and we propose it as a factor in developing a feasible state and/or national policy on abortion.

One is reminded here of Henry de Dorlodot's evaluation of immediate animation made over 50 years ago in his seminal work *Darwinism and Catholic Thought:* "We are not exaggerating in the least when we regard the fact that this theory [of immediate animation] should still find defenders long after the experimental bases on which it was thought to be founded have been shown definitely to be false, as one of the most shameful things in the history of thought."[70]

NOTES

1. Cf. *Donum vitae,* quoting *Gaudium et spes,* in Thomas A. Shannon and Lisa Sowle Cahill, *Religion and Artificial Reproduction* (New York: Crossroad, 1988) 147.

2. We are concerned here especially with victims of rape, incest, or sexual abuse.

3. Philosophers of science have stressed the important difference between the linear growth of scientific data and theoretic conceptions used to interpret them, for important theories have a life of their own that ensures their perenniality. Or, as Santayana put it, those who forget history are condemned to repeat its mistakes.

4. For theologians at the Council of Trent, in contrasting the virginal conception of Christ with the ordinary course of human nature, asserted that normally no human embryo could be informed by a human soul except after a certain period of time: "cum servato naturae ordine nullum corpus, nisi intra praescriptum temporis spatium, hominis anima informari queat" (*Cathecism of the Council of Trent,* Part 1, art. 3, n. 7), cited in E. C. Messenger, *Theology and Evolution* (Westminster, Md.: Newman, 1949) 236.

5. We refer to Dr. Messenger and Canon Henry de Dorlodot.

6. This is the term being used to describe this entity from the zygote state to the beginning of the formation of the primitive streak during the third week (see Keith L. Moore, *Essentials of Human Embryology* [Philadelphia: Decker, 1988] 16). The primitive streak gives rise to other structures which continue the physical development of the embryo. The purpose of using this term, as well as other terms such as zygote, embryo, and fetus, is to integrate scientific descriptions into the moral discussion. These terms, as used in this essay, beg no moral questions but help us clearly identify the entity we are discussing. Cf. Clifford Grobstein, *Science and the Unborn: Choosing Human Futures* (New York: Basic Books, 1988) 62. But see *Donum vitae,* which also uses these terms but attributes "to them an identical ethical relevance, in order to designate the result (whether visible or not) of human generation from the first moment of its existence until birth" (Introduction 1 n.). The text of *Donum vitae* can be found in Shannon and Cahill, *Religion and Artificial Reproduction* 140 ff.; all references will be to this text.

7. Steven B. Oppenheimer and George Lefevre, Jr., *Introduction to Embryonic Development* (2nd ed. Boston: Allyn and Bacon, 1984) 87.

8. Ibid. 87.

9. Bruce M. Carlson, *Patten's Foundations of Embryology* (5th ed. New York: McGraw-Hill, 1988) 134.

10. Oppenheimer and Lefevre, *Introduction* 175.

11. Ibid. 176.

12. Ibid. 175.

13. Moore, *Essentials* 14.

14. Carlson, *Patten's Foundations* 35.

15. Carlos A. Bedate and Robert C. Cegalo, "The Zygote: To Be or Not to Be a Person," *Journal of Medicine and Philosophy* 14 (1989) 642–43.

16. Bedate and Cegalo, "The Zygote" 644.

17. Moore, *Essentials* 16; italics in the original.

18. Carlson, *Patten's Foundations* 186.

19. Moore, *Essentials* 18.

20. Ibid. 24.

21. Carlson, *Patten's Foundations* 296.

22. Ibid. 456.

23. Grobstein, *Science* 47.

24. Ibid. 48.

25. Carlson, *Patten's Foundation* 457.

26. Grobstein, *Science* 48.

27. Carlson, *Patten's Foundations* 458.

28. Michael J. Flower, "Neuromaturation of the Human Fetus," *Journal of Medicine and Philosophy* 10 (1985) 237–51.

29. Ibid. 238–39.

30. Norman M. Ford, *When Did I Begin? Conception of the Human Individual in History, Philosophy, and Science* (Cambridge: Cambridge University, 1988) 176–77. This outstanding and comprehensive analysis of the biological data came to our attention after we had completed much of our own research for this article. We wish to acknowledge how much we have learned from it and to commend it for its exceptionally thorough review of the biological data and philosophical analysis. We also wish to acknowledge the earlier contribution of James J. Diamond, M.D., to this topic: "Abortion, Animation, and Biological Hominization," *TS* 36 (1975) 305–24.

31. *Human Life in Our Day,* par. 84.

32. Grobstein, *Science* 25.

33. *Donum vitae* I, 2, in Shannon and Cahill, *Religion and Artificial Reproduction* 148.

34. An ontological individual is defined as "a single concrete entity that exists as a distinct being and is not an aggregation of smaller things nor merely a part of a greater whole; hence its unity is said to be intrinsic" (Ford, *When Did I Begin?* 212).

35. Grobstein, "Early Development" 235.

36. Carlson, *Patten's Foundations* 23.

37. Ibid. 26.

38. Ford, *When Did I Begin?* 158; italics ours.

39. Although any conclusions should not be laid at his door, Richard McCormick started Shannon thinking about this problem and was suggestive in phrasing the question.

40. *Donum vitae* I, 2, in Shannon and Cahill, *Religion and Artificial Reproduction* 149.

41. Grobstein, *Science* 25.

42. *Donum vitae* I, 2, in Shannon and Cahill, *Religion and Artificial Reproduction* 149.

43. Ibid. I, 2, in Shannon and Cahill, *Religion and Artificial Reproduction* 149.

44. There is much literature on this, but two interesting articles which are extremely useful for their summaries are Joseph Donceel, S.J., "A Liberal Catholic's View," in *Abortion in a Changing World,* ed. Robert E. Hall (New York: Columbia University, 1970), and Carol Tauer, "The Tradition of Probabilism and the Moral Status of the Early Embryo," *TS,* 45 (1984) 3–33. Both articles can be found in *Abortion and U.S. Catholicism: The American Debate,* ed. Patricia B. Jung and Thomas A. Shannon (New York: Crossroad, 1988).

45. Henry de Dorlodot, "A Vindication of the Mediate Animation Theory," in *Theology and Evolution,* ed. E. C. Messenger (Westminster, Md.: Newman, 1959) 271.

46. Dorlodot, "A Vindication" 273.

47. Ibid.

48. Cf. John Connery, S.J. *Abortion: The Development of the Roman Catholic Perspective* (Chicago: Loyola University, 1977) 212.

49. Washington, D.C.: U.S. Catholic Conference, 1977, 4.

50. Archbishop John Roach and Cardinal Terence Cooke, "Testimony in Support of the Hatch Amendment." *Origins* 11 (1981) 357–72; also in Jung and Shannon, *Abortion* 15.

51. *Donum vitae* I, 1, in Shannon and Cahill, *Religion and Artificial Reproduction* 149.

52. *Declaration on Abortion* (Washington, D.C.: U.S. Catholic Conference, 1975) 13.

53. Ibid. 6.

54. See n. 44 above. While many have been unhappy with Carol Tauer's article and have dismissed it, Shannon has not yet seen a substantive refutation of her argument that the "application of the probabilist methods would permit some early abortion" (Jung and Shannon, *Abortion* 79).

55. "Conceptio dupliciter accipi potest; vel enim est activa, in qua Sancti B. Virginis parentes opere maritali invicem convenientes, praestiterunt ea quae maxime spectabant ad ipsius corporis formationem, organizationem et dispositionem ad recipiendam animam rationalem a Deo infundendam; vel est passiva, cum rationalis anima cum corpore copulatur. Ipsa animae infusio et unio cum corpore debite organizato vulgo nominatur Conceptio passiva, quae scilicet fit illo ipso instanti quo rationalis anima corpori omnibus membris ac suis organis constanti unitur" (Benedict XIV, *De festis,* lib. II, c. 15, n. 1, in *Opera omnia* 9, ed. J. Silvester [Prato: Aldina, 1843] 303a).

56. Dorlodot, "A Vindication" 266. It was here that Messenger and Dorlodot recalled that the only theological attempt to define the role of the rational soul as the substantial form of the body was made by the Council of Vienne (DS 481) and that the fathers and theologians of that council did not subscribe to the immediate-animation theory. Dorlodot uses the definition of the council as the major premise of his argument vindicating the mediate animation theory; see Messenger, *Theology and Evolution* 259.

57. Donceel, "A Liberal Catholic" 48 ff.

58. *Quodlibet* 15, q. 13; cited in *John Duns Scotus: Four Questions on Mary*, tr. and intro. by Allan B. Wolter, O.F.M. (Santa Barbara, Calif.: Old Mission, 1988) 6. It is interesting to note that Henry breaks with the tradition and ascribes a longer period of gestation before animation to the male rather than the female as was customary since Aristotle.

59. Anselm of Canterbury, *De conceptu virginali et de originali peccato,* c. 7 in *Anselmi Cantuariensis archiepiscopi opera omnia* 2, ed. F. S. Schmitt (Stuttgart-Bad Cannstatt, 1968) 148 (Anselm of Canterbury 3, ed. and tr. Jasper Hopkins and Herbert Richardson [Toronto: Edwin Mellen, 1976] 152). It is important to keep in mind that the Archbishop of Canterbury is arguing as to when it is possible to contract original sin, something that all theologians in his day agreed required only the existence of a human soul, not any consciousness or voluntary activity on the part of an infant. As he puts it, "Either from the very moment of his conception an infant has a rational soul (without which he cannot have a rational will) or else at the moment of his conception he has no original sin. But no human intellect accepts the view that an infant has a human soul from the moment of his conception. For [from this view] it would follow that whenever—even at the very moment of reception—the human seed perished before attaining a human form, the [alleged] human soul in this seed would be condemned, since it would not be reconciled through Christ—a consequence which is utterly absurd." Today we may have different conceptions as to the nature of original sin and how it is contracted, but we have even less reason than Anselm to believe that there is the remotest possibility of a human will present in what he calls "human seed" at the moment the zygote is formed, or that there is any less rather than a substantially greater amount of "human seed that perishes before attaining a human form."

60. Those who see no insuperable difficulty for the theory of immediate animation in the fact that twins can come from a single fertilized egg should find considerable difficulty in the problem of wastage. To ascribe such bungling of the conceptual process to an all-wise creator would seem almost sacrilegious. One would have to assume that God in His foreknowledge would create souls only for those He foreknew would eventually be born, an argument a prochoice advocate might well apply to aborted fetuses. On the other hand, Catholics, on the basis of rational argument, can hardly hope to argue for anything more than a suitable level of protection warranted by the development stage of the pre-embryo and its sequelae.

61. C. Grobstein, M. Flower, and J. Mendeloff, "External Human Fertilization: An Evaluation of Policy," *Science* 222 (Oct. 14, 1983) 127–33.

62. Bernard Häring, "New Dimensions of Responsible Parenthood," *TS* 37 (1976) 127. This article is also a good review of the scientific literature of that time period and contains references to other articles which discuss our theme.

63. Ford, *When Did I Begin?* 171 ff.

64. Allan B. Wolter, "Chemical Substance," in *Philosophy of Science* (Jamaica, N.Y.: St. John's University, 1960) 108. This citation is an excerpt from a seminal article originally titled "The Problem of Substance." Its primary aim was to present a cosmological account of how mechanical and natural systems differ, why various forms of living substances arise from nonliving matter, and how traditional scholastic philosophical insights and theories such as both the pluriform and uniform hylomorphic conceptions might be helpful as partial insights to a more complex philosophical theory. The psychological role of the rational soul was only discussed peripherally to show how medieval scholastics fitted it into their theories of mediate animation.

65. See J. F. Wippel and A. B. Wolter, *Medieval Philosophy: From St. Augustine to Nicholas of Cusa* (New York/London: Free Press and Collier Macmillan, 1969) 325.

66. Ibid. 320.

67. Wolter, "Chemical Substance" 125–26.

68. For a further discussion of this concept, see James J. Walter, "The Meaning and Validity of Quality of Life Judgments in Contemporary Roman Catholic Medical Ethics," *Louvain Studies* 13 (1988) 195–208. Another discussion can be found in Thomas A. Shannon and James J. Walter, "The PVS Patient and the Forgoing/Withdrawing of Medical Nutrition and Hydration," *TS* 49 (1988) 623–47.

69. We suggest that something of the violence between the extreme prolife or pro-abortionists might be defused, and the political dilemma of Catholic politicians seeking some rational options might be solved, if one were to recognize that the moral status of, and hence the protection appropriate for, a fetus changes with its developmental stages.

70. Quoted by Messenger, *Theology and Evolution* 219.

3 The Choice in "Choose Life"

American Judaism & Abortion

Scott Aaron

Professor Scott Aaron is a teacher of Jewish ethics and values for the Toledo Board of Jewish Education and Temple Shomer Emunim, Toledo, Ohio.

One of the most perplexing questions to Christians interested in the abortion debate is how can Judaism, a religion that celebrates the ethic of "choose life" found in Deuteronomy 30:19, support and condone elective abortion rights in America? Jews support the availability of abortion in far greater numbers than members of any other religion. Some of the leading public figures in the abortion rights movement are Jews. Almost all Jewish politicians have taken a prochoice stand as well. Yet, Judaism reveres as a primary ethical principle the doctrine that no one has the right to put one life before another life. So, is Judaism prolife or prochoice? Paradoxically, it is both, but Christians cannot grasp this without some basic knowledge of American Judaism from both the religious and secular perspectives.

American Jews parallel our Christian neighbors. Of the three main movements within Judaism, the Orthodox community generally opposes nontherapeutic abortion while the Conservative and Reform movements generally support elective abortion. This is comparable to the division between the Catholic church and certain evangelical and fundamentalist Christian denominations which reject abortion under almost all circumstances, and those "progressive" branches of Christianity which generally accept abortion as a moral option at least under some circumstances. The traditional versus modern (i.e., historical vs. contemporary) split in Judaism appears to reflect the division within the Christian community. These appearances, however, are deceiving.

This article first appeared in Commonweal *119 (28 February 1992): 15–18.*

Historically, Judaism is a religion with its own set of laws and standards which, for observant Jews, is as binding as the civil law. Halacha is the body of rabbinical laws (similar to American common law) which are interpretations of how to observe the 613 mitzvot (commandments) in the Torah (five books of Moses traditionally believed to be directly from G-d) in every aspect of daily life. Contrary to general Christian teachings of morality, it has been the traditional belief in Judaism that life does not fully begin until the child is actually born. According to Rabbi David Ellenson, dean of the Hebrew Union College-Jewish Institute of Religion campus in Los Angeles, "basic Jewish rulings on abortion stem from the *Mishna, Ocholot* chapter 7, 6th Halacha, which basically asserts that on a certain level the mother's life takes precedence over the child's life as long as the child is a fetus in the womb." "Once the child enters into the air," however, "then the child's and mother's life take on equal value."

During the first forty days of gestation, the fetus is considered to be in a liquid or unformed state and thus is expendable if necessary because it is not yet alive. After the fortieth day and up until birth, the fetus possesses the status of a limb and is not regarded as a separate and equal life to that of the mother. Thus, the fetus is not a *"nefesh"* (a soul) until its birth. "On the other hand," as Rabbi Ellenson points out, "while it may not be a soul and therefore fully a person, it is not a nonperson either." Just what rights the fetus has and what reasons justify an abortion are the points of conflict on this issue between the traditional and modern Jewish communities.

Orthodox Jews follow the traditional Jewish belief that we do not "own" our bodies because they were created by G-d in G-d's image. Hence Judaism emphasizes that it is incumbent upon Man to take care of and protect his health, and to do everything possible to sustain life. This ethic permeates Jewish law, including the strict prohibitions against murder and reckless activity, the condemnation of euthanasia as murder, and the allowance of exceptions to the sabbath and dietary laws in order to preserve life. The recognized beginnings and potential of life that the fetus possesses are thus held in very high moral esteem, and Orthodox tradition would usually sacrifice the fetus only to preserve the life of the mother.

There is, however, strong precedent within the Orthodox tradition which would allow abortion to preserve the physical health of the mother. Such a situation might arise if the mother had diabetes and the pregnancy would seriously and adversely affect her health to the point that she was unable to function normally, or if she had cancer in remission which the pregnancy might reactivate. Decisions as to whether an abortion would be necessary under these or similar circumstances would be made by an observant Orthodox woman who consulted not only her physician but also her rabbi. Together they would decide if the justification for the abortion was within the moral standards of Jewish law, after weighing the needs and risks to the mother with the moral obligation to create and preserve life.

The key point here is that once a determination is made that an abortion is necessary, the woman is mandated by religious law to preserve her own life and health. To jeopardize her life for that of the fetus would be committing a sin because unlike the child in utero, who may not survive the pregnancy or the trauma of the birth process, the mother's life is already established. Dr. Fred Rosner, a physician and an expert on Jewish biomedical ethics, points out that to traditional Jewish thinking "it's just a mere technicality that says that life begins at birth in Judaism and not at conception the way Catholics have it." The fetus thus occupies a position of developing, not substantiated, life. "Therefore," says Dr. Rosner, "when it's one life against another, you save its mother's life since human life is of infinite value. To save a life you do anything, even if it includes the destruction of an unborn fetus."

This is a hard distinction for many people to accept, Jews and non-Jews alike, but it establishes a necessary guideline for such life-and-death decisions. This is why traditional Judaism, while recognizing and preserving the moral values involved, does not regard abortion as murder. But, as Dr. Rosner points out, "without this saving of a life, you can't touch the fetus just for convenience sake or financial reasons."

Modern Judaism, most notably the Conservative and Reform movements, expands upon the definition of what is permissible abortion. It is important at this juncture to point out the differences in interpretations of the Halacha between the major branches of American Judaism. As noted earlier, the Orthodox follow Halacha literally and rabbis who are recognized by the Orthodox community are bound to handle all issues and questions in strictest conformity with it. Conservative Judaism, although believing that all of the commandments are from G-d and that all Jews are thus bound by them, also believes that there is room for flexible interpretation and application. For instance, Conservative rabbis are very supportive of the use of modern medical technology, such as amniocentesis, in helping resolve these issues. "Since Conservative Judaism believes that Jewish law must be studied and applied historically," writes Rabbi Elliot Dorf, dean of the Conservative movement's University of Judaism in Los Angeles, "it does not say, as some Orthodox rabbis have, that women should never engage in these techniques since that will only encourage them to abort the fetus if they find out it is defective." By way of contrast, Rabbi Dorf writes that "Conservative rabbis . . . maintain that when the physician says that an amniocentesis is advisable, the woman should have one" ("Abortion: Where We Stand," *United Synagogue Review,* Spring, 1990).

Reform Judaism rejects the traditional belief of the revelation of the commandments directly from G-d to Man, and instead believes that divinely inspired men wrote the Torah and that men of equal stature throughout the ages developed the Halacha. Therefore, people today have a choice as to which of the commandments to follow and to what extent, as well as how to interpret the Halacha; it should serve not as law but as guidelines. The emphasis on choice is qualified, however, by the belief that the freedom of choice is meaningless without making religiously based choices in a serious and informed way. Reform Judaism emphasizes that Jews are bound to follow the ethical mitzvot but are free to determine the extent of ritual observance. Therefore, it is natural that in the area of Halacha and abortion, interpretation and compliance differ as well.

Conservative and Reform rabbis differ from their Orthodox counterparts as well in that their advice and counsel is not binding upon their congregants who must choose for themselves what course their lives will take. Rabbis can influence them only through persuasion and education. "I see the role of . . . the rabbi in a case of this sort not as a decisor but as an alter ego," writes Judith Hauptman, associate professor of Talmud at the Jewish Theological Seminary in New York City, "whose job it is to push the mother to think her decision through with painstaking care, to lay the burden of proof on her shoulders, to help her either justify to herself that abortion is the moral choice in her particular case, or if not, to carry the pregnancy to term" (*United Synagogue Review,* Spring, 1990).

Modern Judaism, as can thus be expected from its expansive tradition, can find justification for abortion other than the life or physical health of the mother. Emotional and mental stress may be seen as permissible grounds for an abortion if the mother is seriously affected by them. As it is consistent with Jewish tradition, modern Judaism supports the belief that an abortion is permissible at any time when the mother's well-being is at stake. In contrast, this does not necessarily apply to the child's well-being. Thus, there is general reluctance on the part of many modern rabbis to advise a congregant to abort a child on the basis of a potential birth defect. G-d determines some things beyond human control, and an abortion to spare the child a difficult life is seen as overstepping our control over life and death and intervening into some things that G-d has done for his own incomprehensible reasons.

Other rabbis would advise an abortion under these circumstances if the mother has expressed deep and damaging anxiety over this pregnancy because her well-being, not the fetus's, is in jeopardy. However, as

Dr. Hauptman points out, "a rabbi ought to encourage a woman to en-gage in a serious moral calculus." While a pregnant woman contemplat-ing an abortion for these reasons needs to consider the effect of a greatly impaired child on the needs and responsibilities of her entire family, she needs to weigh that against her own sense of value for the life of that fetus. "If the phrase 'abortion on demand' means that one may choose abortion without thoughtful consideration of all the relevant social and moral issues," says Dr. Hauptman, "then I too am opposed to it." The same logic may also be applied to abortions sought on the grounds of rape and incest.

Abortion as a method of dealing with an unwanted or inconvenient pregnancy is not condoned by any Jewish movement, but modern rabbis often justify the sacrifice of the child as a means of dealing with a realistic threat to the well-being of the mother. The loss of the quality and value and even potential of the mother's life can justify to many the sacrifice of a potential life, especially in cases like teen-age pregnancy. Rabbi Mark Washofsky, professor at the Hebrew Union College-Jewish Institute of Religion's Cincinnati campus and a recognized expert on Reform Juda-ism and abortion, points out that "Moses's exhortation to 'choose life' is a general thrust of Jewish life and observance which, if it means anything, means that we ought to be very careful about life-and-death decisions." He and many modern rabbis see life as definable in more than one way. "If these cases are serious enough that the rabbis have been willing to permit them, perhaps that is choosing life also and perhaps that is also making it possible for women and families to get on with their lives."

The nonclerical Jewish community is often more vocal on its pro-choice position than the religious leadership and for distinctly non-religious reasons. As Rabbi Washofsky clearly says, "I think the average Reform Jew doesn't really think of it in religious terms." For him it is a personal as well as a professional issue, extending beyond his rabbinical position. "Free choice is something I believe in because I'm an American, suburban, urbane, liberal type person and this is what I would believe in if I weren't Jewish. So therefore it's the right thing to do and Judaism believes in doing the right thing, and therefore, Judaism believes in unrestricted access to abortion."

The secular Jewish communal organizations see the issue here as not just one of choice but of protection of constitutional rights. The strongly Catholic and Christian composition of the prolife community, and attempts to legislate what appears to be their religious position, sound alarm bells among secular Jewish leaders. "There is not one Jew-ish position on the abortion question," says Michael Sandberg, Midwest civil rights director of the Anti-Defamation League of B'Nai Brith. Because the potential for diverse views based upon religious orientation is so great, he says, "we regard it as a question of freedom and in large measure a religious freedom." The Anti-Defamation League has a time-honored policy of defending First Amendment issues regardless of which religious belief is being threatened. "We respect the views of the different sides of the controversy and do not say that we are adhering to the Jewish position, but rather regard the prochoice side of the argument as the essential freedom of religion that our organization stands for." Sylvia Neil, director of the Chicago office of the American Jewish Congress, puts it more directly. "If you are looking at this issue in terms of civil liberties or rights for women, a society that is open and is progressive in terms of religious rights most likely is also going to be progressive towards Jews and Jewish rights. Privacy is a religious liberty as well as a civil liberty."

A brief look at the past illuminates the source of these concerns. The United States is the first country in modern times that has allowed Jews to observe freely their religion and participate in every aspect of society without restriction based on faith. However, for much of its history, this country has been influenced by the Christian demographic majority who have incorporated mandatory church attendance, moral purity laws, mandatory prayer in schools, Sunday "blue" laws, public funding of religion, and other Christianity-influenced beliefs into secular law. Only in this century has the Supreme Court declared most of these laws unconstitutional because they violate the First Amendment's prohibition against establishment of a state religion and the freedom of religious exercise for minority religions such as Judaism.

For Jews, there is an underlying fear of losing these hard-won religious freedoms. If we lose the right for a Jewish woman to determine when her religious beliefs mandate an abortion, then next will be prayer in schools, Sunday "blue" laws, public funding of religious institutions: a return to the time of Christian laws for a Christian America as Father Charles Coughlin and William Jennings Bryan among others used to advocate. As Mr. Sandberg points out, "you could argue that if abortion laws should change and become more restrictive or even outlawed, that might pave the way for further efforts by people who argue forcefully that religious teachings ought to have the force of law. We think they shouldn't." This concern is not because Jews want to suppress or neutralize Christianity, but because they want the full protection of the Constitution to value their own varied religious beliefs with equal freedom as all of the other members of the American pluralistic society.

Judaism and Christianity are not analogous on this issue and the legalization of one clearly religious belief, such as life beginning at conception, would conversely outlaw any other. Thus, from a Jewish civil rights perspective, it is understandable that many Jews see the chipping away at *Roe* as the cracking in our constitutional foundation. As Mr. Sandberg emphasizes, "our concern is that none of the religious teachings warrant inclusion by statute or constitutional amendment as part of American life in this democracy. None ought to be adopted as law and any ought to be available as people decide to follow their own religious beliefs on such a difficult issue as this." This concern has become increasingly heightened since the Supreme Court handed back *Employment Services* v. *Smith* during the 1989–90 term which allowed the state of Oregon to make ceremonial use of peyote illegal even though it was an important and historically established part of American Indian religious worship. The Court found banning illegal substances even from religious usage to be overridden by the legitimate secular purpose of controlling drug abuse. The leap from state control of religious observances involving peyote to state banning of a religiously motivated reproductive health decision is not a long one in the eyes of many civil libertarians.

Not every Jew shares Rabbi Washofsky's analysis. The largest Orthodox community organization in America, Agudath Israel, repeatedly sides with the prolife movement in *amicus curiae* briefs in cases dealing with abortion-related issues. Orthodox Jews can regularly be found with Catholics and Christians picketing abortion clinics in their communities. Yehuda Levin, an Orthodox rabbi and president of the Jewish Anti-Abortion League in Brooklyn, resents the shift away from the traditional Jewish respect for fetal life toward nonphysical maternal needs that modern Judaism has initiated. He also believes that modern and secular Judaism's prochoice stance sends false and dangerous messages to the Christian community. "I feel that it's important that the message go out to the hearers of Jerry Falwell or Cardinal O'Connor that there are Jews who keep the traditions." For Rabbi Levin, these traditions mean the allowance of abortion only for severe, therapeutic crises. The abortion disagreement, he believes, reflects the broader fundamental differences between modern and traditional Jews. "We do things the way our grandparents did a thousand years ago," he says, "or to put it in more contemporary terms, we never lost it. The Jews who never lost it have a very prolife view which frankly predates the Christian prolife view."

Overall, it can be said of American Jewry in relation to abortion that while our general secular concern is religious freedom, there is a very clear belief in all the movements of the Jewish religion that fetal development is the beginnings of life and that decisions regarding its possible termination should be treated with the seriousness appropriate to such matters. Still, when the viewpoints range within our community from endorsing elective abortion accessibility because "it's the right thing to do" to opposing it because one believes in living daily life "the way our grandparents did a thousand years ago," no one can say that there is a single Jewish position on abortion or that Judaism itself is prolife or prochoice. This can only be said about individual Jews.

It is thus possible to see how the charge in Deuteronomy 30:19 to "choose life" can be believed to be served by both modern and traditional American Judaism from their respective viewpoints on the abortion issue. Translating this into political support, the majority of American Jewry comes down in favor of some form of abortion availability even if only for life and health purposes because of the mandates of Halacha. Garnering Jewish support for restrictions on abortion that would severely weaken or overturn *Roe* would be difficult. The Jewish community would be concerned that the legalization of one religious viewpoint (i.e., life beginning at conception) would limit or deny decision making according to religious teachings that may differ with the legalized view. This analysis may not always prove true though on related issues such as parental involvement in the abortion decision for minors or public funding for nontherapeutic abortions. Although there is certainly room for discussion and compromise in the moral and legislative debates on abortion, Christians and Jews will never make any mutual progress on this issue until they understand and acknowledge the differences in religious belief systems and the confines of the American Constitution.

4 *HIV and Pregnancy*

BRENDA ALMOND AND CAROLE ULANOWSKY

Brenda Almond is a reader in philosophy and education at the University of Hull, England. Carole Ulanowsky is an instructor for the National Childbirth Trust in England.

R ecently in a hospital in an English provincial town where drugs, HIV infection, and prostitution are problems associated with a distant world of fast city life, a young woman encountered special difficulties with her first pregnancy. Clearly there were problems, but no diagnosis that seemed at all plausible had been offered. Only as she went into labor did a young woman physician make *her* first diagnosis of AIDS.

For the young mother, this was a totally unforeseen disaster—once the diagnosis was made, she was able to identify the source of the infection as a brief sexual encounter preceding the committed relationship in which she had embarked on pregnancy and childbirth. But at this stage, it was too late for the tragedy to be anything other than a double one, for the child was later found to have been born with HIV infection.

At the beginning of pregnancy, normal medical care includes testing a sample of blood for a variety of conditions it might be important for a woman embarking on pregnancy or for those caring for her to know about. These include tests for syphilis, rubella, hepatitis, and other possibilities. Few pregnant women are aware of the list of diseases being ruled out at this stage. There is no need for them to be, since for the vast majority the tests are negative. In addition, most of these conditions can be treated effectively and no stigma is attached to positive findings. HIV infection, however, is seen as a special case, posing a special need for informed consent. At the same time, the notion of informed consent is being given an especially strong interpretation, in which extensive counseling is regarded as a necessary condition if consent is to be considered truly "informed."

The burden of this counseling is, however, likely to be less medical than social and economic. Medically, HIV infection is a condition that can-

---

This article appeared in Hastings Center Report *20 (March/April 1990)* *16–21.*

not be cured, although there is evidence that some approaches to the problem may help maintain health longer. Undoubtedly, however, the social and financial implications of a positive diagnosis are serious. Health and life insurance, mortgages, and house purchase may all be affected. There may be problems for some types of employment and there are clearly likely to be difficulties on the personal level where the question of what to tell sexual partners or close relatives must loom large. A special practical fear on the part of a pregnant woman may be the loss of a sexual partner who is providing home and support for her. These are far from negligible considerations, and it is understandable, therefore, that some people might prefer to avoid knowledge of seropositivity.

Nevertheless, there may be good reasons to establish a woman's HIV status early in pregnancy; and women who might become pregnant may have stronger reasons than others to be sure that they are not seropositive. Our argument is not that testing should be forced on women who genuinely do not want it, but that it is useful and should be recommended to them—indeed, more strongly, that it should be regarded as routine except where special objections are expressed. Respect for objections need not suggest, however, that "consent" should be given a stronger interpretation for HIV than for other tests administered during pregnancy, or that women should be counseled against giving consent.

Because AIDS in the USA and in Western Europe has been particularly associated both in the public mind and in medical reality with certain clearly defined groups—gay and bisexual males, IV drug users, and hemophiliacs—it would be easy to underestimate the problem it poses for young women contemplating or embarked on pregnancy. In New York City, however, the fact is that AIDS is already the leading cause of death for women aged between twenty and twenty-nine and is soon expected to become the leading cause of death for all women of childbearing age in that city. In the UK, there was a 26 percent rise in the discovery of new HIV infection in pregnant women in 1987.[1] (No data exist, however, on the seroprevalence rate for *all* women of childbearing age in the U.K.)

Once the scale of the problem is appreciated, it becomes clear that this is not a problem for a few individuals only. Nevertheless, in considering the wider aspects, it is important to remember that the problem does come back in the end to individuals. This suggests that the issue should be looked at from three interlocking perspectives.

First is the personal perspective, the considerations and concerns of a woman contemplating or embarking on pregnancy. Knowledge of seropositivity is emotionally traumatic for anyone in any situation, but for a woman in the emotionally precarious early stages of pregnancy it may be especially distressing. When counseling is involved, the nature of that counseling is itself an issue to be considered. What advice should others give to a woman in this position? Does she need to know her HIV status? On what grounds should this information be sought or not sought? And, as far as others are concerned, on what grounds should it either not be established or, if available, be withheld?

Second is the perspective of the caregiver. Here a major consideration is the need for safety in perinatal situations. Obstetricians, gynecologists, and midwives have a duty to guard against the spread of infection from mother to baby and from patient to patient. They also have a legitimate concern in relation to the risks they themselves run in perinatal care—risks that may exceed those of other areas of medicine, since in childbirth open wounds are the norm, and practices such as the sampling of cord blood and the draining of mucus present special hazards. Is knowledge of their patients' HIV status essential for caregivers' own security, and how will this knowledge, or lack of it, affect practice in the maternity unit?

Third is the wider community perspective. It would be a narrow ethical perspective that confined attention to the individual patient, for particularly in the case of a pregnant woman two other individuals are liable to be directly involved. One of these is, of course, the child she is carrying. The other is the child's father. His position raises special considerations we will discuss later.

Apart from this immediate small sample, a new issue emerges here. It has been argued that the public interest requires sound epidemiological data on the extent and spread of the disease, and that pregnant women provide the best possible source of this information: they are healthy, sexually active, and provide a core representative sample of the general population than do other groups that have been used for this purpose. Here attention shifts from the interests of the woman to those of the community so that the issue becomes: Should pregnant women be treated as means to other people's ends?

In considering the set of problems that cluster around the issue of HIV and pregnancy, it would be easier to take this last issue first, for the questions involved here are very different from those in the more directly personal areas.

Monitoring HIV Infection by Antenatal Screening

It is important to distinguish between, on the one hand, the collection of epidemiological information that reveals facts relevant to named individuals and, on the other, anonymized testing, in which blood is not tested until all marks of identification other than place, age and patient category have been removed (unlinked). In the latter case, it is difficult to see what valid objection can be raised to the practice.

One objection that is raised, however, by Dutch feminists, British midwives, and the UK-based National Childbirth Trust among others is that the mere use of women for purposes not directly aimed at their personal good is offensive in itself. As a spokeswoman for the Royal College of Midwives put this point: "Mothers should not be used in this way. There is no current justifiable reason to use them as a surveillance group. They attend antenatal clinics for specific reasons to do with the well-being of them and their babies." She went on to say that "Healthy mothers in this situation can hardly be called volunteers; but more as hostages to the need for new initiative to combat AIDS."[2]

This emotive language can scarcely be justified in the case of genuinely anonymized testing. As the British Medical Association Foundation for AIDS has recently argued, the fact that no individual can be identified means that there cannot be any adverse consequences for people whose serum—already taken for other purposes—is exposed to this one extra test. For this reason, they suggest, specific consent for HIV testing is not required.[3]

In fact, many countries do routinely conduct anonymous seroprevalence surveys of this sort; this is why figures *are* available—from the United States and some African countries, as well as Sweden and other European countries. These make it clear that the figures of those affected are significant at a level recognized to justify routine prenatal screening in the case of other illnesses.[4]

The moral argument about the use of women for ends not their own overlooks the way in which the interest of women bearing children is more closely and deeply connected with the community interest than is the case with other patients or populations. To have a child is to commit oneself to society's future. Many women, seeing the issue as one of tackling a threat to that future, will be more than willing to contribute to the knowledge needed to maximize control of AIDS. So while an explicit refusal should of course be respected, explicit consent should not be regarded as a moral requirement where unlinked, anonymous testing is at issue.

THE PERSONAL DILEMMA

The larger question concerns not anonymous surveys, however, but the use of HIV testing in clinical settings: Is ignorance the best policy for the individual? It must be accepted that many people do not want to know if they are seropositive since they are aware that even if they are, they may have a reasonable hope of some years of healthy and satisfying life, which could be blighted by knowledge of seropositivity. But this argument, which raises many questions when it is advanced in connection with testing proposals for homosexuals or for heterosexuals whose sexual lifestyle is varied and active, is particularly inadequate when applied to the case of women who are pregnant or contemplating pregnancy, for a number of reasons unique to this situation.

To begin with, some fear that, because pregnancy may alter cell-mediated immunity, pregnancy and childbirth could be precipitating factors as far as the development of AIDS is concerned, or that if AIDS is already present these factors may operate to accelerate illness.[5] Early diagnosis of opportunistic infections during pregnancy can certainly help prevent both maternal and neonatal morbidity. Most importantly, however, ignorance of a woman's HIV status may lead to the birth of a child with a poor medical prognosis, for there is a very considerable risk of children born to mothers who are HIV-infected being themselves infected, and neonatal morbidity and mortality associated with perinatal HIV is high. Approximately 30 percent of infants born to infected women can be expected to develop AIDS, and over half of these will die during the first year of life.[6]

For all these reasons, for women who are considering pregnancy or who are already pregnant, knowledge of HIV status *can* make a medical difference. In the United Kingdom, the fact of seropositivity is considered sufficient medical grounds for therapeutic abortion,[7] and knowledge will likely deter many women from embarking on pregnancy if they have not already done so.

This is not, however, to preempt the decision about whether to proceed with pregnancy, for this must be the woman's alone. The question is rather whether such a decision is best made in ignorance. On the other side of the balance are more encouraging recent studies that suggest that a woman who is HIV positive but otherwise healthy may give birth to a healthy baby and remain in good health herself.[8] Some women will be prepared to accept the odds. If a woman does not yet have any children, the decision not to proceed is, in the present state of affairs as regards AIDS, a decision to remain childless. Knowing that her own prognosis is bad, or even anticipating a short life expectancy, may provide a very strong reason for a woman to seek fulfillment in motherhood.

One special case may be mentioned here: that of the seronegative woman whose sexual partner is seropositive. In this case, a woman may have to consider incurring the risk of becoming HIV positive herself to become pregnant; but she may judge this risk to be worthwhile to preserve something substantial from a relationship of love cut short by illness.

To make such a decision or to decide responsibly about childbirth, however, an individual needs to know not only the general position but also her own HIV status. If the arguments for personal knowledge are valid, it would clearly also be wrong for a counselor to recommend that the choice be made in ignorance of HIV status. Counseling produces very different results in different contexts, however. In Sweden, for example, where great openness in sexual matters prevails, more than 99 percent of pregnant women accept testing, which is routinely offered them, while in the UK, where there is less openness, figures are dramatically lower. Indeed, in one study in a London clinic only nine out of an estimated 1,500 women deemed of "high risk" agreed to be tested.[9] If we assume that the social consequences and support services for women identified as infected are similar in the two countries, the magnitude of the difference suggests a strong negative bias on the part of UK counselors. The poor acceptance of testing after counseling is even more a matter of concern in view of the Royal College of Midwives' demand for greatly increased expenditures to extend these services.[10]

Two other special points regarding the individual perspective deserve attention. First, if the case for testing at the beginning of pregnancy is accepted, there is a need for speed in diagnosis to allow a maximum of time for the difficult decision about possible termination. It is a disadvantage that HIV may take some time to detect by normal antibody tests, a second test after a three-month interval being recommended to confirm an initial negative finding, while other tests, which are less likely to be falsely negative, are not readily available outside research settings. But this is not a good reason for abandoning any attempt to test at all, since failure to identify the antibody is a problem only for the small minority of cases where the infection has been newly contracted.

Second, it may be argued that tests in these circumstances may be more visible and less confidential than tests taken by individuals in less pressured circumstances. The reason for a termination of pregnancy may emerge, bringing in its train all the consequences of publicity mentioned earlier. But this is not a necessary outcome, and the possibility is in any case not sufficient to outweigh the importance of this information for the woman herself given what is at stake.

THE ISSUES FOR CAREGIVERS

These two last considerations, however, point beyond the predicament of the pregnant woman and toward the surrounding circumstances, the social context within which decisions—decisions about testing, for example, or about termination of pregnancy—must be made. Most directly concerned are those with care responsibilities for pregnant women: physicians, midwives, nurses, counsellors. There are good reasons for beginning with their concern for safety, since as it turns out this has considerable consequences both for patients with HIV infection, for those deemed to be at risk of it, and for patients not thought to be at risk.

This may seem at first sight a surprising claim, but HIV/AIDS is already having a significant effect on antenatal, obstetric, and pediatric care. At the antenatal stage, invasive investigative techniques (such as chorionic villi sampling and amniocentesis) that can give information about the fetus during the early weeks (detecting, for example, such conditions as Down syndrome) are in the case of women who are HIV positive or considered to be "at risk" likely to be avoided for fear of mixing maternal/fetal blood and secretions.[11]

Some clinicians, too, recommend cesarean deliveries for such women to avoid possible transmission of the virus to the baby during normal vaginal birth, pending definitive results of investigations into the relative risks of modes of transmission from mother to baby.[12] Transmission, however, may take place during pregnancy, *in utero*, through the placenta, or during the birth process itself. In the present state of knowledge, then, there is room for doubt as to whether cesarean operations *do* reduce the risk of transmission of the virus.

Because staff must see that other mothers and babies are protected, the Royal College of Obstetricians and Gynecologists' guidelines advise that women who are known to be HIV positive or who are considered to be "high risk" should be looked after apart from other mothers and babies during labor, delivery, and immediately following birth, and that they should not be allowed to handle other women's babies.

The threat of HIV infection means, too, that a baby is likely to be delivered by a team wearing full protective clothing: cap, eye protection, mask, and boots or overshoes since "body fluids may be shed unexpectedly and explosively."[13]

These precautions are recommended also following labor and during the early post-partum period. The use of speedy and efficient mouth-operated suction of mucus at the time of delivery is no longer recommended.[14] Investigative techniques to detect abnormal responses during labor—such as scalp blood sampling, a technique that is highly specific and accurate—are likely to be abandoned in favor of less efficient but safer procedures in terms of avoiding transmission of the virus.

Care of the newborn also involves quite extreme precautionary measures. Babies are to be handled with surgical gloves. These are recommended not only when touching the cord or doing heel pricks, but also when changing diapers or dealing with vomit. Disposable paper tape measures are proposed for measuring the infant's length and head circumference. Breast-feeding by HIV mothers is also discouraged, in view of the evidence of virus transmission by this means.[15]

In the United States, some of these measures are recommended as universal practice independently of the HIV risk as a precaution against all blood-borne infections. In the United Kingdom, however, the natural childbirth movement has long campaigned for less technological management of birth and its aftermath. They would see unmediated human touch as important for both mother and baby.

It may be that informality of approach and setting must now be abandoned in general in maternity care. However, at least in the UK, it seems that RCOG remains ambivalent on this issue, seeing stringent precautions as necessary in the case of women seen as "high risk" for HIV, and unnecessary in other cases.

Yet the question of "high risk" women and how they are to be identified is extremely controversial. Guidelines vary, but include: IV drug-users and their sexual partners; partners of known HIV-positive men, such as some hemophiliacs; the partners of male bisexuals; prostitutes; women from African countries other than those bordering on the Mediterranean; and women who have had sexual relations with men from these places, or whose sexual partners have.[16] In Sweden, the categories are widened to include people from the U.S., and recipients of blood transfusions since 1979.[17] A mere summary of these guidelines is sufficient to show that both many apparently "at risk" women will be wrongly presumed to be so, and also that many genuinely "at risk" will fail to be identified merely by questioning. Sheldon Landesman and colleagues, for example, report a study in an inner city hospital in New York in which self-reporting and interviews failed to identify 42 percent of seropositive women. Without the follow-up testing of all individuals in this sample, five out of twelve women who were in fact HIV antibody positive would have gone undetected. This constitutes a seroprevalence rate of 1.1 percent in a group of women with "no identifiable risk factors."[18]

Compared with actually testing for evidence of HIV infection, it is clear that the risk concept, when used so as to affect significantly a woman's perinatal care and that of her child, is a dubious and unreliable tool. In the case of genuine infection the precautions may unfortunately be necessary. Whether they are is a medical judgment on which we do not embark. But in the face of mere possibility they are undoubtedly distasteful and extreme. Uncertainty about HIV status creates a situation of anomaly and paradox for patients and staff alike. Meanwhile, contradictory messages are sent out: for example, it is recommended that a woman who needs resuscitation should be dealt with by staff who wear the correct clothing and proceed "according to the current recommended practice and standards," but "it must be emphasized that maternal resuscitation should not be delayed whilst awaiting the appropriate equipment."[19] If these measures are essential, then the tension can only be resolved by treating all untested women as infected, or, as the term "universal precautions" suggests, treating all women as potentially infectious.

The conclusion, then, to be drawn from these complex safety considerations points in the same direction as the considerations to be taken into account by the patient herself: accurate knowledge of HIV status is important in the perinatal situation. But what of the broader picture?

THE WIDER CONTEXT

A number of official statements about caregivers' responsibilities have defined these in terms that seem to limit them to the patient directly before them.[20] But a woman on the threshold of pregnancy and childbirth is not an isolate or a unit. Intimately connected with her are child and—in most cases—husband or sexual partner. The narrower perspective has in fact never obtained in the case of maternity care, where mother and baby are regarded as a joint responsibility of the medical team.

As far as the well-being of the child is concerned, most modern societies declare their interest by making it, for example, a legal requirement on a pregnant woman to seek medical care. Without entering into the debate about abortion, it should be stated that the authors of this article have no doubt that a woman who has good reason not to proceed with a pregnancy should not be forced by others to do so. Nonetheless, society does have an interest in women making these choices in a thoughtful and well-informed way. Neither women nor their medical attendants can reach rationally based decisions in relation to HIV issues in ignorance of the facts in a particular situation.

To be taken into account here if the woman is in fact HIV positive are not only the medical risks, but also the question of who is to care for the child if either or both parents are unlikely to survive its infancy.[21] It is important that medical advisors, counselors, or caregivers should not attempt to preempt the patient's right to consider these aspects, although paternalistic attitudes in medicine, particularly in the area of gynecology and obstetrics, are not uncommon. A British gynecologist, for example, writes: "What should *we* do about mothers-to-be with positive tests?" and goes on to argue, "There is at present no effective treatment to offer pregnant women with HIV infection" (emphasis added).[22] Yet clearly there *is* much to be done medically with pregnancies taken to term, even apart from the important issue of termination.

And what, finally, of the sexual partner of an infected woman? He may or may not be the source of her infection and may or may not be HIV positive. If he is not the source of her infection and is HIV negative, then he is clearly at risk, and the question of disclosure to him is more

sharply at issue than it is in the more general cases that have been discussed elsewhere by writers concerned with the question of medical
confidentiality.[23] The pregnancy is in itself evidence of an active sexual
relationship without protection, and would also be seen by most couples
as a time to continue sexual relations without protection.

Clearly in such a case a woman must be urged to tell her sexual
partner, and many women will, in any case, set their partners' health
above their own more narrowly defined interest. (As far as physicians
are concerned, the situation could be regarded as one in which a breach
of confidentiality would be *justified* where a woman was unwilling to
take any kind of action herself, though as a special exception and not as
one in which a new principle of a duty to inform had supplanted the
usual need to preserve confidentiality.)

Such widening implications may lead us to reiterate the position so
far argued for: that women contemplating pregnancy are in a particular
"need to know" situation regarding their HIV status. Once this is more
widely perceived by women, it is possible that they will fill a vital role in
the war against AIDS by bringing this disease out into the open, where it
will be treated as a disease like any other, and not as a social embarrass-
ment or stigmatizing condition.

If this does not happen, the wider picture is bleaker still, as evidence
from other parts of the world suggests. We may expect a dramatic impact
on health and social services with huge economic costs and in the end—
since this is a disease that attacks human beings in their reproductive
function—an impact on birth patterns and a threat to population replacement. In the Third World these consequences, already visible, are beginning to be perceived as a threat to economic and political stability.

What is the way forward? Ultimately, of course, the prevention of
perinatal transmission depends on protecting women of child-bearing
age from HIV infection. In the absence of medical means of doing this, it
is important that those with responsibility for health and sex education
move this issue to the front of education about HIV and AIDS. (Currently, such programs in the UK, for example, give scant attention to the
problem of perinatal transmission, and programs of education for maternity do not mention AIDS.) It is vital for girls to understand the importance of knowing, before becoming pregnant, that they are not HIV
positive. It is important for them to understand that if they are pregnant,
there are good reasons to establish their HIV status at the earliest possible stage.

As far as counseling and medical practice are concerned, those
working in this field should recognize the importance of testing for HIV
infection as another routine procedure except in those cases where a
patient specifically objects. Patients should be notified that HIV screen-

ing will take place, but in-depth counseling should be reserved for those with questions or who later return with positive results.

This is not to set the community or the public interest above that of the individual woman. Far from it. For the worst thing that could happen to any young woman embarking on childbearing is to reach the later stages of pregnancy and childbirth and *then* find out what she would so much have preferred to know earlier: that what would have been a single tragedy has been converted through ignorance into a double one.

REFERENCES

1. John Osborne "Mothers and Babies" in *AIDS: Meeting the Community Challenge,* Vicky Cosstick, ed. (Slough: St. Paul's Publications, 1987), 33. A press report states that the percentage of HIV positive women who have acquired the virus solely through sexual contact has risen from 11 percent in 1985 to approximately 40 percent in 1988; the report adds that the typical profile of a woman diagnosed as HIV-positive in the United Kingdom is that she is white, in her twenties, working, and in a steady relationship. *The Guardian,* 14 December 1988.

2. General Secretary Ruth Ashton quoted in Press Release of Royal College of Midwives, London, 25 May 1988.

3. British Medical Association, "BMA urges anonymous HIV testing," *The Guardian,* 27 August 1988.

4. Howard Minkoff *et al.,* "Routinely Offered Prenatal HIV Testing," *New England Journal of Medicine* 319:15 (1988), 1018.

5. See Howard Minkoff, "Acquired Immunodeficiency Virus," *Journal of Nurse Midwifery* 31:4 (1986), 189–93, at 191; Catherine S. Peckham, Yvonne D. Sentura, and Anthony E. Ades, "Obstetric and Perinatal Consequences of Human Immunodeficiency Virus (HIV) Infection: A Review," *British Journal of Obstetrics and Gynecology* 94 (May 1987), 403–407; see also Minkoff *et al.,* "Routinely Offered Prenatal HIV Testing." However, in the case of asymptomatic women, recent studies would indicate a more optimistic outcome: Dr. Martha Rogers, Chief, Pediatric and Family Studies AIDS Program, CDC, private correspondence.

6. See The National Swedish Board of Health and Welfare, "HIV and AIDS in Care" (1988), 11.

7. BMA, Third BMA Statement on AIDS (1987).

8. Gwendolyne B. Scott *et al.,* "Mothers of Infants with the Acquired Immunodeficiency Syndrome. Evidence for Both Symptomatic and Asymptomatic Carriers," *Journal of the American Medical Association* 253:3 (1985), 363–66.

9. Ministry of Health and Social Affairs (Stockholm, 1988), 36. On the British example, see Raymond B. Heath *et al.,* "Anonymous Testing of Women Attending Antenatal Clinics for Evidence of Infection with HIV," *Lancet,* 18 June 1988, 1394. In the US, testing in a Brooklyn health center was offered to all pregnant women (i.e., not simply those from high risk groups) and was accepted by 40 percent. See Minkoff *et al.,* "Routinely Offered Prenatal HIV Testing."

80   BRENDA ALMOND, CAROLE ULANOWSKY

10. Ashton, Press release.

11. See advice given in The Royal College of Obstetricians and Gynecologists' "Report on Problems Associated with AIDS in Relation to Obstetrics and Gynecology" (UK, 1988), 6, Note 5.

12. See F. Chiodo et al., "Vertical Transmission of HTLV III" Lancet, 29 March 1986, 739.

13. RCOG, "Report on Problems Associated with AIDS in Relation to Obstetrics and Gynecology," Appendix III.

14. RCOG, "Report on Problems Associated with AIDS."

15. Department of Health and Social Security, UK, HIV Infection, Breastfeeding and Human Milk Banking. Guidelines for Doctors, Midwives, Chief Nursing Officers (London: Department of Health and Social Security, April 1988).

16. See Sheldon Landesman et al., "Serosurvey of Human Immunodeficiency Virus Infection in Parturients," Journal of the American Medical Association 258:19 (1987), 2701–2703, at 2703.

17. National Swedish Board of Health and Welfare, "HIV and AIDS in Care" (1988), 19.

18. Landesman et al., "Serosurvey," 2702.

19. RCOG, "Report on Problems Associated with AIDS," 8.

20. The Royal College of Nursing in London, for example, was until recently of the opinion that anonymous screening is an invasion of the integrity and privacy of the human being: testing, even if anonymous, should only be done with consent and with full counseling support. See letter to Chief Nursing Officer, Department of Health and Social Security, "Response of RCN to DHSS Consultative Document on Anonymous Screening" (August 1988).

21. Janine Railton, "Women with AIDS" in AIDS: Meeting the Community Challenge, 52–54, at 54.

22. John Osborne, "Mothers and Babies," in AIDS: Meeting the Community Challenge, 32–35, at 33.

23. See, for example, Grant Gillett, "AIDS and Confidentiality," Journal of Applied Philosophy 4 (1987), 15–20; Raanan Gillon, "AIDS and Medical Confidentiality," British Medical Journal, 27 June 1987, 1675–77.

5 The Argument for Unlimited Procreative Liberty: A Feminist Critique

MAURA A. RYAN, PH.D.

Maura Ryan, Ph.D. is Assistant Professor of Christian Ethics in the Department of Theology at the University of Notre Dame.

As growing numbers of infertile heterosexual and gay and lesbian couples, along with single individuals, seek to parent through techniques that facilitate conception or permit the use of a genetic and/or gestational donor, and the boundaries of the "scientifically possible" enlarge, we are confronted with a host of increasingly urgent questions. Can the components of parenting—genetic, gestational, and social—be separated at will without harm to the participants? Do new forms of noncoital and donor-assisted reproduction threaten the foundations of the family, and hence, social existence as we know it? Are there "natural" limits to human intervention in the procreative process? Ought artificial reproduction be permitted to become a commercial venture? Does the right to engage in coital reproduction, protected for married couples under the U.S. Constitution, extend into a right to engage in noncoital reproduction; if so, for whom, and under what circumstances?

Questions of liberty and individual rights are emotionally charged ones in American public discourse. Moreover, family autonomy has long been held as a value worthy of such firm protection in our courts and legislatures that policies of minimal interference by the state into domestic life have been maintained even where it has meant a certain institutional blindness to the reality of spousal and child abuse. This context explains why the question of procreative liberty is important in

This article first appeared in Hastings Center Report 20 *(July/August 1990): 6–12.*

current public policy debates surrounding the "new reproduction." Decisions with respect to the limits that may be placed on efforts to procreate, on which parties may be permitted to seek technological assistance in procreation, on the amount of public protection or funding to be extended, and on the conditions under which funding or protection might be warranted turn, many legal scholars believe, on the question of whether we have a right to procreate. Some maintain that the Constitution provides for virtually unlimited right of access to reproductive means.

The freedom to decide whether one will bear and nurture children, and under what circumstances, has been a central issue in the women's liberation movement. As persons whose self-identity and social role have been defined historically in relation to their procreative capacities, women have a great deal at stake in questions of reproductive freedom. Early feminists expended significant energy to secure the right to use contraceptive measures and to seek legal abortion, as well as to gain recognition of their rights as consumers of gynecological and obstetrical care. To say that feminism has promoted procreative liberty for women is not, however, to say that contemporary feminists have welcomed recent developments in reproductive technology without reservation.[1] Nor is it to say, despite the central importance given to the protection of women's autonomy in reproductive decisions, that feminists in general would treat procreative liberty as an unrestricted value. Rather, a feminist perspective includes commitments to human relationality as well as autonomy, and attention to the social context of personal choices. Thus questions of individual freedom, even in matters of reproduction, must be raised in conjunction with other equally compelling considerations about what is needed for human flourishing and what is required for a just society.

I want to highlight these themes by attending to the arguments for an unlimited right to procreate raised most cogently by John Robertson.[2] This position, based primarily on the importance of procreation for individuals, contains several elements that are troubling from a feminist perspective. My concern will not be with matters of constitutional law, but instead with the underlying model of procreative liberty, and its consequences for our understanding of reproduction and our attitudes toward human persons in general and children in particular.

The Case for Full Procreative Liberty

Robertson's argument for the protection of a right to reproduce noncoitally or collaboratively (that is, with the participation of a gamete donor or gestator who is not one's spouse) is based on a historical protection of intramarital reproductive rights and the societal interest in safeguarding family autonomy. Since courts have recognized persons' rights to reproduce coitally, and not to reproduce coitally, their right to pursue those ends by noncoital means, if necessary, must also be protected. As a consequence of the natural lottery, infertility ought not prevent some from pursuing what has been recognized as of value to all.

Because childbearing and rearing have been viewed as experiences of great significance to persons, constitutive of individual identity and notions of a meaningful life, the courts have tended to take a position of noninterference in procreative decisions, particularly where married couples were involved. However, while an individual's right *not* to conceive, gestate, and rear has been explicitly protected in cases like *Griswold v. Connecticut* and *Roe v. Wade,* as has the right of parents to rear according to their own beliefs in cases like *Wisconsin v. Yoder,* the right *to* procreate has been addressed only implicitly. Robertson argues that one could and should infer from the right of couples to avoid procreation a correlative right to procreate, and from the unregulated freedom of married couples to add to their families coitally a freedom to do so noncoitally. No clear distinction should be allowed to stand, when procreative means exist, between fertile and infertile couples:

> The reason and values that support a right to reproduce coitally apply equally to noncoital activities involving external conception and collaborators. While the case is strongest for a couple's right to noncoital and external conception a strong argument for their right to enlist the aid of gamete and womb donors can also be made.[3]

Since reproductive rights are derived from the central importance of reproduction in an individual's life and are limited only by a capacity to participate meaningfully and an ability to accept or transfer rearing responsibilities, all those persons meeting this minimum criteria, whether married or not, ought to be free to pursue it.

Having argued that procreative autonomy is finally rooted in "the notion that individuals have a right to choose and live out the kind of life that they find meaningful and fulfilling," Robertson will allow for the use of technology for any reason that would realize the couple's "reproductive goals":

> The right of married persons to use noncoital and collaborative means of conception to overcome infertility must extend to any purpose, including selecting the gender or genetic characteristics of the child or transferring the burden of gestation to another.[4]

Because procreative interests are for some persons dependent on the offspring's having certain gender or genetic characteristics, procreative liberty includes, according to Robertson, the freedom to manipulate egg, sperm, or embryo to achieve the desired offspring, and the freedom to stop implantation or abort a fetus with undesirable characteristics. A couple is not free to alter genetic material in a way that would cause serious harm to the offspring (that is, harm so great as to make life not worth living), but they may do whatever else will facilitate the development of an offspring possessing those characteristics and traits that make having a child meaningful for them.[5] Claims of harm made in the name of society (threats to the ideal of the family, etc.) are not compelling enough in his view to override individual rights.

Many people have taken issue with this position on the grounds that a right to assistance in reproduction simply does not follow from the right not to be compelled to bear a child.[6] It is one thing to say that no one ought to be made to reproduce, or no one ought to be prevented from reproducing by decree; it is quite another to say that society ought to provide whatever is necessary for reproduction to occur.[7]

While sharing these reservations, I wish to raise a different set of objections: The view of offspring presupposed in such a position is unacceptable from a feminist perspective; further, treating the act of reproducing in such a way has serious implications for efforts to bring about a society free of oppression. My concerns lie chiefly in three areas: the tendency in this position to treat children as property; the use of "rights" language and a contract model to define the family; and an imbalance of concern for reproductive ends versus reproductive means.

Attitudes toward Children

The success of Robertson's argument depends upon accepting the view that persons can be the object of another's right. Since he is not arguing for the protection of the right to engage in procreative activities, but the freedom to "acquire that sort of child that would make one willing to bring a child into the world in the first place,"[8] he is asserting the right to acquire a human being (and one with particular characteristics). Nor is Robertson referring simply to the right of persons to share in the experience of child nurture (since ability to adopt would satisfy that), but to have a genetically related child. As a feminist, I would agree that persons ought to be protected in their right to determine when and in what manner they will reproduce, and that they should be free to shape familial life in a way meaningful for them. But such a right should not be understood as unlimited, as extending as far as the acquisition of a concrete human being. Every exercise of freedom has a history and a context; our liberty is thus conditioned both by our potential for causing harm to others and by our responsibility for the quality of our common lives. A view of unlimited procreative liberty does not give sufficient attention to the ways in which not only individual offspring could be harmed, but the human community. Nor does it take seriously enough the possibilities for conflicts between claims.

First, such a position fails to respect offspring as autonomous beings, as ends in themselves. While a child's special dependency requires a condition of compromised autonomy vis-à-vis his or her caretakers, still that child comes into this world as a human person with the potential for self-determination. Although we might grant that the experience of reproduction appropriately fulfills needs and desires for the adults involved, advocating a model where children are brought into this world *chiefly* for that purpose gives too much weight to parental desires and too little to the protection of the offspring's essential autonomy. I am not saying that the desire to reproduce must be altruistic to be morally acceptable, nor that the experience of reproduction ought to be, or even could be, free of parental hopes and expectations for that offspring. My challenge is to a framework wherein the basis for unlimited procreative liberty is an individual desire for a particular type of child, a desire that is seldom weighed appropriately against the reality of the child-to-be as a potential autonomous human being. At what point does a being, who has been conceived, gestated, and born according to someone's specifications, become herself or himself? And if a child comes into the world primarily to fulfill parental need, are there limits to what a parent may do to ensure that the child will continue to meet the specified expectations?

With others, I share the fear that this understanding of procreative liberty incorporates a notion of children as products, on the assumption that individuals have a right to a particular kind of child and ought to be free, insofar as it is possible without causing grave physical harm, to manipulate the reproductive process so as to acquire the desired offspring. Currently, collaborative reproduction is a lengthy, arduous, and quite costly experience. How might parents look upon offspring when they enter the process with the belief that a certain kind of child is *owed* to them, and after they have paid a high price for that child? Certainly well-meaning people can bring children into the world through artificial reproduction and value them highly because of what they have gone through to have them. But this view of reproduction carries nonetheless the sense of "ordering" or "purchasing" children in accordance with specific parental desires, which in the end objectively devalues the child.

Not unlike, and just as dangerous as the thinking that makes women the property of their husbands, is the underlying view that children are not first and principally autonomous persons who also function as members of families and societies but rather the proper object of a parental right. We place our children at serious risk when we fail to see them first as existing for their own sakes and when we allow ourselves to think of them as malleable goods.

There are, in addition, serious problems in accepting as the standard for deciding how technology will be used to intervene in the reproductive process the adult initiator's definition of "procreative excellence." Since we are talking about a potentially autonomous human being, questions about the manipulation of genetic features, etc., ought to be asked first from the point of view of the offspring's best interests, not the prospective parents' desires. The decision then would be whether a certain genetic characteristic ought to be altered to facilitate that child's flourishing rather than whether a feature ought to be manipulated to make that offspring more acceptable to the parent.

A position of unlimited procreative liberty rooted in individual desire risks harming as well the quality of our lives together in community. Since reproduction in this view is tied so closely to one's private conception of a meaningful life, we are never talking about offspring per se, but a very specific type of offspring—a child with those genetic and gender characteristics that allow it to be incorporated into and contribute to the initiator's overall life project.

In a world where mixed-race and handicapped children are not now being adopted because they are "undesirable" we need to ask who determines, and should be permitted to so determine, what human characteristics are "desirable." My claim is not that parents are wrong to want a healthy, and genetically similar, child nor that persons may not have any good grounds for intervening in a pregnancy, for example one in which it is obvious that given certain characteristics the child will place great burdens on the parent or the family. My criticism is directed at an implied yardstick of acceptability, and the determination of reproductive standards based on personal whim. Such a model stands at odds with a feminist vision of community where all are welcome and persons are challenged to deal creatively with differences.

In addition, we need to weigh the consequences of using a model of reproductive desirability which includes choices about the preferred sex of one's offspring, for efforts to promote equality between persons in society. This is not to suggest that such a practice, if widespread, would result in more boys being chosen than girls. We have no way to know that nor reason necessarily to assume it. What is dangerous, in light of the reality of sexism in our society, is the perpetuation of the belief that an offspring's gender should be a determinative factor in her or his value to parents, or to anyone else. The primary question is whether the project to provide the subjectively desirable child is where social energies and resources in reproductive medicine ought to be directed.

The underlying ideal of perfection shaping this perspective and the belief that all so-called imperfection, even in so complex a process as reproduction, can or should be eliminated, needs thus to be questioned seriously. Reproduction and nurture are processes that are never totally within our control, no matter how sophisticated our technology. The formation of a child's character and personality, the development of his or her talents, have to do with a great deal more (such as education, historical events, significant role models) than genetic blueprint. A genetically normal, or "genetically perfect" offspring in this model can for a variety of reasons turn out to be the sort of person his or her parents would not have objectively speaking "been willing to bring into the world." Thus the claim that a parental right to a satisfying reproductive experience justifies the manipulation of genetic material is flawed, for the sort of guarantee sought cannot be provided by control of conception.

The attempt to exert this level of control over the creation of offspring is not only an illusory project but a mistaken one. I do not want to advocate a total passivity toward nature or to suggest that the use of technology in altering the conditions of conception and gestation is always inappropriate. But the feminist value of cooperation with and humility toward nature suggests a middle road between technical domination of the natural reproductive process and passivity. This middle road entails, at least, some attention to the essential elements of particular personhood, and thus a weighing of which features of our offspring we ought to attempt to determine in advance and which we should accept as characteristics of that unique being.

It is not only the sense of "reproducing for excellence" that is troubling about the case for unlimited procreative liberty but the presupposition that since children are property, all relationships between offspring and interested adults can be wholly a matter of contract. This way of thinking about the family is in some ways reflective of an old and familiar pattern, one about which feminists ought to be very cautious.

THE CONTRACTUAL MODEL OF FAMILY

Robertson admits that when we begin to have multiple participants in reproduction "it becomes unclear which participants hold parental rights and duties and will function socially and psychologically as members of the child's family."[9] Such confusion can be alleviated, however, by a presumption that the contract between the parties will determine obligations and entitlements toward the child, rather than the commonly held definitions of paternity and maternity. Whether collaborative arrangements can or will result in family disruption and identity confusion for the offspring or in productive and satisfying "alternative" family experiences will depend in part on the clarity and quality of these contracts. Experience with donor sperm, Robertson argues, suggests that the contract between parties will play the decisive role in determining rearing rights and duties to the offspring. Generally speaking, the presumption of rightful parentage ought to go to the initiating couple according to the agreements made prior to conception.

If these practices become institutionalized, there is no doubt that well-constructed contracts will be enormously helpful for clarifying parental rights and duties and that all the parties, including potential offspring, would benefit from legal protection. There are serious problems, however, with accepting a simple contract solution to the confusion of collaborative reproduction; it is both inadequate and perpetuates an ideologically dangerous model of the family. For example, claiming that the pre-conception contract can be sufficiently clear as to determine parental relationships in advance denies the complexity of reproduction as an affective and social experience as well as a biological one. Accounts of surrogate mothering, for example, suggest it can be quite difficult to decide the shape of one's reproductive role beforehand when we are engaged in a project about which we can come to have very deep feelings. In addition, the nature of what reproductive initiators are contracting about is qualitatively different than the object of ordinary contracts. We do not have at this time, and may never have, a good way to determine the value of specific reproductive contributions or to weigh conflicts between contributors (for example, what is the market value of gestation versus gamete donation?) At the very least, to use sperm donation as a paradigm for workable contracts reflects inattention to the vast differences, emotional as well as physical, in the nature of various collaborative roles. Moreover, it masks inequalities between parties with respect to risk and benefit. A contract that may well be sufficient to determine rearing duties and rights with respect to a sperm donor may not address at all the complex physical and affective situation of the surrogate mother.

Our understanding of the experience can perhaps be reinterpreted as Robertson suggests, so that what comes to count as reproduction is the donation of genetic material for one person, or the experience of gestation for another. Yet while there are very good reasons for preserving the freedom of individuals to choose their level of participation in procreation, to say that the meaning of reproduction can be reduced to one of these partial roles is to perpetuate an impoverished notion of what it means to be a parent. Assigning various rights and obligations to abstract roles may facilitate the execution of collaborative contracts, but risks treating the various components of reproduction as though they fit into neat compartments, and as though the conception-gestation-rearing relationship is entirely negotiable. Feminists do not want to affirm a view of reproduction that makes the moral connections between conception, gestation, and rearing such that conception generates an absolute duty to rear; at the same time, however, concerns for embodiment and thus for reproduction as a whole process mitigate against treating parental obligations and entitlements in isolation from the experiences of conception, pregnancy, and birth.

There is, of course, a kind of tacit agreement, at least in our society, involved in every gestation and birth with respect to the resultant offspring's nurture (and in a sense, also with respect to parental entitlements). Whatever model has been used thus far to understand the relationship, however, has not taken the form of an entirely free contract. Prior to the development of technology, we identified the mother as the woman giving birth to the child and the father as the man whose sperm initially fertilized the egg—those persons with biological and experiential connection, rather than those who have contracted for parental rights and duties. Even when we describe situations where another individual has taken over rearing responsibilities for a child not his or her issue, we continue to refer to that person as an "adoptive" or "foster" parent. We do this not to say anything about the quality of rearing, but to preserve a truer sense of identity and biological continuity for the child, acknowledging that no matter what function the rearing adult serves, he or she cannot ever become the child's father or mother in the traditional sense. I do not want to hold that there could be no legitimate reasons for separating genetic, gestational, and rearing components of reproduction, or that persons who conceive a child will always be the best rearers of that child and that they must therefore be the rearers in all cases. Experience shows that children can be raised well in situations other than the traditional biologically related family. However, the genetic-gestation-rearing connection in procreation ought not be disregarded a priori in the way suggested by the contract model, both for the sake of protecting the offspring's sense of identity as a value and for preserving an awareness of the importance of the task involved when human life is created.

While "rights" and "entitlements" in childbearing do have much to do with an agreement to accept responsibility, the biological parent-child relationship is still deeply significant, particularly if we are speaking of the intimate mother-child bond in a normal gestation experience. It may be acceptable to say that a woman who has conceived, carried, and birthed a child may legitimately choose to transfer rearing obligations to another, but it does not seem correct to say then that this experience of procreation places *no* claim on her as a mother unless she chooses to assume one under the terms of a contract, or that her claim to this child is identical to the claims of all other contracting parties prior to the contract. Both the experience of having conceived and carried a child and the implicit agreement to nurture ground parental entitlements; these two dimensions must be seen as elements of the same experience even where a decision is made to separate them. Given the significant burdens and challenges of childbearing and the length of time the commitment ordinarily encompasses, this interconnection is important to protect when possible. Implicit in my critique is the great irony of collaborative reproduction: it is precisely the value of this biological connection, which must be open for renunciation on the part of the donor or gestator, that drives the search for new methods and justifies the infertile party's right to assistance.

The Involuntary Nature of Kinship

The authority of the collaborative contract, coupled with a property view of children, generates a troubling picture of the parent-child bond. One of the false notions perpetuated in such a model of parental entitlement is that we are free to choose all obligations, and able to formulate all the conditions of our lives to meet our expectations. While most contracts and commitments are based on things such as shared purpose, equal benefit, common attraction, etc., and are entered into and terminated voluntarily, until recently, the agreement to conceive, gestate, and rear a child has been of a different nature. While in the best of circumstances we make a choice to parent, and a series of choices about how children will be raised and the shape our family life will take, a great deal of the experience of reproduction is not in our control. The common expression "This child has a face only a mother could love" speaks, of course, to the fact that a parent's bond to her child transcends all cultural standards of beauty, etc., but also alludes to a deeply entrenched understanding of the "givenness" and duration of parental responsibilities. These have included acceptance of a relatively unknown outcome, of inequalities in benefits and burdens, and also of a certain irrevocability. "A face only a mother could love" says something as well about acceptance and fidelity to children, even to those whose looks or gender or genetic characteristics are not what the parent would have desired or what meets society's standards. We have accepted the fact that, unlike a product in the market, children cannot be returned or exchanged if found to be other than what was expected.

The commitment a parent undertakes is not dependent on that child's behavior or the return of like affection or the fulfillment of expectations in life, although those factors can certainly influence a parent's subjective experience and may at times modify obligations. A child does not enter into a committed relationship with his or her parents in the same way that a parent, by virtue of the decision to bear offspring, does with the child; still, there is some measure of givenness in the child-parent relationship as well. We are free throughout life to choose friends, a mate, employers, etc. but not our family of origin. One of the things that family life can teach us is that we are born into some obligations, and some are born to us, and life includes the acceptance of those kinds of indissoluble and predefined obligations as well as the ones we freely incur. The involuntary quality of kinship can also teach us how to accept others as intimately connected to us, even when they fail to live up to our standards or when they do not possess the physical or personal qualities most attractive to us. To image reproduction as primarily a contractual process, where all the elements are open for negotiation, threatens to lose sight of this sense of transcendent commitment.

From the perspective of feminist ethics, the contractual view of procreative liberty assumes and perpetuates a traditional patriarchal model of the family (centered around rights and ownership), a model that has proven oppressive and sometimes dangerous for persons, especially women. A contract approach is initially attractive as it appears to bring about greater flexibility in the definition of family and the protection of procreative liberty (among the values feminists want to promote). But when persons are treated primarily as the object of another's right, and significant relationships are defined wholly according to legal arrangements rather than the experiences of nurture, the symbolic framework is that of the patriarchal family. Janet Farrell Smith has argued that this property model of parenting, having at its center a notion of rights, is inherently gender-biased and is protective of dangerous authority patterns. It is problematic in her view both because its structure of relationship is "male" in form and because males have traditionally been the exclusive holders of familial rights.[10]

What makes such a model destructively gender-biased, according to Smith, is its rootedness in an extractive view of power rather than a developmental one and its relation to the authority patterns of the traditional patriarchal family. The major elements of such a property model of human relations,

> namely ownership and proprietary control, have had more to do with fathering than with mothering. The realities of motherhood, on the other hand, have had more to do with care, nurturance and day-to-day responsibility. These represent a very different set of moral and political ideals.[11]

The concepts of right and entitlement used in the contractual model correspond to the values preserved in traditional notions of patriarchal fathering (control and ownership) rather than to those of care and responsibility associated with mothering. While many feminists would not want to posit "distinctively female" values or ideals, most would reject familiar structures that treat persons as property and would call instead for a style of parenting that is respectful of a child's autonomy and encourages individual flourishing. They would, as well, reject models of the family that attach authority to rigidly defined roles in favor of models based on equality between partners and cooperation in the performance of family tasks.

As Smith argues, promoting a property (or "rights-centered") model, whether through vigorous protection of familial autonomy or by the rhetoric of "right to procreate" can only reinforce an ideal of the family that not only does not encourage more respectful and cooperative parenting styles but may further facilitate the abuse of parental power. In the context of Robertson's argument, familial autonomy means a protection of parental control as rightful parent (owner) over minor children (a control that in the past has extended to wives). But this sort of familial autonomy underlying arguments for clarity of contract serves largely to protect proprietary interests rather than to facilitate intimacy or the development of creative, more humane forms of parenting for women and men.[12] Since the problem is not only that males have been the exclusive holders of rights to property (including their wives and children) but that this way of imaging the family denies the reality of women and children as fully human, it may not be enough simply for feminists to argue for equality between women and men in the holding of these rights. Rather, the very language of rights, implying as it does some exclusive access to property, must be seen as inappropriate when describing the structure of the family.

REPRODUCTIVE ENDS AND MEANS

One of the weaknesses of the argument for unlimited procreative liberty is a tendency to split ends from means, to overemphasize goals while giving little moral consideration to the methods employed to achieve them or to the price paid. Robertson's concern to promote the procreative initiator's interests is not adequately balanced, for example, by a concern for the persons who will participate as the means to the stated reproductive goals. Except where he discusses contract stipulations (requirements for informed consent, freedom from coercion, screening procedures, etc.) Robertson does not speak of donors and gestators as though they really have interests to be weighed; he argues, in fact, that unless grave harm is being done, their interests cannot override individual procreative liberty. As we saw earlier, the offspring as a particular child is treated not as an end in himself or herself, but as the means to a goal (a fulfilling parenting experience). The question of how such treatment may affect that child's quality of life, sense of identity, or development is hardly raised.

The problem is not that the holding of a reproductive end is wrong in itself, but that it may be mistaken to assume that an end-state can be clearly demarcated from the processes that lead up to it.[13] The primary assumption that reproduction is highly valued by individuals and therefore that freedom of access should be promoted treats reproductive freedom for the most part as a value that could be pursued in isolation of other claims (except the minimal obligation not to do grave harm to an offspring). Feminists reject such thinking as inadequately attentive to the reality of events as processes and to the fact that the means we use to bring about any end are part of the total reality of the event in question. Thus it is not enough to assert that providing genetically related children to infertile individuals is a good to be promoted; questions must be raised about the nature of the arrangement by which that might occur, the impact of that project on the individuals involved and on the larger human community, and the claims other goods are simultaneously exerting.

It is wrong to suppose that an individual procreative right can be posited and its unlimited exercise upheld without careful consideration of the moral nature of the means necessary to attain its end. Interest in a genetically related child cannot be seen as an independent end, the value of which automatically discounts concerns for the present and future state of the offspring, for the physical and emotional safety of the collaborators, or for the place of the experience of reproduction in our collective value system. In addition, the particular techniques used in collaborative reproduction need separate evaluation. We might accept the use of artificial insemination by a donor, for example, on particular grounds (as that the risks to donor are small and the benefit great), but have serious reservations about the practice of surrogacy. An adequate argument for procreative liberty as a good would have to include a fair description of the necessary means since they cannot be separated from the end-state.

Because reproduction has a social dimension, and reproductive practices have profound real and symbolic impacts on the community, the promotion of individual procreative liberty can never be an abstract end. The value of collaborative reproduction for individuals needs to be weighed against the costs these practices may exact, not only in the lives of those individuals directly involved, but also with respect to the promotion of full human community. An assessment of procreative liberty that takes seriously the contextual nature of our choices asks, in addition to whether the "new reproduction" is good for individuals, how it relates to social concerns (to efforts to secure an adequate standard of living for all persons, to progress in the quality of class, gender, and race relations, etc.).

A commitment to the creation of a just society requires that an individual desire for a genetically related child cannot be held up as an end commanding significant public resources and energy if as a "good" it encourages the exploitation of vulnerable persons or fosters negative attitudes toward persons or groups of persons. At a minimum, questions need to be raised about the influence of institutionalizing these practices on our views toward women: will opportunities to serve as egg donors or gestators facilitate progress toward equality with men for women, or does this type of service further identify women in an oppressive way with their reproductive capabilities? If individuals have a right to a genetically related child, do others have an obligation to donate genetic material, and how will the extent of the obligation be determined? What are the potential consequences of medicalizing reproduction in terms of women's right to control over their own bodies? And who will the women be who serve as donors?—will the poor, who have always been exploited by the rich, be used to perform even this form of domestic service?

To take account of the context in which individual procreative liberty is pursued, we also need to weigh the expense and energy channelled in the direction of these reproductive services against the realities of poverty and overpopulation. We need to ask whether we should support the right of individuals to go to any length to acquire the type of child they want when there are so many children already living who are not being taken care of. And, recognizing that collaborative reproduction ordinarily has as its object a white child, we need as well to examine the kind of racial attitudes being perpetuated. We cannot treat the pursuit of a genetically related child, or the protection of individual procreative liberty, as though they are abstract goods that are never in conflict with other relevant goods, nor can we consider procreative liberty from the point of view of its end alone. Given the nature of the procreative task, *how* we reproduce is as significant as *whether* we do.

PROMOTING FULL HUMANITY
The promotion of women's right to self-determination, especially in matters of reproduction, has indeed been a critical item on the feminist political agenda. But for most feminists, protection of individual autonomy is never treated as the single value to be considered in the analysis of a situation. A commitment to viewing persons as embodied and relational, as well as autonomous, mitigates against an abstract notion of freedom that does not take seriously enough the way in which personal

choices alter the shape of the world in which they occur. Questions of personal liberty, including how far our right to procreate extends, can only properly be asked from the point of view of our reality as relational beings whose power for reproduction is a capacity with profound personal and social implications. It is never even theoretically unlimited.

The objectification of children, impoverishment of meaning in the experience of reproduction, damage to notions of kinship, the perpetuation of degrading views of women—all these concerns may be deemed "symbolic harms" that are not compelling enough to override personal liberty. But attention to women's experience has taught feminists that there are no "merely symbolic" harms; we interpret and shape experience through our symbols and therefore how we think about persons, events, and biological processes has a great deal to do with how we behave toward them. We need, then, to pay careful attention to what is being said of personhood, of parent-child relationships, of reproductive capacities, and so on in arguments for unlimited procreative liberty. If we hope to use reproductive technology in a way that promotes the full humanity of all persons, in a manner that is truly creative rather than destructive, then we must be attentive to the potential for harm on all levels. We have an ever-expanding power to reshape the experience of reproduction; whether we will prove in the future to have done so in the service of human life or not will have more than a little to do with how we came to think about it and what we allowed to be of value today.

ACKNOWLEDGMENTS

The author would like to thank Professors Margaret Farley and Richard L. Fern for helpful comments on earlier drafts.

REFERENCES

1. While a few feminists have heralded developments in technology as the ground of possibility for women's true liberation, most have remained more cautious, foreseeing potential for further oppression as clearly as hope of equality. See Shulamith Firestone, *The Dialectic of Sex: The Case for Feminist Revolution* (New York: Bantam Books, 1971), 238; Christine Overall, *Ethics and Human Reproduction: A Feminist Analysis* (Boston: Allen and Unwin, 1987).

2. John Robertson, "Procreative Liberty and the Control of Conception, Pregnancy and Childbirth," *Virginia Law Review* 69 (April 1983), 405–462; "Embryos, Families and Procreative Liberty: The Legal Structures of the New Reproduction," *Southern California Law Review* 59 (1986), 942–1041.

3. Robertson, "Embryos, Families and Procreative Liberty," 961.

4. Robertson, "Procreative Liberty," 450.

5. Robertson, "Procreative Liberty," 432.

6. See Overall, *Ethics and Human Reproduction,* chapter 8; also Richard L. Fern, "The Fundamental Right to Marry and Raise a Family," unpublished manuscript (1987).

7. The parallel would be marriage, that is, there is a recognized right to noninterference in the decision to marry but no obligation on society's part to provide a mate. See William J. Daniel, "Sexual Ethics in Relation to IVF and ET: The Fitting Use of Human Reproductive Power," in *Test-Tube Babies,* William Walters and Peter Singer, eds. (Melbourne: Oxford University Press, 1982), 73.

8. Robertson, "Procreative Liberty," 430.

9. Robertson, "Procreative Liberty," 424.

10. Janet Farrell Smith, "Parenting and Property," in *Mothering: Essays in Feminist Theory,* Joyce Treblicott, ed. (Totowa, NJ: Rowman and Allanheld, 1983), 199–210.

11. Smith, "Parenting," 208.

12. Smith, "Parenting," 206.

13. For a discussion of a feminist critique of dualistic means-ends reasoning, see Jean Grimshaw, *Philosophy and Feminist Thinking* (Minneapolis: University of Minnesota Press, 1986), 187–226.

6 Therapy or Tampering: The Ethics of Reproductive Technology and the Development of Doctrine

RICHARD A. MCCORMICK, S.J.

Jesuit Father Richard A. McCormick is the John A. O'Brien Professor of Christian Ethics at the University of Notre Dame.

In this chapter I will consider five points: (1) the factual background, (2) standard in vitro fertilization, (3) third-party involvement, (4) the moral status of the pre-embryo, (5) the Instruction of the Congregation for the Doctrine of the Faith.

On September 8, 1986, the Ethics Committee of the American Fertility Society (AFS) released its report under the title *Ethical Considerations of the New Reproductive Technologies.*[1] The report is the result of eight arduous meetings beginning February 1–2, 1985. As a member of that committee, I would not qualify as its best critic. Yet if past experience with similar reports (e.g., the Ethics Advisory Board, 1979; the "Warnock Report," 1984; the "Waller Report," 1982–1984) is any indication, the AFS report will prove highly controversial. For instance, when the Ethics Advisory Board's final report was published in the *Federal Register* on June 18, 1979, it generated some 13,000 public comments, and they were overwhelmingly negative.[2] The Secretary of the then Department of Health, Education and Welfare received fifty letters, signed by twenty senators and seventy-three representatives. Most argued that "*in vitro* fertilization research was immoral and unethical, that the future impli-

---

This chapter appeared in The Critical Calling: Reflections on Moral Dilemmas Since Vatican II *(Washington, D.C.: Georgetown University Press, 1989): 329–352.*

cations were grave, that adequate guidelines to prevent abuses had not yet been developed, and that the rights of the embryo would be compromised."[3]

I have no doubt that the AFS report will continue to enjoy similar tender mercies. Even though time and clinical practice have taken the novelty and surprise out of in vitro fertilization, still there is an uneasy sense that a powerful technological dynamic is loose here, one with a capacity for considerable abuse. I doubt that the AFS report will allay such fears. Let me cite a single example. Chapter 15 of the report deals with "Artificial Insemination-Donor" (AID). After listing the indications for the procedure, it details some key reservations (e.g., possible psychological problems in the husband, wife, donor; risk of transmitting serious genetic disease; effect on child, etc.). The report then states: "Because of the general concern over the use of third party gametes, the use of A.I.D. remains controversial. However, the Committee finds the use of A.I.D. ethically acceptable." Some may see an act of the will in such leaps of logic. I did and wrote the following dissent.

> One member of the Committee argued that the use of third parties—whether by donor sperm, donor ovum, or surrogate womb—was ethically inappropriate. First, it seems violative of the marriage covenant wherein exclusive, non-transferable, inalienable rights to each other's person and generative acts are exchanged. Thus it fundamentally severs procreation from the marital union. Second, by premeditation—in contrast to adoption—it brings into the world a child with no bond of origin to one or both marital partners, thus blurring the child's genealogy and potentially compromising the child's self-identity. Third, once conceded the moral right to be inseminated by the sperm of another man, wives might easily conclude (and it would be difficult to reject their logic) that it is preferable to be inseminated in the natural way. Thus adulteries might be multiplied to the detriment of marriage. Fourth, the stud-farm mentality is supported with its subtle but unmistakable move toward eugenics. Fifth, the use of third parties tends to absolutize sterility as a disvalue and childbearing and rearing as a value, thus distorting—and potentially threatening—some basic human values: life, marriage, and the family.
>
> Taken cumulatively, such considerations suggest that the use of third parties to overcome sterility is not for the good of persons integrally and adequately considered. It involves risks to basic dimensions of our flourishing. Such risks to basic values outweigh, in a prudential calculus, individual procreative

desires or needs. In summary: when calculus involves *individual* benefit versus *institutional* risk of harm, the latter should take precedence.[4]

This concern could be worded much more subtly and carefully, I am sure. For instance, one of my graduate students at the University of Notre Dame pointed out to me that if what I suggest about third parties is true, then the calculus does not really involve individual *benefit.* A genuine benefit should not involve institutional or social risk of harm. A putative one might. My point, however, is the types of concern raised by the new reproductive technologies. They touch on some very basic human values: marriage and the family, parenting, genealogy and self-identity of the child, human sexual intimacy and even the sanctity of life itself. It is perhaps understandable, then, why these discussions generate a heavy load of emotion and rhetoric about "playing God," "tampering with nature," "immoral means to good ends," "procreative privacy," etc. Such slogans do not analyze problems. They simply promulgate solutions that have been arrived at on other grounds.

Before raising some of the key ethical issues, I think it appropriate to supply a brief factual background.

On July 25, 1978 Louise Brown was born in Oldham, England, from in vitro fertilization (IVF). She was the first so-called "test-tube baby," the culmination of years of pioneering research by Patrick Steptoe and Robert Edwards. Since that time and as I write, some five thousand babies have entered this world via this procedure, most of them in Australia, England and the United States. The number changes almost daily.

IVF is relatively simple and straightforward. The ovaries are stimulated (by clomiphene citrate, human menopausal gonadotropin or combinations of these) to produce multiple eggs since pregnancy rates increase with transfer of more than one embryo. The eggs are ordinarily recovered by laparoscopy and follicle aspiration, though transvaginal retrieval (not involving general anesthesia) is increasingly used. They are then coincubated with sperm for around twelve to eighteen hours to allow fertilization to occur. After an additional forty-eight to seventy-two hours, the embryo (many scientists prefer the term "pre-embryo") is transferred to the uterine cavity by a catheter. If the procedure is successful, implantation in the uterus will occur in two to three days and a pregnancy will be detectable at about ten to fourteen days following transfer.[5]

Based on the experience of the past seven years, in vitro fertilization is both safe and relatively efficient. There is no known increased risk to parents or offspring and the success rate (depending on team-experience and technique) can approach that of the natural process (20–25% per cycle of treatment).

There are several reasons why couples might consider in vitro fertilization. The most common is tubal (fallopian) damage or destruction due to inflammatory disease. Other pelvic factors that have failed conventional therapy (e.g., pelvic endometriosis) could also be indications. The same could be said of simple unexplained or idiopathic infertility.

If the story ended here, there would be little cause for concern. Many ethicists and moral theologians (not all, as we shall see) have no problem with the procedure if the gametes (egg, sperm) come from husband and wife, and if the procedure is safe for mother and child-to-be. Indeed, LeRoy Walters (Kennedy Institute of Ethics) refers to the morality of in vitro fertilization as a "stagnant issue."[6] Nearly ten years ago (May 4, 1979) the Ethics Advisory Board reported to the Secretary of Health, Education and Welfare that IVF is "acceptable from an ethical standpoint." The Board insisted that this was to be understood as "ethically defensible but still legitimately controverted" because it acknowledged genuine concerns about the moral status of the embryo and the potential long-range consequences as "among the most difficult that confronted the Board." The Board did not wish to wave the magic wand of its fiat at such concerns.

And this is where the story continues. Now that laboratory culture conditions for fertilization and continued development have been refined, clinicians are being confronted with requests for all kinds of variations of the basic technology: donor sperm, donor ova, donor embryo, surrogate mothers (with sperm and/or ova from donors), surrogate carriers, single women, lesbian couples, frozen sperm, frozen embryos etc. For instance, when the husband is sterile with irreversible azoospermia (dead or weakened sperm) or has some genetic disorder that would constitute an unacceptable risk to progeny, donor sperm is suggested. Or again, if the wife lacks ovaries because of surgical removal or suffers from ovarian failure, donor eggs are sought. If both partners are afflicted with one or more of the medical indications mentioned, they might look for a donated embryo.

The possibilities and variants are mind-boggling. As George Annas has pointed out, it is now possible for a child to be born with five distinct parents: a genetic father, a rearing father, a mother who provides the egg, the woman in whose womb the embryo gestates, the mother who rears the child.[7] Or again, an embryo could be frozen for a generation, then thawed and transferred to its now adult sister—thus becoming the daughter of its sister. Variations like this are not mere fantasies. The first case of a surrogate carrier (woman's egg fertilized in vitro by husband's sperm, then placed in another woman) was reported in 1985.[8] In another case, a lesbian was fertilized by donor sperm.[9] Clearly, the separation of genetic, gestating and rearing roles raises complex ethical and legal problems underlined by *Time*'s question "which one gets the Mother's Day card?"[10] and by Red Foxx's throwaway aphorism "Mama's baby, Poppa's maybe."

Then there is the question of the embryo itself. International attention was focused on this issue when an American couple (Mr. and Mrs. Mario Rios) died in an airplane accident after leaving two frozen embryos in an Australian clinic. Are such embryos children, and in this case orphans? Or are they something less? To whom do they belong? What should be done with them? Should they be thawed and allowed to die, or should they be adopted? And more generally, is it ever permissible to experiment on spare embryos? Indeed, may they be produced precisely for this purpose?

Responses to questions like these are likely to be sharply divided. There have been any number of groups that have made reports or submissions (e.g., Medical Research Council [Great Britain], 1982; Royal College of Obstetricians and Gynecologists, 1983; Catholic Bishops of Victoria, 1982; British Medical Association, 1983; Catholic Bishops' Joint Committee on Bio-Ethical Issues, 1983; American Fertility Society, 1984). The two best known reports are British and Australian: the so-called "Warnock Report" named after chairperson Dame Mary Warnock ("Report of the Committee of Inquiry into Human Fertilisation and Embryology," 1984) and the "Waller Report" named after chairperson Louis Waller ("Interim Report," 1982; "Report on Donor Gametes in I.V.F.," 1983; "Report on the Disposition of Embryos Produced by In Vitro Fertilization," 1984).[11]

Both of these reports accept standard (between husband and wife) IVF, freezing of embryos, donation of oocytes, and donation of embryos in IVF. Both reject surrogate motherhood. Where research on the embryo is concerned, majorities of both the Warnock and Waller groups approved it in principle, the Waller Report specifying that only spare embryos are to be used. Both groups put a fourteen-day limit on such research because after this point there is present the "primitive streak" indicating developmental individuation. Prior to this point, the cell-mass (fertilized ovum—technically zygote) has a kind of totipotentiality. That is, it may divide (or be severed) and become twins. Two cell masses may recombine to become a single individual known as a chimera or mosaic. Indeed, animal studies indicate that individual blastomeres of the zygote can be removed without compromising future growth potential and can themselves become full-fledged individuals.

With this brief factual sketch, let me now turn to the moral issues. There are many moral issues that adhere to the new reproductive technologies. For instance, Clifford Grobstein and Michael Flower have listed the following aspects: the IVF process itself, freezing of embryo, marital status of patients, third-party involvement, embryo adoption, embryo research, fertilization across species boundaries, extended embryo culture, commercialization.[12] Obviously, I cannot discuss all of these.

Here I would like to review the issues from the perspective of recent Catholic formulations. There are three key issues that constantly surface and lie behind those mentioned above: (1) IVF itself; (2) third-party involvement; and (3) the moral status of the embryo.

1. Standard IVF. By "standard" I refer to the simple procedure minus any accompaniments or variations that might alter moral evaluation. Concretely, this means that sperm and ovum come from husband and wife and the pre-embryo is implanted in the uterus of the wife.

The analytic history in the Catholic community begins in 1897. On March 24 of that year, the Holy Office gave its response to the question "May artificial fecundation of a woman be done?" Its answer: "It is not permissible."[13]

Obviously, this is not a cut-through to clarity. Specifically, it remained unclear whether the artificiality of the procedure was being condemned or only the manner of obtaining semen (masturbation). Many authors (among them the American Gerald Kelly, S.J.) opted for this latter view and continued to defend artificial insemination if the semen could be licitly obtained.

It was against this background that Pius XII entered the picture. In 1949, in an address to the Fourth International Congress of Catholic Doctors, Pius XII stated: "The simple fact that the desired result is attained by this means does not justify the use of the means itself; nor is the desire to have a child—perfectly lawful as that is for married persons—sufficient to prove the licitness of artificial insemination to attain this end." He referred to "procreation of a new life according to the will and plan of the Creator" and concluded that artificial insemination by husband (AIH) "must be absolutely rejected."[14] This exclusion, to which Pius XII repeatedly returned, must be put into its proper context. Apparently, the congress which he addressed had factions that were supporting an *uncritical* use of AIH ("uncritical" meaning that they had glossed over too quickly the problem of obtaining semen).

Again, on October 29, 1951, in his famous address to the Italian Catholic Union of Midwives, the pope argued that AIH converts the home into a biological laboratory. He worded it as follows:

In its natural structure, the conjugal act is a personal action, a simultaneous and immediate cooperation on the part of the husband and wife which by the very nature of the agents and the propriety of the act is the expression of the mutual gift which according to Holy Scripture brings about union "in one flesh only." This is something more than the union of two seeds which may be brought about even artificially without the natural action of husband and wife.[15]

On May 19, 1956 (Second World Congress on Fertility and Sterility), he spelled this out in even greater detail. After condemning contraception, he continued:

And the Church has likewise rejected the opposite attitude which would pretend to separate, in generation, the biological activity from the personal relation of the married couple. The child is the fruit of the conjugal union when that union finds full expression by bringing into play the organic functions, the associated sensible emotions, and the spiritual and disinterested love which animates it. It is within the unity of this human activity that the biological prerequisites of generation should take place.[16]

In summary, then, Pius XII was insisting that the child (for the good of the child and the marriage) must be the fruit of the conjugal union. But it is the fruit of the *conjugal* union only when it is conceived *in a conjugal way,* that is, by sexual intercourse. Therefore, to be the fruit of the conjugal union the child must be conceived by sexual intercourse. But a child conceived by artificial insemination by husband is not conceived by sexual intercourse. *Ergo.* Pius XII, then, viewed the conjugal act as having a natural and God-given design which joins the procreative (life-giving) and unitive (love-making) dimensions. On this basis, he excluded both contraception and AIH. This approach would, of course, constitute a strong a fortiori argument against IVF. But Pius XII immediately added: "On the subject of the experiments in artificial human fecundation 'in vitro,' let it suffice for us to observe that they must be rejected as immoral and absolutely illicit." That seems clearer than it really is. The basis of the rejection could be (most likely) the mere unnaturalness, or it could be that the pontiff saw this as experimental and dangerous tampering with embryonic life. Whatever the case, Pius XII would certainly have rejected IVF.

I believe it accurate to say that Pius XII, especially in his 1956 analysis, was foreshadowing the analysis of Paul VI in *Humanae Vitae*.[17] Paul VI asserted in that encyclical the inseparability, in the conjugal act, of the unitive and procreative dimensions of the act. This inseparability ("willed by God and not to be broken by men on their own initiative") was repeated in John Paul II's *Familiaris Consortio*.[18]

What are we to make of all of this in so far as it touches in vitro fertilization? At first blush, it might seem to commit the magisterium to a rejection of in vitro fertilization. But before that conclusion is drawn, several points should be weighed carefully.

First, there is the authoritative character of Pius XII's interventions. Pius was addressing a problem at the official level for the first time (the 1897 response of the Holy Office was interpreted by many as centering its rejection of artificial insemination on masturbation to obtain semen). Furthermore, his pronouncements are almost never cited by subsequent popes and by bishops around the world. In other words, the Church— to borrow from Ladislaus Orsy, S.J.—was in the initial stages of its reflection on this matter.[19] That being the case, it would be a disservice to attribute anything like a definitive character to Pius' conclusions.

This point is reflected in the attitude of two Roman theologians, consultors of the Congregation for the Doctrine of the Faith, and "teachers at prestigious Roman institutions in the very shadow of the Holy See."[20] They are Marcellino Zalba, S.J., and Jan Visser, C.S.S.R. Both have challenged Pius' condemnation of artificial insemination by husband. Zalba regards the papal analysis as too "physicist," leaning too heavily on the materiality of the act and not enough on its moral significance.[21] Visser acknowledges that we have come a long way from the days when a papal allocution would forever end a discussion. He believes that the argument of Pius XII retains its value as a general principle but doubts its absoluteness where insemination by husband is involved.[22]

The second point is the very meaning of the inseparability of the unitive and procreative. Some see this inseparability as excluding in vitro fertilization. Thus the Catholic Bishops of Victoria, in their submission (1983) to the Waller Committee stated: "In pursuit of the admirable end of helping an infertile couple to conceive and have their baby, I.V.F. intervenes in their supreme expression of mutual love. It separates 'baby-making' from 'lovemaking'."[23] Similarly, Carlo Caffarra, head of the Pontifical Institute for the Family, appeals to the inseparability of the unitive and procreative to reject IVF. "The moral problem is that procreation can no longer be said to be—and in fact is not—dependent upon the sexual act between two married people."[24] This is also the position taken by F. Giunchedi, G. Pesci, D. Tettamanzi and others.[25]

But the matter is simply not that clear. To the assertion that *Humanae Vitae* and *Familiaris Consortio* exclude procreation without the unitive act, William Daniel, S.J., notes:

> All we learn from this passage [of *Humanae Vitae*], however, is that *if the conjugal act is performed* it should have these qualities: it should not be falsified in either of its essential "significations." This does not necessarily imply that if there is to be procreation it should be by means of a unitive act.[26]

This very same point is made by G. B. Guzzetti.[27] He notes that the inseparability of the unitive and procreative is *of the conjugal act*. We may not extend or transfer this to an inseparability between the conjugal act itself and the generative process. In other words, the inseparability of the unitive and procreative in the conjugal act does not rule out generative acts outside of it. It must be remembered that Paul VI and John Paul II, in asserting the inseparability of the unitive and procreative, were directly concerned with rejecting contraception in marriage. Artificial reproductive procedures were not of immediate concern to them.

This is a technical, textual point, and in this sense Daniel is correct. What one says about the conjugal act does not necessarily apply when there is no question of the conjugal act. However, it seems clear that official formulations such as those of *Humanae Vitae* viewed the matter in more sweeping terms (the procreative process). Any lingering doubts about this were dissipated by the Congregation for the Doctrine of the Faith's 1987 "Instruction on Respect for Human Life in its Origin and on the Dignity of Procreation." The CDF sees in in vitro fertilization a separation of the unitive and procreative analogous to that found in contraception.

Other supportive arguments are marshalled against IVF. For instance, infertility is not a life-threatening disorder and IVF does not correct it, but only bypasses it. Use of a "therapeutic" modality for a condition that is not medically harmful and is not itself corrected tends to medicalize more basic human problems. But this type of consideration is far too general to exclude IVF. If applied consistently, it would exclude many medical interventions, e.g., cardiac bypass surgery.

Or again, Carlo Caffarra has stated:

> *In vitro* fertilization . . . establishes between the one performing the fertilization and the one to be born a relationship of "production of an object." Herein lies the intrinsic illicitness: the person cannot be an object produced by human labour, but a subject willed by a personal act of love.[28]

A child, it is argued, should be begotten, not made. Anything else is literally a misconception. In other words, IVF is more tampering than genuine therapy.

Many other theologians reject this line of reasoning. They do not see IVF as "manufacture" of a "product." Fertilization *happens* when sperm and egg are brought together in a petri dish. The technician's "intervention is a condition for its happening: it is not a cause."[29] Furthermore, the attitudes of the parents and technicians can be every bit as reverential and respectful as they would be in the face of human life naturally conceived.

So where does this leave us? Prior to the CDF's "Instruction," matters seemed to be as follows. The pivotal consideration on IVF from the perspective of magisterial statements is the inseparability of the unitive and procreative dimensions of sexuality. (Obtaining sperm by masturbation does not present a formidable obstacle because many theologians regard this as a different human action from the type of masturbation rejected as ipsation or self-petting.) This inseparability can be understood in either of two ways, the narrow sense or the broad sense. A word about each.

The narrow sense. This refers to the inseparability of the unitive and procreative *in the conjugal act.* The sense is: if the conjugal act is performed, these dimensions may not be separated. The more narrow sense states nothing and implies nothing about artificial reproduction beyond the marital act. As William Daniel puts it: "It is about the way a couple present themselves to one another: that no inner contradiction be introduced into their bodily language."[30] This is all that the principle need mean as we find it in Paul VI (*Humanae Vitae*) and John Paul II (*Familiaris Consortio*). Understood in this way, the principle does not exclude in vitro fertilization. (I leave aside for the moment the validity of the principle, that is, whether blocking procreative potential via contraception involves introducing a contradiction into the bodily language of spouses. I think that it need not.)

The broad sense. This understands the inseparability of the unitive and procreative in such a way that procreation ought not occur in marriage except as the result of a sexual act. This represents an understanding of the principle that returns to the perspectives of Pius XII. On this reading, IVF would be excluded.

Many theologians do not see things in this way. They argue that Pius XII was excessively influenced by the theology of F. Hürth, S.J., who explicitly stated that the moral law and the biological law coincide on these matters. They further argue that Vatican II shifted the criterion of judgment—away from faculties and their purposes to a strong emphasis on the centrality of the person. More in detail, they view IVF not as a sub-stitution for sexual intimacy, but as a kind of prolongation of it, and therefore as not involving the total severance of the unitive and procrea-tive. Not everything that is artificial is unnatural.[31]

I agree with this view. Indeed, I believe it has sufficient theological authority behind it to be regarded as what was traditionally referred to as "a solidly probable opinion." But the issue at stake should be clear. It is the meaning of the inseparability of the unitive and procreative. If this inseparability must be read *in the broad sense* in *Humanae Vitae* and *Familiaris Consortio*—as Caffarra and others argue—then clearly, both contraception and IVF must be excluded. If, however, inseparability can be understood differently, then IVF would not necessarily be excluded. Specifically, it might be sufficient if the *spheres* of the unitive and procre-ative are held together so that there is no procreation apart from mar-riage, and no full sexual intimacy apart from a context of responsibility for procreation.

This matter is somewhat academic because it is possible to justify IVF without modifying the understanding of the inseparability of the unitive and procreative if this inseparability is read in the narrow sense—as applying only to the conjugal act *if it occurs*. In this way one could approve standard IVF without, for example, approving contra-ception. What is not possible, however, is to approve IVF and be consis-tent with Pius XII's understanding of things and with the Caffarra–Tettamanzi–Giunchedi reading of the inseparability of the unitive and procreative.

The departure from Pius XII means that IVF is at some point inex-tricably bound up with the notion of the development of doctrine. It is clear that many theologians—even some regarded as quite conservative, such as Zalba and Visser—have moved beyond the formulations of Pius XII. It is also clear that in doing so they must, in some way or another, modify the understanding of the inseparability of the unitive-procreative dimensions of sexual expression as Pius XII would have seen it and as Caffarra–Tettamanzi–Giunchedi see it. That raises the interesting ques-tion of the development of doctrine in moral theology. That such devel-opment has occurred in the past is unquestionable. For instance, Walter J. Burghardt, S.J., states the conviction of many when he asserts that "I am convinced that Vatican II's affirmation of religious freedom . . . is discontinuous with certain explicit elements within the Catholic tra-dition."[32] That such development can occur in the present ought to be unquestionable.

In the present instance we may well be confronted with a doctrinal development. If this is the case, such a development would probably have a recognizable structure. Using the emergence of *Dignitatis Humanae (Declaration on Religious Freedom)* as a vehicle, I would tentatively suggest attending to a three-step process: (a) the earlier formulation and the reasons and circumstances that explain it, (b) a change in the circumstances and reasons that supported the earlier formulations, (c) experience and reflection leading to an altered formulation.

Concretely, there were cultural and historical circumstances that led to Gregory XVI's *Mirari Vos* (which rejected religious liberty) and made it quite intelligible in those circumstances. But the circumstances had gradually changed by 1965 and "the American experience" had been reflected upon sufficiently to generate efforts at a new formulation of the Church's concerns.

This is only to admit that the Church's formulations of her moral convictions are historically conditioned. This should surprise no one, for even dogmas are historically conditioned. The Congregation for the Doctrine of the Faith acknowledged a fourfold historical conditioning. Statements of the faith are affected by the presuppositions, the concerns ("the intention of solving certain questions"), the thought categories ("the changeable conceptions of a given epoch"), and the available vocabulary of the times.[33]

Could an evaluation similar to the one that led to *Dignitatis Humanae* be occurring with regard to procreative technologies? One who defends that thesis could point at rather clearly identifiable circumstances that led Pius XII to reject all AIH. Specifically, as already noted, there was the influence of F. Hürth, S.J.[34]

In the nearly forty years since Hürth's influential essay, there has been a change in the basic categories of understanding surrounding the discussion. One such change was that the centuries-old primacy given to procreation over other meanings of sexual expression was, as John Mahoney, S.J., notes, "publicly and definitively abandoned" by Vatican II.[35] Another principal change is the criterion to be used in judging the rightfulness or wrongfulness of human conduct. Vatican II proposed as the criterion not "the intention of nature inscribed in the organs and their functions" but "the person integrally and adequately considered." Furthermore, to discover what is promotive or destructive of the person is not a deductive procedure.

This is not to blame Pius XII in any way. His achievement was magnificent. He was, after all and as it should be, dependent on his theologians. Similarly today, the pope must depend on theological advisors who, like all of us, are pilgrims and see only darkly. There are two points to emphasize in saying this. First, when teaching on doctrinal questions, the pope must be careful to prevent his circle of advisors narrowing so as to exclude legitimate currents of theological thought, as Rahner has repeatedly noted. Second, even with the broadest and best consultation, authoritative teaching will unavoidably be time and culture-conditioned. A certain form of ecclesiastical fundamentalism tends to forget this.

Is an evolution occurring with regard to the understanding of the unitive and procreative dimensions of sexuality? If Pius XII's conclusions are the measure, then it has already occurred, as much contemporary theological writing testifies. The really interesting and bound-to-be controversial question is: to what extent has the principle itself of the inseparability of the unitive and procreative been affected by this development? Will not the acceptance of IVF lead to a long second look at the inseparability principle as it is used to reject contraception? If a doctrinal development has indeed occurred since Pius XII, does it not very likely go deeper than the instantial acceptance of reproductive technologies?

Development usually involves both continuity and change. If doctrinal development is occurring, one might guess that the thread that yields both continuity and change is the notion of the inseparability of the unitive-procreative dimensions of sexuality. The continuity: the *general* validity of the insight. The change: a broadened understanding away from an act-analysis of this inseparability. This is certainly the understanding of any number of non-Catholic Christian groups. Whatever the case, the aforementioned inseparability principle must promote the person "integrally and adequately considered." When it becomes an obstacle to that promotion, it loses its (generally operative) normative force; for it is subject to and judged by the broader criterion.

In conclusion, then, from this perspective I see no insuperable theological obstacle to standard IVF. I will return to this below.

2. Third party involvement.   Most often this will take the form of donor sperm. Sometimes it could involve donor eggs, donor embryos, donor wombs. Each has distinctive dimensions and problems that cannot be collapsed and overlooked. Yet all share a common denominator, even if in different ways: third party involvement. What is to be thought of that?

In 1949, Pius XII expressed himself unequivocally. "Artificial insemination in marriage, with the use of an active element from a third person, is equally immoral and as such is to be rejected summarily. Only marriage partners have mutual rights over their bodies for the procreation of new life, and these rights are exclusive, nontransferable and inalienable."[36] By this "active element from a third person" Pius meant donor insemination. But his argument would apply equally to donor eggs. Furthermore, he viewed such third party involvement as opposed to the good of the child because between the child and at least one rearing parent there is "no bond of origin, no moral and juridical bond of procreation."

By and large, theologians (even many non-Catholic ones) have supported Pius XII in his conclusion. Many of these are the very ones who parted company with him on AIH. Thus Karl Rahner argued that AID "fundamentally separates the marital union from the procreation of a new person."[37] Rahner also faults the anonymity of the donor, which represents a refusal of responsibility as father and an infringement of the rights of the child. It should be remembered that when Sweden passed legislation (1984) giving children conceived by AID the right (at eighteen years of age) to know the identity of their genetic fathers, donor insemination came to a virtual standstill. The same thing seems to be happening in parts of Australia. Obviously, donors want neither recognition nor responsibility.

Those who take a different point of view (and a few Catholic theologians have done so)[38] would argue that genetic lineage, while of value psychologically, legally and medically, does not have an absolute primacy. In some context, trade-offs to protect other values could be appropriate. Furthermore, they would argue that sexual exclusivity is not violated because there is no sexual activity.

There are two key issues here on which there is likely to continue to be strong disagreement: (1) Does third party involvement (via gametic donation or surrogate gestation) infringe on conjugal exclusivity? (2) Does having a jointly raised child justify such infringement? My own answer is yes to the first, no to the second. I hold these positions because I believe the notion of conjugal exclusivity should include the genetic, gestational and rearing dimensions of parenthood. Separating these dimensions (except through rescue, as in adoption) too easily contains a subtle diminishment of some aspect of the human person. Others, including very responsible persons, will see this matter quite differently, indeed would vigorously oppose these points of view. Given this situation, I believe that IVF with donor gametes (I do not include surrogacy here) is probably not feasible for prohibition by public policy. In addition to this, a legal ban might well be judged unconstitutional.

To insist that marital exclusivity ought to include the genetic, gestational and rearing components can be argued in at least two different ways. First, it might be argued that any relaxation in this exclusivity will be a source of harm to the marriage (and marriage in general) and to the prospective child. For instance, the use of donor semen means that there is a genetic asymmetry in the relationship of husband and wife to the child, with possible damaging psychological effects. If a surrogate mother is used, conflicts could arise that damage both the marriage and the surrogate.

William J. Winslade and Judith Wilson Ross recently raised some of the questions I have in mind.

> Is the child to know about the method of its birth? If so, how much information should the child have—only that which is deemed to be health-related data, or all of the other biological information about its heritage that most of us value? Whose interests, whose preferences, whose needs count here? Born into a society that is already fragmented by divorce and confused about alternative life styles, morals and sexual choices, the child may well have serious identity problems at a later time. Does such a possibility have to be seriously considered by those who want to undertake unusual reproductive methods?

The Winslade–Ross essay concludes:

> The interests and well-being of the baby-to-be-made seem to be the last issues considered, and sometimes (when physicians promise anonymity to the donor or parents require it of the surrogate) seem not to be considered at all.[39]

Another form of this first approach is the assertion that third party involvement separates procreation from marriage *in principle.* That opens the door, both by human proclivity and the logic of moral justification, to a litany of worrisome problems such as single-woman insemination and insemination of a lesbian couple. Furthermore, as I noted above, it might lead the wife of a sterile husband to conclude that the natural way (sexual intercourse) is less expensive and more convenient than donor in vitro fertilization or AID. Thus adultery would be fostered. The *Chicago Tribune* recently headlined a story as follows: "Unmarried, Pregnant and Proud of It." It went on to describe one mother as follows: "One night with a stranger gave ____ the baby she'd wanted for a year."[40] When sterility gets absolutized as a disvalue in our practices and thought patterns, strange things can happen.

An argument built on possible harmful consequences is one subject to empirical verification. It must be admitted in all honesty that the data is thin at best, often even conjectural. Fears of what might happen once marital exclusivity is relaxed are legitimate even if they do not always lead to clearly established absolute prohibitions. In the past I have argued that the risks and potential harms involved would support a safeside moral rule (procreation should be restricted to marriage) against the slide to abuse. This is a prudential calculus which gives greater weight to *institutional* risk of harm than to *individual* benefit, as I noted in my dissent statement cited above. I see no compelling reasons to modify this judgment.

A second form of argument is that third party involvement is itself violative of the marriage covenant independent of any potential damaging effects or benefits. This would appear to be the view of Pius XII. The view might be argued by appeal to Christ's union with the Church, or God's union with God's people. Such appeals root in the sources of faith and to that extent might not be shared by those of other faiths. For instance, the distinguished Paul Ramsey writes: "To put radically asunder what God joined together in parenthood when He made love procreative, to procreate from beyond the sphere of love . . . or to posit acts of sexual love beyond the sphere of responsible procreation (by definition, marriage) means a refusal of the image of God's creation in our own."[41] While many Christians might find this analysis quite persuasive, I do not believe it could be urged as a basis for public policy.

However, there is a simpler way of making this point. Many couples regard in vitro fertilization not as a *replacement* for their sexual intimacy, but as a kind of *continuation* or *extension* of it. On that view, third party presence (via egg or sperm) is presence of another in the intimacy itself, a thing that ought not to be.

3. **The moral status of the embryo.** The difficulty and delicacy of this issue may be highlighted by two references. Speaking to a distinguished group of scientists meeting in Rome in 1982, John Paul II stated: "I condemn, in the most explicit and formal way, experimental manipulations of the human embryo, since the human being, from conception to death, cannot be exploited for any purpose whatsoever."[42] On the other hand, the highly respected Karl Rahner came to a different conclusion. Admitting that the personhood of the embryo is highly doubtful, he stated: "It would be conceivable that, given a serious positive doubt about the human quality of the experimental material, the reasons in favor of experimenting might carry more weight, considered rationally, than the uncertain rights of a human being whose very existence is in doubt."[43] This is also the position of other reputable theologians.

Catholic formulations have for decades spoken of the human being "from the moment of conception." The underlying supposition is that from the moment (or process) of the union of sperm and ovum there is present a fully protectable human being. Yet this supposition has been seriously challenged by contemporary embryology, particularly the lack of developmental individuality in the early days after conception. Surely the pope is aware of these facts as Rahner was; yet he draws a different practical conclusion. It is possible to argue that the pontiff was drawing a kind of safeside rule against abuse. Such rules are as valid and persuasive as the dangers they envisage are unavoidable. In other words, if clear lines can be drawn that block this slide toward abuse, the rule is less persuasive.

Whatever the case, the difference between Rahner and John Paul II is reflected in the varying evaluations of the embryo found in the wider community. Some regard the embryo as a fully protectable humanity; others qualify that status. This latter was the position of the Ethics Advisory Board in 1979. It stated: "The human embryo is entitled to profound respect; but this respect does not necessarily encompass the full legal and moral rights attributed to persons."[44] The EAB went on to accept research that is designed to assess the safety and efficacy of clinical IVF.

Very similar approaches are to be found in the Warnock Report and the Waller Report. This should be of no little significance to the Church that holds that "in fidelity to conscience, Christians are joined with the rest of men in the search for the truth, and for the genuine solution to the numerous problems which arise in the life of individuals and from social relationships."[45]

What is at stake in our assessment of the moral status of the embryo? Several things. First, our attitude toward "spare" and/or defective embryos. May they simply be allowed to perish? Is even the possibility of such "spares" sufficient to interdict the entire undertaking? Second, our attitude toward cryopreservation of embryos. Embryos can be frozen and kept at the ready should an attempted transfer fail. Thus the need for a second or third invasive laparoscopy is prevented. Yet the thawing process is not all that benign. Some 30–40% of embryos do not survive it. Is that itself an abuse? Finally, there is experimentation. Researchers will undoubtedly want to divide embryos with a view to preimplantation genetic diagnosis. They may also eventually want to attempt gene repair in early embryos.

One thing should be clear: the status of the preimplanted embryo is an *evaluative* question, not a directly scientific one. One cannot, of course, prove evaluations one way or another. One can, however, assemble information that suggests or leads to an evaluation. I believe that there are significant phenomena in the preimplantation period that suggest a different evaluation of human life at this stage. Therefore, I do not believe that nascent life at this stage makes the same demands for protection that it does later. In this sense I agree with Rahner.

However, other conscientious persons will hold different evaluations. Evaluations ought not be decreed. The Supreme Court in its *Wade* and *Bolton* decisions for all practical purposes decreed its own evaluation of nascent life as the morality and law of the land. What, then, is to be done? I raise this question with regard to *public policy*; for I believe that the underlying moral question is as yet unsettled.

When there are no shared convictions about substantive outcomes, there is public wisdom in turning to procedures. Specifically, I believe that there should be a policy presumption against experimentation on embryos and exceptions to this should be allowed only after scrutiny and approval by an appropriate authority. In my judgment, the matter is of such importance that the body should be national in character.

At present, as I write, there is a policy stalemate. Congress imposed a moratorium on fetal research in 1974. In 1975, regulations were promulgated that required that fetal research and human in vitro fertilization research, in order to be federally funded, must be approved by an Ethics Advisory Board. The EAB reported to the Secretary of DHEW that in vitro fertilization and embryo transfer (and certain research necessary to it) are ethically acceptable. No Secretary of DHEW or HHS acted on this report, and the Ethics Advisory Board no longer exists. Hence there is a policy vacuum.

The American Fertility Society's *Ethical Considerations of the New Reproductive Technologies* moved into this vacuum. It should be studied very carefully and critically.

And that brings us finally to the CDF's Instruction. It was dated February 22, 1987, but was actually released somewhat later.[46] The Instruction is a rambling, repetitious document numbering forty pages. Much of its material, however, is excellent and will elicit agreement from a broad constituency. This is especially true of its first ten pages, where its anthropological assumptions are spelled out. It proposes a general criterion for the uses of science and technology: the integral good of the human person. This is a splendid beginning. The Instruction also acknowledges the constructive role science and medicine can play in aiding human persons. It cautions against a blanket rejection of newer technological possibilities on the grounds of mere artificiality and it expresses appropriate sympathy for the suffering of the infertile couple.

It is when the Instruction enters the realm of detailed applications that it is likely to encounter stormy weather. For instance, when it deals with the status of the pre-embryo, its conclusions are unambiguous. It refers to: "unconditioned respect"; "treated as a person from the moment of conception"; "rights as a person must be recognized." Finally, the CDF asks: "How could a human individual not be a human person?" The wording of the Instruction seems to me to vacillate between two assertions: the pre-embryo *must be treated as* a person; the pre-embryo *is* a person. These are remarkably different statements. It is, I believe, easier to defend the first assertion than the second.

More specifically, the Instruction fails to distinguish between *genetic* individualization and *developmental* individualization. The former is certainly present from the very earliest beginnings (a phrase I use instead of "moment of conception" since fertilization is now known to be a process, not a moment). The latter, however, is not. Developmental individualization is completed only when implantation has been completed, a period of time whose outside time-limits are around fourteen days.[47] Practically, then, to the CDF's question "How could a human individual not be a human person?" the proper answer is: by not being—yet— a human individual. The CDF states that it is "aware of the current debates concerning the beginning of human life, concerning the individuality of the human being." Yet it takes no account—other than genetic— of the phenomena that lead outstanding reproductive biologists such as Clifford Grobstein to deny developmental individualization to the pre-embryo. Charles Krauthammer summarized this as follows: "Where the report fails is in its refusal to draw lines, or rather in its insistence on drawing lines at such enormous protective distance from the hellish center that the exercise loses its power to persuade."[48]

The Instruction rejects third-party involvement in procreative technologies. My own agreement with such a rejection is clear from what I have written above.

What is likely to prove much more controversial is the rejection of the so-called "simple case"—artificial reproduction (AIH and in vitro fertilization) with the gametes of husband and wife. On my own reading, this rejection would have to apply also to GIFT (gamete intrafallopian transfer). Why? The Instruction states that artificial insemination cannot be justified within marriage "except for those cases in which the technical means is not a substitute for the conjugal act." In the GIFT procedure, technical means are clearly a "substitute for the conjugal act."

Four Catholic institutions (Nijmegen, Lille, and the two Louvains) announced, shortly after the appearance of the Vatican's Instruction, that they would continue to provide in vitro fertilization with embryo transfer to otherwise infertile married couples (the "simple case"). That should be a tipoff about the persuasiveness of the position taken by the Congregation for the Doctrine of the Faith when it rejected any technology that replaces sexual intercourse for procreation.

I have discussed this "simple case" with physicians, moral theologians, healthcare personnel, married couples, and priests. Although my discussants are certainly not exhaustive, *no one* I spoke with accepts the Vatican's rejection of the "simple case." This informal consensus is underlined in the many committee reports from around the world. Such a consensus must give pause to those who maintain that the document is the Church's final word on this matter.

More to the point, such consensus forces our attention on the analysis that led the congregation to reject in vitro fertilization even when the gametes of husband and wife are used. What is that analysis? It is stated succinctly as follows: "The Church's teaching on marriage and human procreation affirms the 'inseparable connection, willed by God and unable to be broken by man on his own initiative, between the two meanings of the conjugal act: the unitive meaning and the procreative meaning'."[49]

The document goes on to point out that just as contraception separates the unitive and procreative dimensions of sexual expression, so also, in an analogous way, do technological interventions such as in vitro fertilization and artificial insemination by husband. The congregation's rejection of such procedures rests ultimately on the inseparability principle adduced by the document. Indeed, in a remarkable statement, the congregation notes that its rejection of in vitro fertilization between husband and wife "is strictly dependent on the principles just mentioned." In other words, if those "principles just mentioned" can be shown to reveal a weakness, the conclusion will have the same weakness; that is what "strict dependence" means. The statement is remarkable because in the past ecclesiastical documents have asserted that the conclusion's validity is not strictly dependent on the analyses given or available to support it.

It should not be overlooked that the congregation views the principle in question as applying both to contraception and to reproductive interventions. Thus, if that principle is modified, then the very analytical basis for the Church's rejection of contraception has been modified or rejected. In this sense, I believe that the document is more concerned with contraception than with reproductive technologies. If the Church's analysis of contraception were different than it is, the document would be substantially different.

What, then, is to be said of this inseparability principle? Other Christian groups have supported a similar principle, but they have interpreted it differently, as I noted earlier. They have asserted that the unitive and procreative dimensions should indeed be held together, that married love should be generously life giving, and that procreation should occur in the context of covenanted love. But they have viewed such inseparability as something to be realized in the *relationship, not in the individual act.*

Thus the document insists that the unitive and procreative be held together *in every act*—no contraception and, on the other hand, no in vitro fertilization. Others, asserting a similar inseparability, argue that the unitive and procreative should be held together *within the relationship*; or, in more practical terms, just as contraceptive intercourse can be life giving (as nourishing the couple's life giving relationship), so in vitro fertilization can be unitive (as strengthening the relational good, the bond between the couple).

Above, I referred to the "principles just mentioned." Really a single principle is in question here: the inseparability of the unitive and procreative dimensions *understood as applying to every act.* Modify that understanding and the conclusion does not follow.

What, then, is to be said of this understanding? I want to raise several points here to show why many theologians—to say nothing of others—have had and will continue to have serious problems with the official Catholic understanding of the inseparability of the unitive-procreative dimensions of sexuality (as expressed in the Instruction, *Humanae Vitae* and *Familiaris Consortio*).

First, there is the very notion of the procreative dimension of *every act* of sexual intercourse. The idea that in *every act* of sexual intercourse the unitive and procreative dimensions must be inseparable implies that every act of intercourse is in some sense procreative. What does it mean to attribute a procreative dimension to sexual union when it is known to be infertile (e.g., because of age)? It is simply and in every respect a nonprocreative act. What does it mean to attribute a procreative dimension to sexual union during periods (e.g., during natural family planning) when it is known to be and intended to be infertile? To maintain that such an action is "open to procreation" and maintains the inseparability of the unitive-procreative dimensions makes no sense. The action is unobstructed, to be sure. But to argue that it must (morally) be unobstructed is to attribute an overriding moral value to physical unobstructedness. That is why many theologians see in this analysis a form of "physicalism."

Some years ago, John C. Ford, S.J., and Gerald Kelly, S.J., wrote: "The marriage act has other natural and intrinsic ends in addition to procreation which are separable from actual procreation or any intention of actual procreation."[50]

If such separation of "other intrinsic ends" (the unitive) "from actual procreation or any intention" of it is achieved by nature itself in individual acts, in what sense is the act procreative? In what sense are the unitive and procreative held together in the individual act?

Second, I readily admit that the inseparability principle (as applied to every act) contains a germ of truth, but that germ is arguably a legitimate aesthetic or ecological (bodily integrity) concern. All artificial interventions, whether to promote or prevent conception, are a kind of "second best." They involve certain disvalues that, absent sterility or fertility, respectively, we would not entertain. In this sense, we can agree with the congregation that conception achieved through in vitro fertilization is "deprived of its proper perfection." Much the same can be said of the use of contraception. However, a procedure "deprived of its proper perfection" is not necessarily morally wrong in all cases—unless we elevate an aesthetic-ecological concern into an absolute moral imperative. It seems to me that insistence on the inseparability of the unitive and procreative in every act does precisely this.

Third, what is responsible for this elevation of an aesthetic-ecological concern into an absolute moral imperative? For centuries Catholic theological thought viewed procreation as the *only* legitimate meaning and purpose of sexual intercourse. The contemporary teaching that every act of intercourse must be open to procreation (thus no artificial contraception) is a linear descendant of that earlier view and of the inadequate biology on which it rested.[51]

Fourth, the congregation correctly notes that "the one conceived must be the fruit of his parents' love." No one would deny that. Indeed, that is precisely what many Christians mean when they say that the unitive and procreative must be held together *in the relationship.* But to move from that general premise to the conclusion that the child must be conceived through sexual intercourse involves a leap in logic whose implication is that sexual intercourse is the only loving act in marriage.

This gap is underlined in the congregation's attitude toward technology. It states: "The one conceived must be the fruit of his parents' love. He cannot be desired or conceived as the product of an intervention of medical or biological techniques."

Obviously, technology can be abused. And just as obviously, the form of this abuse is to make the prospective child a consumer item on a shopping list—"Give me blue eyes this time." But technology need not be so abused. Ultimately, then, the citation above involves a false opposition. Being a product of a medical intervention is not opposed to being "the fruit of his parents' love." If experience is our guide—and I think it clearly is not in the congregation's document—accepting medical interventions to overcome sterility between husband and wife is, or can be, precisely a concrete manifestation of their love. I have seen this repeatedly. In this sense, it is easy to understand why many physicians regard in vitro fertilization and embryo transfer not as a replacement for sexual intercourse, but as a help to it, a kind of extension or completion of it.

In summary, then, I find the congregation's analysis and reasoning on "the simple case" unpersuasive. So do many others. It is understandable, therefore, why several Catholic institutions have already indicated they intend to continue to perform in vitro fertilization for married couples. It is also understandable why individual couples and physicians might draw the same conclusion.

Finally, let me say that I find myself in agreement with French bio-ethicist Patrick Verspieren, S.J. He states:

> The techniques of artificial procreation thus contain an imper-fection and undeniable risks; but this determination, by itself, allows only with difficulty the conclusion that any recourse to these procedures is immoral. The ultimate reasons that led the Congregation for the Doctrine of the Faith to pronounce every form of artificial procreation "illicit" are to be found elsewhere: in my opinion, in the arguments of authority and in the posi-tions taken by the previous popes.[52]

In a sense, therefore, the CDF faces the future by looking backward, and in doing so it has to live with the assumptions that make "begotten, not made" an absolute moral imperative. In my judgment, that is not an easy theological life.

NOTES

1. "Ethical Considerations of the New Reproductive Technologies," *Fertility and Steril-ity* 46 (1986), Supplement 1.

2. Susan Abramowitz, "A Stalemate on Test-Tube Baby Research," *Hastings Center Report* 14 (1984): 5.

3. Abramowitz, loc. cit., 5.

4. Cf. note 1, at 825.

5. For this basic information, cf. "Ethical Considerations" as in note 1.

6. LeRoy Walters, as in Abramowitz (cf. note 2), 6.

7. *Washington Post,* 14 April 1985.

8. *Philadelphia Inquirer,* 28 August 1985.

9. *Archives of Internal Medicine,* March 1985.

10. *Time,* 31 July 1978. Charles Krauthammer has summarized the issue at stake as synthetic children, synthetic families and synthetic sex (*New Republic,* 4 May 1987, 18).

11. Cf. LeRoy Walters, "Human in Vitro Fertilization: A Review of the Literature," *Hastings Center Report* 9 (1979): 23–43; also Walters, "Ethical Issues in Human in Vitro Fer-tilization and Embryo Transfer," in *Genetics and the Law III,* ed. Aubrey Milunsky and George J. Annas (New York: Plenum Publishing Co., 1985).

12. Clifford Grobstein and Michael Flower, "Current Ethical Issues in IVF," *Clinics in Obstetrics and Gynecology* 12 (1985): 877–91.

13. AAS 29 (1896–97), 704.

14. AAS 41 (1949), 559–60.

15. AAS 43 (1951), 835–54.

16. AAS 48 (1956), 467–74.

17. AAS 60 (1968), 488–89.

18. AAS 74 (1982), 119.

19. Ladislaus Orsy, S.J., "Reflections on the Text of a Canon," *America* 154 (1986): 396–99. For further confirmation of this, cf. G.B. Guzzetti, "Magistero della chiesa e fecundazione in vitro," *Scuola cattolica* 113 (1985): 284–99. Guzzetti is primarily concerned with responding to the rather expansive claims of Dionigi Tettamanzi, "Gli interventi del magistero dell chiesa sulla fecondazione in vitro," *Scuola cattolica* 113 (1985): 67–113. See also Guzzetti, "Debolezza degli argomenti contro l'embryo-transfer," *Revista di teologia morale* 17 (1985): 71–79.

20. Guzzetti, "Magistero," 291.

21. M. Zalba, S.J., "Aspetti morali e giuridici circa l'inseminazione artificiale," *Palestra del clero* 58 (1979): 438 ff.

22. Jan Visser, C.S.S.R., "Problemi etici dell' embryo-transfer," in *Ricerca scientifica ed educazione permanente 7–9* (1982–1983): 47 ff.

23. Catholic Bishops of Victoria (Australia), *Submission to the Committee to Examine in Vitro Fertilization,* unpublished document, 6 August 1982.

24. *Catholic Chronicle,* 16 November 1984. Caffarra has expressed himself frequently on this matter. Cf. *L'Osservatore Romano,* 4 July 1984, 5.

25. L. Leuzzi, "Il dibattito sull'inseminazione artificiale nella riflessione medico-morale in Italia nell'ultimo decennio," *Medicina e morale* 22 (1982): 343–71.

26. William Daniel, S.J., "In Vitro Fertilization: Two Problem Areas," *Australasian Catholic Record* 63 (1986): 21–31, at 31. Cf. also Daniel, "The Morality of in Vitro Fertilization," in *Moral Studies,* ed. Terence Kennedy, C.S.S.R. (Melbourne: Spectrum Publications, 1984), 47–71.

27. Guzzetti, "Debolezza" (cf. note 19), at 72–73.

28. Carlo Caffarra, *L'Osservatore Romano* (English edition), 30 July 1984. This interview was also published in *The Advocate* (Melbourne), 23 August 1984. For a response to this form of argumentation, cf. William Daniel, "In Vitro Fertilization: Two Problem Areas" (cf. note 26), 27 ff.

29. Daniel, loc. cit., 27.

30. Daniel, loc. cit., 31.

31. P. Verspieren, S.J., "L'Aventure de la fécondation in vitro," *Etudes* (November 1982): 479–92.

32. Walter J. Burghardt, S.J., in *Religious Freedom:* 1965 and 1975 (Mahwah, N.J.: Paulist, 1977), 72.

33. *Catholic Mind* 71 (October 1973): 58–60.

34. F. Hürth, S.J., "La fécondation artificielle: Sa valeur morale et juridique," *Nouvelle revue théologique* 68 (1946): 416.

35. John Mahoney, S.J., *Bioethics and Belief* (London: Sheed and Ward, 1984), 28.

36. AAS 41 (1949), 557–61. For an English version, cf. *Catholic Mind* 48 (1950): 250–53, at 252.

37. Karl Rahner, "The Problem of Genetic Manipulation," *Theological Investigations* 9 (New York: Herder and Herder, 1972), 225–52, at 246.

38. For example, Louis Janssens, "Artificial Insemination: Ethical Considerations," *Louvain Studies* 8 (1980): 3–29.

39. William J. Winslade and Judith Wilson Ross, *New York Times,* 21 February 1986, 27.

40. *Chicago Tribune,* 3 October 1985.

41. Paul Ramsey, *Fabricated Man* (New Haven: Yale University Press, 1970), 88–89.

42. *Origins* 12 (1982), 342.

43. Karl Rahner, S.J., "The Problem of Genetic Manipulation," *Theological Investigations,* as in note 37, 236.

44. *Federal Register* 35033–58, 18 June 1979.

45. *Documents,* no. 16, 214.

46. Congregation for the Doctrine of the Faith, "Instruction on Respect for Human Life in its Origin and on the Dignity of Procreation" (Vatican City: Vatican Polyglot Press, 1982).

47. A recent example of the fourteen-day rule is "Richtlinien zur Forschung an frühen menschlichen Embryonen," *Deutches Ärzteblatt-Ärztliche Mitteilungen* 50 (1985): 3757–64.

48. Charles Krauthammer, as in note 10.

49. "Instruction," 26.

50. John C. Ford, S.J., and Gerald Kelly, S.J., *Contemporary Moral Theology: Marriage Questions* (Westminster: Newman, 1963), 405.

51. Cf. Richard A. McCormick, S.J., "Begotten, Not Made," *Notre Dame Magazine* 15 (Autumn 1987): 22–25. Shortly before his death, the renowned Bernard Lonergan, S.J., noted of birth control: "The traditional views [on contraception] to my mind are based on Aristotelian biology and later stuff which is all wrong. They haven't got the facts straight. A conception is not intended by every act of insemination" (*Catholic New Times,* 14 October 1984, 15).

52. Patrick Verspieren, S.J., "Les fécondations artificielles. A propos de l'Instruction romaine sur le don de la vie'," *Etudes* 366 (May 1987): 615. For a critique of the recent literature on the Instruction, cf. Edward Vacek, *Theological Studies* 49 (1988): 110–31. See also the response of the Ethics Committee of the American Fertility Society in *Fertility and Sterility* 49 (no. 2, Supplement 1, 1988), 1S–7S.

7 Ethical Issues in Manipulating the Human Germ Line

MARC LAPPÉ, PH.D.

Marc Lappé, Ph.D. is a professor in the Department of Medical Education at the University of Illinois at Chicago.

1. INTRODUCTION

Germ line engineering embraces any of several techniques which permit the alteration of germinal epithelium, sperm or eggs, or early products of conception such that genetic changes become permanently encoded in the sex cells of the resulting adult. Germ cell alterations can be distinguished from somatic cell ones by virtue of their intergenerational consequences. In theory, only changes directed at the germ line can produce heritable changes. In practice, some somatic cell alterations may also become transmissable, as will be discussed below.

Germ line engineering of the human genome may become technically feasible within a decade, particularly since specific techniques for directing genetic changes in somatic cells already exist (Anderson, 1985, pp. 55–63). Genomic alteration of germ cells has already been demonstrated in animal models (Hammer *et al.*, 1986, pp. 269–278), and has been proposed as a rapid method for accelerating the genetic improvement of livestock (Van Raden and Freeman, 1985, pp. 1425–1431).

While such techniques mark a major advance in our ability to manipulate and control genetic material in animals, the prospect of their application to humans raises fundamental questions about the limits to human control over genetic destiny. Although few convincing rationales have been promulgated which justify using germ line engineering in humans (cf. Fowler *et al.*, 1989, pp. 151–165), vociferous objections to

---

This article first appeared in The Journal of Medicine and Philosophy *16 (December 1991): 612–639.*

using this technology have appeared (Rifkin *et al.*, 1983, pp. 1360–1361). It remains important to consider germ line engineering because it can provide great benefits as well as harm.

Potential justifications for germ line alterations include the correction of genetic defects not otherwise amenable to somatic cell treatment; permanent stabilization of genetic material in offspring of high risk matings (e.g., fragile X syndrome); or the elimination of the need for repeated prenatal diagnosis and selective abortion in genetically at-risk families. Germ line interventions could also permit increases in the frequency of desirable genes and/or the decrease of deleterious ones (*eugenic* changes) and can thereby lead to the selection and perfection of lineages of organisms with improved genetic characteristics. The present essay will examine the arguments for and against working towards such objectives in humans.

2. State of the Art

Germ line changes can be produced by any of three techniques, each with technical strengths and limitations of its own (Anonymous, 1989, p. 107; Tam, 1986, pp. 187–194). The first technique entails the direct microinjection of specific sequences of DNA (cloned DNA) into the pronucleus of a one-celled fertilized egg. This procedure has been perfected in laboratory animals, and leads to a variable percentage of successfully integrated embryos (usually on the order of 10–30 percent). The second utilizes an embryonic stem cell derived from the blastocyst stage which is manipulated in tissue culture by direct transfection with raw DNA or by using a retrovirus to carry genetic material into the cell. Effectively transfected cells can then be reintroduced to a developing embryo during the blastocyst period of development. The third technique involves the use of retroviruses to carry DNA sequences into four cell embryos, the blastocyst or the midgestation embryo. This technique is in theory the most precise, but is presently limited to experimental animals. A fourth technique in which sperm is treated directly with raw DNA appeared to promise a rapid method for achieving permanent genetic change, but it has not proven to be reproducible to date (Barinagg, 1989, pp. 590–591).

3. Distinguishing Somatic from Germ Line Engineering

The multifarious methods which can alter the germ line highlight a common misconception about germ line engineering: germ line changes need *not* be accomplished by direct alteration of the sperm or ova prior to fertilization.

As a result of early genetic engineering, the traditional modes of genetic engineering may result in alterations of *both* somatic and germ line cells. This is so because any genetic change made to the embryo theoretically can be incorporated into its germ line, as long as the change was done prior to the differentiation and segregation of the sex cells from the body of the early embryo proper. Thus, if performed early enough in embryonic development, any gene-modifying technique can lead to germ line alterations. A genetically altered cell which is introduced prior to the segregation of the cellular precursors of the germinal epithelium in the neural crest (in the early somite stage embryo) has the prospect of being permanently incorporated in the sex cells. It is only after the neural plate has folded to form the neural crest that these sex cells migrate to their sites in the primordia of the germinal epithelium to assume their function as stem cells. In females, the primary oöcytes (oögonia) are fixed in number, while germ cells in males are continuously replenished on a fixed cell cycle.

In theory, therapy could also be targeted exclusively to the germ cells of either parent without producing somatic cell genetic changes or effecting a therapeutic change in the phenotype of that adult. Conversely, most somatic cell therapies are directed at a patient and are not presently intended to alter the germ line.

These three modalities can usefully be put into the following typology:

A. "Mixed" germ line/somatic cell therapy.
B. "Pure" germ line therapy.
C. "Pure" somatic cell therapy.

The category of greatest interest in this essay is A. Previous discussions have fairly exhaustively treated pure germ line therapy (category B.) The ethical objections to traditional germ line therapy have centered on the limits of non-consensual research and the unacceptability of manipulations done on embryos (Fowler et al., 1989, pp. 151–165). Broader theological objections to altering the heritable genetic material transgenerationally have also been broached (Walters, 1986, pp. 225–227).

Much more complex ethical issues are generated when the subject is an existing patient with a bona fide need for a genetic intervention which may indirectly alter his germ cell lineage. This prospect is raised by the realization that many forms of somatic cell genetic engineering are contemplated for early treatment of embryos or fetuses. With systemic genetic disorders like adenosine deaminase deficiency, the therapeutic goal will be to convert as many autologous or transplanted cells as possible in a newborn, also raising the possibility that germ line cells in the same individual will be affected by transformed or transfected cells. The first experimental subjects may receive either transfected cells, viral vectors or primitive stem cell populations that may simultaneously convert or seed germ line precursors with the same genetic changes intended for body cells. Stem cell treatment of young children and, hypothetically, even young adults may also colonize the germinal epithelium. This possibility must be considered, for example, in somatic cell engineering of males whose own spermatocytes have been depleted or destroyed by congenital disease or chemical toxicity, since recovery of functionally azoospermic males has been demonstrated (see Lipschulz *et al.* 1980, pp. 464–468). This finding suggests that primary spermatocytes may regenerate from as yet unknown precursors. The eventuality of concomitant germ cell transfection or seeding may be seen as either an unintended "risk" or secondary "benefit" of the somatic cell intervention, depending on the nature of the resulting heritable change. This is so in cases of concomitant germ line change because any therapeutic achievement (or errors) achieved by somatic gene therapy will then be perpetuated in future generations.

4. PROXY CONSENT

Because changes in the germ line potentially affect someone in addition to the recipient of the prospective germinal tissue (i.e., the offspring and future descendants of the treated individual), germ line experimentation raises novel questions of traditional research ethics. Foremost among these is the adequacy and acceptability of proxy consent. Little guidance exists for others assuming the risks for future persons of potentially flawed manipulations of the germ line. By definition, germ line alterations place irreversible changes into the genetic material. Any qualitative alterations to the phenotype that results from such changes may prove to be highly desirable or undesirable to future persons depending on the adaptive value of the resulting traits in unknown future environments. To discover whether or not such changes are in fact beneficial thus requires that we know with some certainty what the future holds and can faithfully convey those probabilities in a discussion of informed consent by proxy. Germ line interventions may therefore subject at least one or probably two generations of future persons to experimentation before the phenotypic effects of the germinal change can be said to "test out". As will be discussed below, such an exercise in predictive science is fraught with uncertainties.

5. TARGETS OF GERM LINE ENGINEERING

The range of therapeutic options possible with germ line engineering includes two distinct end-points: (1) *correction,* in which researchers would identify and repair or replace defective genes in the germ line (i.e., those whose products generate serious pathological or physiological consequences); and (2) *enhancement,* in which researchers alter the genetic makeup of the sperm or egg or their precursors to improve characteristics of offspring in "favorable" ways (Walters, 1986, pp. 225–227). Only the first is squarely within the domain of orthodox medicine. Note that recent improvements in cosmetic surgery and biotechnology-facilitated cloning of human genes like those for human growth hormone increase the likelihood that genetic techniques may find a place in selective improvement in physiological or physical characteristics not strictly pathological in nature.

Arguments for repair or correction of genetic defects have traditionally been justified on the basis of a moral duty to relieve human suffering when we have the capacity to do so. Using somatic gene therapy to achieve such ends raises special problems in that the treatment results in a universal and probably irreversible change in the individual's cells (as compared to a drug which may be discontinued). This problem is compounded where attempts are made to program a person's germ cells with the same genetic change targeted for somatic cell therapy. These problems are less evident when germ line changes occur secondarily.

From an ethical viewpoint, the eventuality of secondary germ cell conversion raises more intergenerational problems than does pure germ line therapy. While there would be no basis in theory to restrict procreation for a somatically engineered individual, the uncertainty of *what* genetic alterations had actually occurred in a secondarily impacted germ line would make procreation of such a person more risk-laden than when there was reasonable foreknowledge of just how the germ line was likely to have been changed.

From animal models, we know that transgenic mice can have multiple gene insertions, higher mutation rates, and greater propensity to cancer than their normally generated counterparts (see Orian *et al.,* 1990, pp. 393–397). These possibilities might make the first experimental subjects of mixed somatic cell-germ line therapy reproductive pariahs until we had a basis to vouchsafe the genetic integrity of their reproductive cells.

The converse situation, wherein a person receives no benefit himself from germ line engineering but is treated only to assure his descendants are free from some genetic defect, comprises a different ethical circumstance. In principle, a carrier of deleterious genes who accepted a risk for himself in germ line therapy to permit the well-being of his offspring and future generations is morally more acceptable than when offspring were inadvertently jeopardized. Obviously, since nonprocreation of a carrier of deleterious genes assures a similar outcome, the ethics are not straight-forward.

6. Typology of Germ Line Alterations

At least four different outcomes can be evaluated as shown in Table 1. While all previous critiques of the acceptability of germ line therapy have dealt with Type III of interventions (i.e., those in which germ line therapy is the intended outcome), the present one considers the consequences of the Type I therapy where germ line alterations are unintended consequences of "standard" somatic cell engineering. Consider the ethical conundrum raised by the prospect of an otherwise ethically acceptable Type I somatic cell protocol. What if the only limitation of the protocol were that it required conditions which *might* lead to implantation of stem cells in the germ line (e.g., it had to be made early in embryonic or fetal development to correct a basic hemoglobinopathy)? Would we find the experiment ethically suspect? I think not, especially if the primary beneficiary of the intervention would be a healthy, genetically "normal" child. If secondary germ line changes would be acceptable as a secondary effect of an otherwise acceptable protocol, what makes them less acceptable if they were the *primary* objective of a Type III intervention?

Consider the circumstance where the sole objective of an intervention in an otherwise healthy individual is to correct a germ line defect and *not* to treat his underlying condition (e.g., the gene coding for retinoblastoma in a still asymptomatic carrier). Assuming other conditions are met (e.g., that risks are knowable or known, and that informed consent can be given, etc.), such a procedure would be ethically questionable only to the extent that treatments to affect future persons are less justified than those to correct problems in present ones.

Table 1.   Differences in Outcome and Intent in Genetic Engineering

Intended target of intervention	Germ line consequences
1. Somatic cells	3. Germ line altered
2. Germ cells	4. Germ line unaltered

These four possible outcomes comprise a typology of interventions:

I.   somatic cells are targeted but germ lines are inadvertently affected [1 → 3]

II. somatic cells are altered but germ lines are not (conventional somatic gene therapy) [1 → 4]

III. germ cells are targeted and altered [2 → 3]

IV. germ cells are targeted but unaltered [2 → 4]

However, ethical acceptability is eroded where germ line therapy is intended to achieve a *eugenic* effect in the person's descendants irrespective of *any* therapeutic objective in the host or his immediate offspring. This is so because it is morally suspect to use the parent (and subsequently his children) as means to achieve societally directed ends that are not necessarily those shared or desired by the family.

7. Arguments Against Germ Line Therapy

The major ethical arguments about germ line engineering thus turn on whether persons can be used as means to uncertain, or morally questionable, ends. It matters whether the objective *and* consequence of the intervention are intended to affect only a single individual, that individual and his family, future lineages from that family line, or whole groups of persons. Medical ethicists generally consider that competent persons may give consent for interventions for which they and they alone assume risks but that they are less justified in giving consent for their own offspring when the benefit/risk ratio is closer to unity.

Because this germ line research also presupposes direct experimentation on embryos, the whole ethical debate of the acceptability of research on fertilized eggs and embryos may have to be rejoined. The core of this debate turns on the acceptability of killing genetically altered but defective embryos or allowing their creation in the first place. The related question of fetal experimentation has already received much attention and is beyond the scope of the present inquiry. These questions are part of the broader issues of assuming risks for future generations.

In one view, germ line research comprises unethical experimentation on the unborn because the early embryo can never be an acceptable subject of experimentation. Not only can it not give informed consent, but it is exquisitely vulnerable to some interventions and experimental incursions which can produce lasting harms. But with the demonstrated success of *in vitro* fertilization, the objection to using normal *gametes* under experimental conditions has been largely overcome.

A further argument against Type III research is that researchers designing germ line strategies would likely be required to sample or, in an extreme, to destroy embryonic tissue to ensure that errors would not be perpetuated into a fully developed human fetus. This assurance would either require wholesale destruction of failed attempts while still in embryo stages, or at an extreme, the killing of abnormal fetuses whose phenotypes did not correspond to initial expectations. These difficulties might be minimized if reasonably close animal models existed. If it could be shown that germ line alterations were successful in permanently correcting a major genetic defect common to a certain familial lineage, and if non-destructive sampling (e.g., via the polar body) were possible, germ line therapy in humans would be technically feasible although still morally questionable.

In the end, objectors to germ line engineering presume that it may fail (i.e., that it will project potential harms into the future), while supporters argue that any potential good of the intervention would be multiplied by their future projection. In this view, the benefits of successful germ line engineering would enjoy a longevity unachievable by somatic cell manipulation.

8. Application of the Law of Double Effect

These issues appear less vexing in the context of Type I interventions which are expressly designed to assure a better physiological state of the organism through somatic genetic therapy. As I have noted, many somatic gene therapy programs entail the use of stem cells which are introduced to a young infant or child in the hope of replacing some or all of the cells of a major organ system such as the liver or bone marrow, making it conceivable that such cell grafts could also enter the germinal epithelium, especially in males. Were this to occur, some sperm might be produced that carried the genetically altered instructions intended to correct the somatic cell defect in the genetically diseased individual.

This possibility makes it important to consider the achievement of germ cell engineering as a secondary consequence of somatic cell therapy under the "law of double effect". Under this provision of Catholic Doctrine, an act which is otherwise ethically objectionable may be morally acceptable if it is the inevitable and unavoidable consequence of carrying out primary morally desirable intervention. Thus, if it is necessary to terminate a tubal pregnancy to save a mother's life, the fact that a fetus is by necessity also destroyed is considered a tragic but acceptable moral consequence. By analogy, if some forms of somatic cell engineering were also to alter the germ line as an indirect consequence of an ethically approved attempt at genetic engineering, there might also be an instance of double effect. Obviously, before such an inadvertently altered person would be encouraged to reproduce, careful appraisal of the genetic composition of his sperm would be mandatory. It would be unlikely, however, that all eventualities of his reproduction could be anticipated without having an embryo produced in which gene expression could be assessed. This manipulation would bring us once again to the problems entailed with research on the products of germ line engineering.

Were the technique of somatic cell therapy plus indirect germ line alteration to prove successful to both the parent *and* his offspring, it would provide appreciable impetus to do more such experimental manipulations irrespective of the ethical nuances raised by non-consenting experimentation and embryo research. (This is exactly what happened with *in vitro* experimentation.) In theory, it would be difficult to object to germ line changes arising as a consequence of somatic cell therapy since they will reduce the likelihood of future transmission of the genetic defect in question, in itself a morally praiseworthy goal.

9. Risks to Future Generations

The acceptability of such radical departures from normal procreative decisions turns to a large extent on the duty of the present generation to protect or to enhance the genetic quality of the next. The technology of genetic engineering which is now being contemplated for somatic cells is intended to affect only the present individual. Any genetic damage which is indirectly caused by manipulations of the germ line will be perpetuated independently of what is done to the phenotype of the genetically engineered patient. In this sense, it is valid to speak of intergenerational consequences of genetic engineering of the germ line.

As we have seen, Type III germ line engineering may be critiqued because it makes irrevocable decisions for future generations without a reasonable proxy or mechanism of consent, and because it alters the genetic makeup of subsequent generations in ways that by definition have unforeseeable consequences (Weatherall, 1988, pp. 13–14). Consideration of such long-range risks is outside the purview of most formal ethical review boards. For instance, Institutional Review Boards are limited in their ability to consider long-range implications and risks of proposed experimentation (45 CFR 46). Presumably, such issues would have to be discussed at other levels of review of genetic experimentation.

While valid, the argument that we cannot know enough to secure the well-being of genetically modified individuals who become part of future generations is insufficient to ban germ line engineering. To reject all germ line alterations as "unethical" because not all germ line-engineered individuals will be assured normal protective options or that they may be genetically unsuited to future environments is tantamount to saying no one should have children. Even the terminally impaired may accept their salvation from genetic disease as a tradeoff for their non-reproduction, a position argued previously to justify encouraging rescued female phenylketonurics to be sterilized. These arguments show the extent to which some people might go to justify germ line engineering. For this reason, it is critical to review the concept of intergenerational responsibility to determine if germ line manipulations can be justified for future persons.

10. Intergenerational Ethics

Intergenerational ethics can be broken into two subsets: those that pertain to the immediate descendants of individual couples, and those that relate to the more global impact of a wider application of the technology. For the purposes of this essay, the prospect of germ line engineering for couples at risk of transmitting serious genetic disease is considered more likely than that of systematically altering genes on a large scale. Nonetheless, the ethical issues are sufficiently similar to treat them both together. Sufficiently compelling reasons for introducing genetic changes to the germ line exist. As we have discussed previously, germ line engineering provides a vehicle for blocking the transmittal of heritable forms of debilitating illness from one generation to the next. If germ line engineering were accomplished on a scale sufficiently large to affect whole populations, it could also have eugenic effects by reducing the frequency of dominantly inherited or X-linked conditions in future generations.

The root of ethical concerns about such otherwise desirable interventions hinges on the limits of eugenics generally and of experimentation to achieve long-term genetic changes. Some of these limitations have been imposed by various bodies (e.g., that on experimental manipulation on embryos recommended by the Ethics Committee of the American Fertility Society [Ethics Committee, 1986, pp. 35–945]). Others are more diffuse, and constitute the basic ethical precepts on which pure (Type III) germ line therapy is based.

11. Experimentation for Future Benefits

Foremost among these precepts are the ethical duties imposed by what Sumner Twiss of Brown University has termed, "the ethic of long-range responsibility" (Twiss, 1976, pp 28–30). This ethic requires that we acquire relevant predictive knowledge (about the expression of germ line implants, for example) before we implement the technology to effect such changes. Thus, before we were to bring a germ line altered person into being, we would have to know what that person would look like both phenotypically and genetically. Unfortunately, as I have shown the nearest model for such a person, the transgenic mouse has *not* shown the necessary degree of uniformity or regulatory control after being manipulated. Some germ line altered animals fail to express their genotypes or have altered gene control mechanisms (see Orian, 1990, pp. 393–397). This situation means that "to get to know" how germ line therapy will work in humans will more likely than not require that we experiment on human embryos and perhaps fetuses with extreme uncertainty. Only in this way could we discover, for instance, how well genes that are inserted into germ cells function. But we would still not know how such genes act *transgenerationally*.

To make that discovery would require that we perform a second generation of experimentation on the germ cells of the first experimental subjects (i.e., the F1 generation before it reproduced to produce the F2 generation). Such an eventuality implies that we must be able to predict future consequences with sufficient certitude to give a valid consent for such manipulations. Given present limitations, I consider this possibility unlikely. We also cannot know without experimentation if the handling and control of sex cells and the products of conception will produce harms that are ethically unacceptable. All of these uncertainties mean that we cannot meaningfully assure an extant parent the outcome of manipulation of his progeny. Moreover, it will be morally problematic to get parental consent to abate any damage which the intervention may do to his or her progeny since this requires the intentional conception of a human embryo which may need to be destroyed or will bear initially invisible cellular harm. This eventually argues for respecting the minimalist duty to ensure that we refrain from acts which create unresolvable difficulties for as yet unborn persons.

These problems underscore a second limitation posed by intergenerational ethics to germ line therapy. When we are ignorant about indirect or delayed second-order consequences to any intervention, particularly when these consequences may be harmful and/or irreversible, we are obliged to exercise "responsible restraint" in developing and implementing that technology (Twiss, 1976, pp. 28–30).

Together, these two conditions circumscribe germ line therapy and limit the weight given to the claim that we have a moral imperative to improve future generations. Advocates of so-called "transgenerational ethics" insist that we have a duty to at least not leave subsequent generations worse off than we are at present. However, such a requirement does not demand that we use germ line engineering to assure genetic equality for the future, since we cannot know now what their phenotype requirements will be in their contemporary environments. Simply ensuring that we do not allow deterioration of the gene pool through an infusion of new mutations (e.g., through faulty germ line interventions or exposure to mutagens) would suffice to meet this minimal requirement.

12. Genetic "Improvement"

These last arguments anticipate a more complex issue: whether or not we have a duty to improve on the present generation to ensure "better" genotypes in the future. Many ethicists concur that we have a

minimal duty to ensure that the legacy we bequeath to the next generation leaves them at least no worse off than we were at the onset of our
generation. But our obligations for future generations are much less
clear than are those for present ones. Do we have a duty to promote the
good of what Martin Golding calls a "distant futurity" (Golding, 1978,
pp. 507–512)? Under this construction, we have a duty to selectively
reduce the genetic load passed on to future generations. This argument
has formed part of the rationale for the crude attempts at eugenics over
the last five decades, culminating in Hitler's notorious "Lebensborn"
movement in the early 1940s. In the Lebensborn program, selective
breeding between so-called "Aryan" couples was conducted to perpetuate "desirable genotypes". This program produced no evidence of
benefit to society. Hitler's eugenic program and similarly misguided
attempts at eugenic sterilization in this country underscore how readily
we may do harm in attempting to "improve" the genetic makeup of
future generations. Some researchers have none the less noted that certain genetic diseases are almost certainly disadvantageous for future
generations. In Martin Golding's view for instance, we have a duty to "do
what we can, consistent with reason and morality, to eliminate them"
(Golding, 1978, pp. 507–512).

Some commentators stop short of advocating eugenic interventions
because of the difficulty in defining the gray zone of a marginally deleterious recessive disorder. It is clearer that we do have a duty to reduce
the likelihood of the perpetuation of clearly undesirable dominant or
X-linked traits like Lesch-Nyhan disease or neurofibromatosis. Germ
line interventions could in theory ensure that neither the birth nor the
procreation of an individual with such powerfully undesirable, dominantly inherited conditions or traits would occur.

But other less technologically controversial or intrusive measures
already exist to achieve the same ends. Both zygote selection (via polar
body analysis) and prenatal diagnosis with selective abortion exist
and could obviate the need for germ line interventions for treating individuals with such dominantly inherited conditions. The selective
destruction of affected early embryos or fetuses to save their "normal"
counter-parts will still raise serious ethical issues about taking human
life. Importantly, these consequences would be minimized by the ability
to select—or genetically engineer—the sperm or eggs.

13. "Selective" Elimination and Germ Line Engineering

Because virtually all of the technologies now available to *select* desired from undesired genotypes entail killing a potential human being
through genetic diagnosis and selective abortion for instance, interventions at the level of germ cells may paradoxically be more morally ac-

ceptable than are those done later in embryogenesis. (This assumes of course that a germ line engineering can be perfected without killing or destroying human embryos in the first place.) Moreover, while screening and selective abortion of genetically abnormal fetuses suffice for "eliminating" most Mendelian disorders in the immediate offspring, they do not protect against fetuses which carry recessive disorders in the heterozygous state, nor against the constant reintroduction of X-linked and dominant traits by spontaneous mutation.

For many conditions, notably classic hemophilia and Duchenne muscular dystrophy, such spontaneous mutations are the dominant modes of reintroduction of the genes each generation. To ameliorate the impact of these conditions on future generations, a technique would be needed that could screen germ line cells for defective genes prior to fertilization.

If it were possible to screen such sperm (or less likely, eggs) and use only those with small numbers of deleterious mutations, it would be possible to achieve "germ line" ends without genetic engineering. In the event that most or all sperm carried deleterious mutations, germ line engineering might be used to stabilize the genome or buttress the genome against mutations. Such futuristic models could be achieved by providing extra copies of the "good" genes (so that mutations would have to affect *both* copies to produce a defect).

For recessive traits, prenatal diagnosis and abortion are even more problematic from a eugenic sense, since these techniques can lead to reproductive compensation and still higher gene frequencies in future generations of the deleterious genes. Neither mass genetic screening to find the at-risk population for recessive disorders nor the screening of each of their pregnancies to eliminate the 50% of the embryos which were carriers and the 25% which were homozygotes would be morally acceptable, since no one has defined heterozygotes for any recessive condition as warranting selective abortion. Thus, none of the conventional techniques used to identify high risk pregnancies or to selectively abort affected fetuses are either universally acceptable or very efficient methods for manipulating the genome over the long run.

In theory germ line engineering could provide a method for efficient elimination of deleterious, recessive disorders. Presumably, universal genetic screening at birth for the genetic load each individual carries would permit the identification of those whose germ line bore an unduly high proportion of deleterious lethal or abnormal genes. Selective engineering of such germ lines, through isolation of primordial germ cells or stem cells for at-risk individuals (e.g., atomic bomb casualties or radiation-exposed workers), could in theory permit the preferential selection of "high quality" (i.e., low genetic load) sperm, and the subsequent use of this improved population for inseminating appropriate mates. Such eugenic uses of germ line *selection* fulfill the presumptive ethical obligation to leave future generations at least as well off as our own.

By contrast, other techniques are fraught with problems. Even after successfully correcting a known genetic defect, late arising tumors in treated animals have been reported. Alterations in the germ line may also not be faithfully perpetuated in future generations because of failures in integrating at appropriate sites in the host genome. Germ line changes by insertional mutagenesis are particularly problematic, since such techniques disrupt the integrity of resident cellular genes. About 10–20 percent of transgenic mice can carry *new* deleterious recessive mutations in essential genes (Palmiter and Brinster, 1985, pp. 343–345).

Thus, germ line engineering may generate hidden genetic damage in one generation that may only show up in subsequent ones. Disrupting the normal mechanism of genetic homeostasis, creating recessive mutations, or upsetting the normal control mechanism are but three ways that genetic engineering could result in distant harms leading to disease, disability or death in the offspring of an ostensibly genetically "cured" individual.

Given these likelihoods, germ line engineering may only be justified if germinal changes occur secondary to otherwise morally supportable interventions.

14. THEOLOGICAL CONCERNS

Germ line alterations come closer to playing God than have any other manipulations so far construed for the new genetic technologies. Since creation is considered by some to be sacrosanct and inviolate to the point of disallowing destruction of even seriously defective fetuses, obvious parallel concerns might be voiced at germ line interventions. But not necessarily. The Roman Catholic Pontiff's permissive response to somatic cell engineering would appear to leave open the possibility of considering interventions which would allow an individual who had a dominant lethal condition that would express itself say by the age of 10 to have *both* germ line and somatic cell engineering to prevent its occurrence. These steps would not only preserve one life, but would permit the fulfillment of the divine plan to permit procreation for an individual who might not otherwise have that opportunity. At the same time, the intervention would allow the affected individual free reign in his own reproduction, without fear of reintroducing the deleterious gene to yet another generation.

15. Long-term Implications

Would not the same consequential ethics eventually permit the widespread proliferation of germ line engineering if the first experimental manipulations proved successful? The ethical requirement requires showing that a germinal intervention provides the sole method of rescuing an otherwise hopeless, ethically deserving developmental circumstance.

Is there a condition amenable only to germ line intervention which would qualify? Even the most serious genetically determined traits are rarely if ever perpetuated with 100% expression in the offspring. Balanced translocations, dominantly inherited disorders, homozygous recessive conditions, and X-linked traits are passed on to only some offspring, and then only (as in the case of recessive conditions) if the partner is heterozygous for the same defect. Homozygous/homozygous crosses are extremely rare in humans, as are matings in which all offspring will invariably die (cf lethal yellow or W phenotypes in mice). In all other circumstances, careful gamete embryo *selection* (e.g., through examination of the polar body of the newly fertilized egg) can identify the at-risk versus the normal embryo. Judicious detection and elimination of genetically defective sperm, eggs or embryos all but vitiates the need for germ line engineering.

16. Conclusions

Germ line changes which result as a secondary consequence of otherwise well designed and ethically acceptable manipulations of somatic cells (e.g., to cure an otherwise devastating or fatal disease) can be seen as acceptable. More serious objections apply to intentional germ line interventions because of the unacceptability of using a person solely as a vehicle for creating uncertain genetic change in his descendants. It is also morally unacceptable to use the promise of future benefit to experiment on fetuses or embryos for whom other technologies exist to achieve the end of being free of major genetic defect. Although most of these technologies entail destruction of the affected embryo or fetus, others (e.g., genetic tests done on the polar body) do not.

The more difficult question of the use of germ line engineering as a technique of last resort to both somatically and germinally "cure" an individual of a major hereditary disorder (e.g., Huntington's chorea or retinoblastoma) is more problematic. Here, one must weigh the benefits and risks of the timing of the intervention. Earlier interventions, such as injecting genetically engineered cells at the blastocyst stage, may paradoxically leave the host still afflicted by the disorder, but with germ cells that are "cured". The creation of such chimeric hosts in which the primary attempt is to relieve them of suffering is again a case of "secondary effect" and is morally defensible.

While it is ethically questionable to assume risks for future generations, it is not clear that altering the germ line to offset a near certainty of adverse consequences of normal procreation is morally contraindicated, especially if this can be achieved by zygote selection and *not* genetic modification. Similarly, the lack of assurance that the changes made to germ line cells will be faithfully expressed in offspring becomes a simple problem in experimental ethics. Where risks are profound for normal procreative choices, as in the situation where known mutagenic damage or intrinsic defective genes are involved, germ line engineering will have strong adherents. The difficulties inherent in performing the technology in addition to the risks posed by its inaccurate application are problems which could be resolved with adequate experimentation and preparation. Thus, such objections to germ line tampering or engineering (to use two pejoratives) are temporizing and insufficient to warrant the present ban on experimentation on embryos or fetuses.

It is also theoretically possible to limit the effects of germ line manipulation to a single generation, either through concurrent manipulations that limit fertility or by committing the conceptus to abstain from reproduction as one of the trade-offs of his genetic alteration. These somewhat draconian devices to limit the intergenerational impact of germ line engineering do not obviate the other major ethical concerns discussed in this paper. Germ line engineering as a directed attempt to change the genotype of future generations cannot ethically be justified. However, when such changes arise as an indirect and otherwise unavailable consequence of an approved form of somatic cell engineering, they are morally acceptable.

REFERENCES

Anderson, W.F.: 1985, "Human gene therapy: Scientific and ethical considerations", *Recombinant DNA Technical Bulletin* 8, 55–63.

Anonymous: 1989, "Making mice with designer genes", *Journal of NIH Research* 1, 107.

Barinagg, M.: 1989, "Making transgenic mice: Is it really that easy?" *Science* 245, 590–591.

Code of Federal Regulations 45, 46.III.

Ethics Committee of the American Fertility Society: 1986, "Ethical considerations of the new reproductive technologies", *Fertility & Sterility* 46 Suppl 1, 3S–94S.

Fowler, G., Juengst, E.T., and Zimmerman, B.K.: 1989, "Germline gene therapy and the clinical ethos of medical genetics", *Theoretical Medicine*, 151–165.

Golding, M.: 1978, "Obligations to future generations", in W. Reich (ed.), *Encyclopedia of Bioethics*, Macmillan, New York, pp. 507–512.

Hammer, R.W., Pursel, V.G., and Rexrood, C.E., Jr., *et al.*: 1986, "Genetic engineering of mammalian embryos", *Journal of Animal Science* 63, 269–278.

Lipschulz, L.I., *et al.*: 1980, "Dibromochloropropane and its effect on testicular function in men", *Journal of Urology* 124, 464–468.

Muller, H.: 1987, "Human gene therapy: Possibilities and limitations", *Experientia* 43, 375–378.

Orian, J.M., Tamakoshi, K., Mackay, I.R., *et al.*: 1990, "New murine model for hepatocellular carcinoma: Transgenic mice expressing metallothionen-ovine growth hormone fusion gene", *Journal of the National Cancer Institute* 82, 393–397.

Palmiter, R.D., and Brinster, R.L.: 1985, "Transgenic mice", *Cell* 41, 343–345.

Rifkin, J., *et al.*: 1983, "Theological letter concerning the moral arguments against genetic engineering of human germline cells", reported in C. Norman, "Clerics urge ban on cells", *Science* 220, 1360–1361.

Twiss, S.: 1976, "Ethical issues in setting priorities", *Annual of the New York Academy of Science* 245, 28–30.

Van Raden, P.M., and Freeman, A.E.: 1985, "Potential genetic gains from producing bulls with only sires as parents", *Journal of Dairy Science* 68, 1425–1431.

Walters, L.: 1986, "The ethics of human gene therapy", *Nature* 320, 225–227.

Weatherall, D.J.: 1988, "The slow road to gene therapy", *Nature* 331, 13–14.

8 *Human Gene Therapy: Why Draw a Line?*

W. FRENCH ANDERSON

Dr. W. French Anderson is Chief of the Laboratory of Molecular Hematology, National Heart, Lung, and Blood Institute, National Institutes of Health, in Bethesda, Maryland.

On January 19, 1989, the Director of the National Institutes of Health (NIH), Dr. James A. Wyngaarden, approved our clinical protocol to insert a foreign gene into the immune cells of cancer patients (Roberts, 1989). Although our protocol does not represent gene therapy *per se*, the techniques used are identical to those required for gene therapy (Anderson, et al., 1988). The technology for inserting genes into humans has arrived.

Somatic cell gene therapy (i.e., the insertion of a normal gene into somatic, or body, cells of a patient) has the potential for reducing or eliminating the suffering and death caused by genetic as well as other types of diseases (Anderson, 1984). A large number of individuals and groups have presented persuasive arguments that such therapy would be a moral good and even a moral responsibility.[1] And yet, even those of us who are the most enthusiastic proponents of gene therapy have deep-seated concerns about the possibilities of misuse and, therefore, a hesitancy about taking the first step. In this essay I try to get at the roots of these concerns.

UNEASINESS WITH GENE THERAPY

One element of our hesitation is a concern about the slippery slope. Once we begin and are successful at somatic cell gene therapy, we then open the door for the next logical step: germline gene therapy, that is, the correction of the disorder in the gamete cells of the patients so that

This article first appeared in The Journal of Medicine and Philosophy *14 (December 1989): 681–693.*

children of the patient would receive the normal gene. I have argued elsewhere (Anderson, 1985) that germline therapy would be ethically appropriate once several specific criteria are satisfied.[2]

Successful somatic cell gene therapy also opens the door for enhancement genetic engineering, i.e., the supplying of a specific characteristic that individuals might want for themselves (somatic cell engineering) or their children (germline engineering) which would not involve the treatment of a disease. The most obvious example at the moment would be the insertion of a growth hormone gene into a normal child in the hope that this would make the child grow larger. I have drawn my own "line" at enhancement engineering (Anderson, 1985). But why should a line be drawn here? Perhaps parents should be allowed to choose (if science should ever make it possible) whatever useful characteristics they wish for their children. Is our nervousness about this possibility simply fear of the unfamiliar? Is there really any reason why we should be cautious about moving into human applications of genetic engineering? I believe that there is.

A Basis for Our Uneasiness

At the core of society's concern about beginning the human application of genetic engineering may be our sense that we are developing a capability to *change* who and what we are. Might the procedure be able to produce alterations in the fundamental structure of our existence—our humanness? We do not really understand what makes up our humanness,[3] nor do we know precisely what role genes may play. But whatever our humanness is, we fear the possibility of its being tampered with.[4]

Granted we now influence the genes present in our population by our choice of a mate, by our use of genetic counseling, prenatal screening, and selective abortion, by our exposure to environmental mutagens, radiation, etc. The side effects of some forms of present therapies can lead to genetic damage (e.g., chemotherapy, radiotherapy) or overt changes in our bodies (e.g., surgery, hormone therapy). Some therapies introduce cells with their genetic material from one individual into another (e.g., bone marrow and organ transplants, blood transfusions). But the benefits or damages that may result to the gene pool from these events are unintended. What we are now considering is to take intentional steps to alter the human genome. We do not understand how a thinking, loving, interacting organism can be derived from its molecules, but we are approaching the time when we can change some of those molecules. How then can we derive the benefits made possible by gene transfer technology while protecting ourselves from its potential risks?

Drawing a Line

As with any other powerful technology, we should examine human genetic engineering from two aspects:

(1) What is technically feasible now or in the near future (versus what will only be possible in the distant future or not at all)? What are the benefits and risks of the technology now; how will these benefits and risks change over time?

(2) What are the ethical implications for society as each new step of genetic engineering technology becomes possible? What are the fundamental moral principles that should guide our considerations? Can "lines" be drawn or will any application of genetic engineering in humans put us on an irreversible slippery slope that leads to undesirable consequences? If lines can be drawn, where and how should they be drawn?

I will attempt to provide answers for each of these questions.

What Is Technically Feasible?

Below is an updated summary of what was examined in detail elsewhere (Anderson, 1985).

Somatic cell gene therapy: is now technically feasible for a number of diseases. Efficacy still needs to be improved in all cases, but present progress strongly suggests that within ten years many diseases will be treatable, at least partially, by means of gene transfer. Besides genetic defects, other serious diseases are candidates for therapy including some types of cancer, AIDS, some forms of heart and vascular diseases, etc. What still remains untreatable are dominant disorders where the problem is not the absence of an activity, but the synthesis of a harmful product (for example, Huntington's chorea). Until it is possible to correct a defect *in situ*, some diseases will remain untreatable. All that is possible for the foreseeable future is the insertion of a normal gene into the genome. Therefore, only the loss of an activity can be corrected. Furthermore, genetic defects that produce damage during early embryonic life are not treatable at present. As for risks, insertional mutagenesis (damage caused by non-specific insertion of the added gene) will remain a source of potential risk until site-specific insertion is possible. Site-specific insertion of genetic material can be done to a limited extent in lower organisms and progress is being made in accomplishing the task in mammals, but a clinically useful procedure is still several years away.

Germline gene therapy. The ability to perform this procedure is not closer now than at the time of the previous review (Anderson, 1985), and is unlikely to be available in a clinically useful form for a number of years.

Enhancement Engineering

Somatic: is now technically feasible. The same technology that provides somatic cell gene therapy can be used for somatic cell enhancement engineering; the potential risks, however, are greater (see below).

Germline: is not technically feasible now. The same technical considerations hold here as for germline gene therapy although as for somatic cell enhancement engineering, the risks are greater.

What Are the Ethical Implications?

I will argue that a line can and should be drawn between somatic cell gene therapy and somatic cell enhancement engineering.

Lines can be drawn. Our society has repeatedly demonstrated that it can draw a line in biomedical research when necessary. The Belmont Report (National Commission, 1978) admirably illustrates how guidelines were formulated to delineate ethical from unethical clinical research and to distinguish clinical research from clinical practice. Our responsibility is to determine how and where to draw lines with respect to genetic engineering.

We cannot anticipate what society will or will not accept a few decades from now. Nor can we predict what society a millennium from now might have wanted us to do; the people of that time may want re-engineered bodies (Glover, 1984). Indeed, it can be argued that, considering how fluid the gene pool is, the random insertion of one or two specific genes is exceedingly unlikely to cause any harm, and therefore any application of genetic engineering that appears useful ought to be allowed and might, in fact, become routine in a few decades. Regardless of what our culture might decide for itself in the future, our immediate concern ought to be how to approach the initiation of gene therapy with some degree of confidence that we, as a society, are proceeding reflectively.

Fortunately, this careful approach is what is now taking place. The Human Gene Therapy Subcommittee of the NIH's Recombinant DNA Advisory Committee has already established a *de facto* line (Department of Health and Human Services, 1986): proposals for deliberate germline alteration will not be considered; protocols for somatic cell gene therapy must justify why the disease selected is a good candidate, including the seriousness of the disease and the lack of effective alternative therapy. The Subcommittee has rejected requests from public interest groups to provide specific guidelines for defining the "line". This is wise, since

written criteria from a government committee could become inappropriately restrictive. It is possible, however, to draw lines.

Lines should be drawn. Somatic cell gene therapy for the treatment of severe disease is considered ethical because it can be supported by the
fundamental moral principle of beneficence: It would relieve human suffering. Gene therapy would be, therefore, a moral good. Under what circumstances would human genetic engineering not be a moral good? In
the broadest sense, when it detracts from, rather than contributes to, the
dignity of man. Whether viewed from a theological perspective or a secular humanist one, the justification for drawing a line is founded on the
argument that, beyond the line, human values that our society considers
important for the dignity of man would be significantly threatened.

I suggest that somatic cell enhancement engineering would threat-
en important human values in two ways: first, it could be medically
hazardous, i.e., the risk could exceed the potential benefits and could
therefore cause harm, and second, it would be morally precarious, i.e., it
would require moral decisions that our society is not now prepared to
make and which could lead to an increase in inequality and an increase
in discriminatory practices.

Enhancement engineering could be medically hazardous. Medicine is a
very inexact science. Every year new growth factors, new regulatory
mechanisms, and new metabolic pathways are discovered. There are
clearly many more to be discovered. Most impressive is the intricate way
that all of the hundreds of pathways in each cell are coordinated. Likewise, the body as a whole carefully monitors and balances a multitude of
physiological systems. Much additional research will be required to elucidate the effects of altering one or more major pathways in a cell. To add
a normal gene to overcome the detrimental effects of a faulty one is
probably not going to produce any major problems, but to insert a gene
to make more of an existing product might adversely affect numerous
other biochemical pathways. In other words, replacing a faulty part is
different from trying to add something new to a normally functioning,
technically complex system. Correcting a defect in the genome of a human is one thing. But inserting a gene in the hope of "improving" or
selectively altering a characteristic might endanger the overall metabolic
balance of the individual cells as well as of the entire body.[5]

To illustrate the difference between correction and improvement,
consider as an example a television set. Most of us know very little about
the insides of a TV. If our set were to stop working and we looked inside
and saw a broken wire, it would not be unreasonable to think that by
replacing the broken wire the operation of the set would be corrected.
But what if our set merely does not have as sharp a picture as our neigh-

bor's? Suppose we note that his set has an extra part inside. Without knowing anything about the makes and the engineering requirements of the two sets, would our set be "improved" if we simply inserted his extra part into our set? The chances are great that we would do more harm than good. At least we could take the part back out if it did not help. But once a gene has been inserted into a person's cells, it is not possible to take it back out. Even though in most cases a gene insertion would probably cause no significant disruption, we possess insufficient knowledge of the human body at present to understand the effects of attempts to alter, rather than simply to correct, the genetic machinery of a human.

In summary, it could be harmful to insert a gene into humans. In somatic cell gene therapy for an already existing disease, the potential benefits could outweigh the risks. In somatic cell enhancement engineering, however, the risks would be greater while the benefits would be considerably less clear.

Enhancement engineering would be morally precarious. But even aside from the medical risks, somatic cell enhancement engineering should not be performed because it would be morally precarious. Let us assume that there were no medical risks at all from somatic cell enhancement engineering: that the technology had arrived whereby any gene could be safely inserted into the appropriate somatic cells of an individual and we knew how to insure that no disruption of the cell's metabolism would occur. There would still be reasons for objecting to this procedure. To illustrate, let us consider some examples. What if a human gene were cloned that could produce a brain chemical which would result in markedly increased memory capacity in monkeys after gene transfer? Should a person be allowed to receive such a gene on request? Should a pubescent adolescent whose parents are both five feet tall be provided with a growth hormone gene on request? Should a worker who is continually exposed to an industrial toxin receive a gene to give him resistance on request? What if it were a time of national crisis and the worker was in an industry which was critical for the national security? What if it was the industry that wanted the worker to receive the gene rather than the worker himself?

The problems suggested by these scenarios are three: 1) how to determine what genes should be provided; 2) how to determine who should receive a gene; and 3) how to prevent discrimination against individuals who do or do not receive a gene.

(1) *How to determine what gene should be provided.* We allow that it would be ethically licit to use somatic cell gene therapy for treatment of serious disease. But what distinguishes a serious disease from a "minor" disease from cultural "discomfort"? What is suffering? What is significant suffering? Does the absence of growth hormone that results in a

growth limitation to two feet in height represent a genetic disease? What about a limitation to a height of four feet, to five feet? Where does one draw the line? Each observer might draw the lines between serious disease, minor disease, and genetic variation differently. But all can agree that there are extreme cases that produce significant suffering and premature death. Here then is where a line should be drawn for the initial use of human genetic engineering: treatment of serious disease. There will, of course, be disagreement about certain cases but at least we have narrowed the scope of uncertainty. Some will argue that establishing the line at significant suffering and premature death is too restrictive. As we become more experienced with gene therapy (assuming that it is successful), then the line should and undoubtedly will be moved to include more classes of diseases.

(2) *How to determine who should receive a gene.* If the position is established that only patients suffering from serious diseases are candidates, then the issues are no different from any other medical decision: Who receives a liver transplant, who receives kidney dialysis, etc.? The decision is based on medical need within a supply and demand framework. But if the use of gene transfer extends to allow a normal individual to acquire, for example, a memory-enhancing gene, then profound problems would result. On what basis is the decision made to allow one individual to receive the gene but not another: To those best able to benefit society (i.e., the smartest already)? To those most in need (i.e., those with low intelligence? But how low? Will enhancing memory help a mentally retarded child?)? To those chosen by a lottery? To those who can afford to pay? As long as our society lacks a significant consensus about the answers, the best way to make equitable decisions in this case should be to base them on the seriousness of the objective medical need, rather than on the personal wishes or resources of an individual.[6]

(3) *How to prevent discrimination.* Discrimination can occur in many forms. If individuals are carriers of a disease (for example, sickle cell anemia) would they be pressured to be treated? Would they have difficulty in obtaining health insurance unless they agreed to be treated? Or be required to pay much higher premiums? These are ethical issues raised also by genetic screening and by the human genome project. But the concerns would become even more troublesome if there were the possibility for "correction" by the use of human genetic engineering. In times of national crisis might workers in a dangerous industry be encouraged to protect themselves by means of genetic engineering as a patriotic act? What if a person refused? Our society's belief that a person has a fundamental right of autonomy would be threatened in these various circumstances.

If there are only limited resources, would those "fortunate" individuals who received a "favorable" gene be discriminated against by those left out? A report of the Office of Technology Assessment indicates that society's attitude would be positive towards an individual, suffering from a serious disease, who received a gene in order to return towards normal health (U.S. Congress, 1987). It is quite another matter to know what our society's attitude would be towards persons who used genetic engineering to try to make themselves or their children "better" than normal. Finally, we must face the issue of eugenics, the attempt to make hereditary "improvements". The abuse of power that societies have historically demonstrated in the pursuit of eugenic goals is well documented (Ludmerer, 1972; Kevles, 1985). Might we slide into a new age of eugenic thinking by starting with small "improvements"? Once started, would we then truly find ourselves on a slippery slope that would lead to an attempt to re-engineer humans? Jeremy Rifkin (1983, pp. 14, 23, 228, 231–234) and Nicholas Wade (1982a, 1982b) sound alarmist in their strident warnings. But are they really that far off the mark? It would be difficult, if not impossible, to determine where to draw a line once enhancement engineering had begun. Therefore, gene transfer should be used only for the treatment of serious disease and not for putative improvements.

In summary, our society is comfortable with the use of genetic engineering to treat individuals with serious disease. Once we step over the line that delineates treatment from enhancement, a Pandora's box would open. On medical and ethical grounds a line should be drawn excluding any form of enhancement engineering.

CONCLUSION

Because our knowledge of the human body and mind is so limited, and because we do not know what harm we might inadvertently cause by gene transfer technology, the use of genetic engineering to insert a gene into a human being should first be used only in the treatment of serious disease. In order to proceed judiciously, the classes of disease that would be the first ones considered for treatment by gene therapy should be determined in advance. The initial "line" should be those diseases that produce significant suffering and premature death. As experience is gained, the line should be moved to include a wider range of diseases and, possibly, germline gene therapy for specific diseases (depending on the efficacy and safety data that become available). Gene transfer should not be used for enhancement engineering.

NOTES

1. For reports from groups see: President's Commission, 1982; U.S. Congress, 1982; Manipulating Life, 1982; Parliamentary Assembly of the Council of Europe, 1982 (there have now been 16 statements—all favorable—from a range of international bodies [L. Walters, personal communication]); U.S. Congress, 1984; for papers by scientists see: Anderson, 1971; Friedmann and Roblin, 1972; Anderson and Fletcher, 1980; Mercola and Cline, 1980; Williamson, 1982; Davis, 1983; Motulsky, 1983; Miller, 1983; Grobstein and Flower, 1984; Williams and Orkin, 1986; Ledley, 1987; Weatherall, 1988; for papers by theologians, ethicists, philosophers, and others see: Shinn, 1978; Pope John Paul II, 1982; Pope John Paul II, 1983; Fletcher, 1983; Capron, 1983; Nelson, 1984; Gorovitz, 1984; Fletcher, 1985; Walters, 1986; Nichols, 1988; Fowler et al., 1989. In addition, in national surveys sponsored by the U.S. Congress's Office of Technology Assessment (OTA), the majority of Americans favor somatic cell gene therapy (U.S. Congress, 1987, pp. 69–77).

2. Three criteria are: first, there should be considerable previous experience with somatic cell gene therapy that clearly established the effectiveness and safety of treatment of somatic cells; second, there should be adequate animal studies that established the reproducibility, reliability, and safety of germ line therapy, using the same vectors and procedures that would be used in humans; and third, there should be public awareness and approval of the procedure (Anderson, 1985; cf. editorial, 1988, and Fowler et al., 1989).

3. I have used the word "humanness" in the manner discussed in detail by Joseph Fletcher (1979). The term refers to "the very nature of man" as opposed to human nature; i.e., to an ill-defined "humanhood inventory" or "profile of man". Joseph Fletcher is one of the few authors who has attempted to provide such an inventory/profile. He lists fifteen positive attributes and five negative ones. His positive elements include, for example, minimum intelligence, self-awareness, a sense of futurity, etc. B.M. Ashley has also discussed "What does science say we are" in Ashley (1985).

4. I do not believe that the widespread public uneasiness about human genetic engineering that I have found in talking with diverse groups throughout the country over the past 20 years is founded solely in worries about cancer, toxic side effects, or random mutations. People smoke, drink, overeat, use drugs, drive recklessly, pollute the environment with mutagens, etc., with only moderate expressions of concern. Anxiety about genetic engineering strikes deeper than this. And even though individuals cannot usually express in words why they are nervous, they know that they are. An element here is that, as studies of risk perception have shown (Fischhoff et al., 1981), the public tends to underestimate familiar risks and overestimate risks that are unfamiliar, hard to understand, invisible, involuntary, and/or potentially catastrophic. Recombinant DNA and gene therapy fall into this latter category. Nonetheless, as stated above, even some of us who are highly knowledgeable and enthusiastic about genetic engineering are uneasy about it.

5. Someday we should be able to insert a gene into a precise location in a chromosome of a cell (site-specific integration), have the gene engineered so that it will function exactly as predicted, or even change the nucleotide sequence of a gene in vivo (gene surgery). Although these procedures can be carried out to a limited degree in lower organisms now, they are not possible in mammals. When we have obtained that degree of sophistication, then the scientific concerns expressed in this essay would be considerably less relevant. Since it will be many years before we reach that point, however, we can leave the question of the moral correctness of human genetic engineering in the presence of adequate knowledge to that future society.

6. Our Western culture is very pluralistic and permissive. We, ourselves, might not want to smoke, use krebiozen to treat our cancer, or ride a rocket over the Snake River canyon, but we allow others to do what they wish with their own lives and bodies, within broad limits, short of suicide or hurting others. Thus, our society may want to allow some-

day somatic cell genetic engineering by a competent adult for him/herself. But until we have acquired considerable experience with regard to the safety of somatic cell gene therapy for severe disease, and society has resolved at least some of the ethical dilemmas that this procedure would produce, non-therapeutic use of genetic engineering should not occur.

REFERENCES

Anderson, W. F.: 1971, "Genetic therapy", in M. P. Hamilton (ed.), *The New Genetics and the Future of Man*, William B. Eerdmans, Grand Rapids, Michigan, pp. 109–124.

Anderson, W. F.: 1984, "Prospects for human gene therapy", *Science* 226, 401–409.

Anderson, W. F.: 1985, "Human gene therapy: Scientific and ethical considerations", *Journal of Medicine and Philosophy* 10, 275–291.

Anderson, W. F., Blaese, R. M., and Rosenberg, S. A.: 1988, "N2 transduced tumor infiltrating lymphocytes", *Recombinant DNA Technical Bulletin* 11, 153–182.

Anderson, W. F. and Fletcher, J. C.: 1980, "Gene therapy in human beings: When is it ethical to begin?", *New England Journal of Medicine* 303, 1293–1297.

Ashley, B. M.: 1985, "What does science say we are?", in B. M. Ashley, *Theologies of the Body: Humanist and Christian*, The Pope John XXIII Center, Braintree, Massachusetts, pp. 19–50.

Capron, A. M.: 1983 (June 16): "Don't ban genetic engineering", *Washington Post*, p. A26.

Davis, B. D.: 1983, "The two faces of genetic engineering in man", *Science* 219, 1381.

Department of Health and Human Services: 1986, "National Institutes of Health points to consider in the design and submission of human somatic-cell gene therapy protocols", *Recombinant DNA Technical Bulletin* 9, 221–242.

Editorial: 1988, "Are germ-lines special?", *Nature* 331, 100.

Fischhoff, B., Lichtenstein, S., Slovic, P., Derby, S. L., and Keeney, R. L.: 1981, *Acceptable Risk*, Cambridge University Press, Cambridge.

Fletcher, J. C.: 1983, "Moral problems and ethical issues in prospective human gene therapy", *Virginia Law Review* 69, 515–546.

Fletcher, J. C.: 1985, "Ethical issues in and beyond prospective clinical trials of human gene therapy", *Journal of Medicine and Philosophy*, 10, 293–309.

Fletcher, Joseph: 1979, "Humanness", in *Humanhood: Essays in Bioethics*, Prometheus Press, New York, pp. 7–19.

Fowler, G., Juengst, E. T., and Zimmerman, B. K.: 1989, "Germ-line gene therapy and the clinical ethos of medical genetics", *Theoretical Medicine*, 10, 151–165.

Friedmann, T. and Roblin, R.: 1972, "Gene therapy for human genetic disease?", *Science* 175, 949–955.

Glover, J.: 1984, *What Sort of People Should There Be?*, Penguin Books, Middlesex, England.

Gorovitz, S.: 1984 (December 9), "Will we still be 'human' if we have engineered genes and animal organs?", *Washington Post,* pp. C1, C4.

Grobstein, C. and Flower, M.: 1984, "Gene therapy: proceed with caution", *Hastings Center Report* 14(2), 13–17.

Kevles, D. J.: 1985, *In the Name of Eugenics,* Alfred A. Knopf, New York.

Ledley, F. D.: 1987, "Somatic gene therapy for human disease: Background and prospects", *Journal of Pediatrics* 110, 1–8, 167–174.

Ludmerer, K. M.: 1972, *Genetics and American Society,* The Johns Hopkins University Press, Baltimore.

Mercola, K. E. and Cline, M. J.: 1980, "The potentials of inserting new genetic information", *New England Journal of Medicine* 303, 1297–1300.

Miller, H. I.: 1983 (June), "Gene therapy: Not to be feared or over-regulated", *Bio/ Technology,* p. 382.

Motulsky, A. G.: 1983, "Impact of genetic manipulation on society and medicine", *Science* 219, 135–140.

National Commission for the Protection of Human Subjects of Biomedical and Behavioral Research: 1978, *The Belmont Report,* U.S. Government Printing Office, Washington, D.C.

Nelson, J. R.: 1984, "From genesis to genetics: A theoretical-ethical exercise", in *Human Life—A Biblical Perspective for Bioethics,* Fortress Press, Philadelphia, pp. 155–173.

Nichols, E.: 1988, *Human Gene Therapy,* Harvard University Press, Cambridge.

Parliamentary Assembly of the Council of Europe: 1982 (33rd ordinary session), Recommendation 934.

Pope John Paul II: 1982, "Biological research and human dignity", *Origins* 12, 342–343.

Pope John Paul II: 1983, "The ethics of genetic manipulation", *Origins* 13, 385–389.

President's Commission for the Study of Ethical Problems in Medicine and Biomedical and Behavioral Research: 1982, *Splicing Life,* U.S. Government Printing Office, Washington, D.C.

Rifkin, J.: 1983, *Algeny,* Viking Press, New York.

Roberts, L.: 1989, "Human gene transfer test approved", *Science* 243, 473.

Shinn, R. L.: 1978, "Gene therapy: Ethical issues", in W. T. Reich (ed.), *Encyclopedia of Bioethics,* Free Press, Macmillan, New York, pp. 521–527.

U.S. Congress Subcommittee on Investigations and Oversight of the Committee on Science and Technology: 1982, *Human Genetic Engineering,* U.S. Government Printing Office, Washington, D.C.

U.S. Congress Office of Technology Assessment: 1984, *Human Gene Therapy—A Background Paper,* U.S. Government Printing Office, Washington, D.C.

U.S. Congress Office of Technology Assessment: 1987, *New Developments in Biotechnology. Volume 2: Background Paper: Public Perceptions of Biotechnology*, U.S. Government Printing Office, Washington, D.C.

Wade, N.: 1982a (July 22), "Whether to make perfect humans", *New York Times,* p. A22.

Wade, N.: 1982b (December 29), "The rules for reshaping life", *New York Times,* p. A26.

Walters, L.: 1986, "The ethics of human gene therapy", *Nature* 320, 225–227.

Weatherall, D. J.: 1988, "The slow road to gene therapy", *Nature* 331, 13–14.

Williams, D. A. and Orkin, S. H.: 1986, "Somatic gene therapy: Current status and future prospects", *Journal of Clinical Investigation* 77, 1053–1056.

Williamson, R.: 1982, "Gene therapy", *Nature* 298, 416–418.

World Council of Churches: 1982, "Manipulating life: Ethical issues in genetic engineering", *Church and Society,* World Council of Churches, Geneva.

DEATH AND DYING

Hans Jonas
Timothy E. Quill
Thomas A. Shannon
James J. Walter
William A. Gray, M.D.
Robert J. Capone, M.D.
Albert S. Most, M.D.
The Atlanta Archdiocese
Ezekiel J. Emanuel, M.D.
Linda L. Emanuel, M.D.
Albert R. Jonsen

9 The Burden and Blessing of Mortality

HANS JONAS

Hans Jonas served, until his death in February 1993, as the Alvin Johnson Professor Emeritus of Philosophy at the New School for Social Research in New Rochelle, N.Y.

Since time immemorial, mortals have bewailed their mortality, have longed to escape it, groped for some hope of eternal life. I speak, of course, of human mortals. Men alone of all creatures know that they must die, men alone mourn their dead, bury their dead, remember their dead. So much is mortality taken to mark the human condition, that the attribute "mortal" has tended to be monopolized for man: in Homeric and later Greek usage, for example, "mortals" is almost a synonym for "men," contrasting them to the envied, ageless immortality of the gods. *Memento mori* rings through the ages as a persistent philosophical and religious admonition in aid of a truly human life. As Psalm 90 puts it, "Teach us to number our days, that we may get a heart of wisdom."

Over this incurably anthropocentric emphasis, not much thought was spent on the obvious truth that we share the lot of mortality with our fellow creatures, that all life is mortal, indeed that death is coextensive with life. Reflection shows that this must be so; that you cannot have the one without the other. Let this be our first theme: mortality as an essential attribute of life as such—only later to focus on specifically human aspects of it.

Two meanings merge in the term *mortal:* that the creature so called *can* die, is exposed to the constant possibility of death; and that, eventually, it *must* die, is destined for the ultimate necessity of death. In the continual possibility I place the burden, in the ultimate necessity I place the blessing

---

This article appeared in Hastings Center Report 22 *(January/February 1992): 34–40.*

of mortality. The second of these propositions may sound strange. Let me argue both.

I begin with mortality as the ever-present *potential* of death for everything alive, concurrent with the life process itself. This "potential" means more than the truism of being destructible, which holds for every composite material structure, dead or alive. With sufficient force, even the diamond can be crushed, and everything alive can be killed by any number of outside causes, prominent among them other life. However, the inmost relation of life to possible death goes deeper than that: it resides in the organic constitution as such, in its very mode of being. I have to spell out this mode to lay bare the roots of mortality in life itself. To this end I now beg you to keep me company on a stretch of ontological inquiry. By this, we philosophers mean an inquiry into the manner of being characteristic of entities of one kind or another—in our case, of the kind called "organism," as this is the sole physical form in which, to our knowledge, life exists. What is the way of being of an organism?

Our opening observation is that organisms are entities whose being is their own doing. That is to say that they exist only in virtue of what they do. And this in the radical sense that the being they earn from this doing is not a possession they then own in separation from the activity by which it was generated, but is the continuation of that very activity itself, made possible by what it has just performed. Thus to say that the being of organisms is their own doing is also to say that doing what they do *is* their being itself; being for them consists in doing what they have to do in order to go on to be. It follows directly that to cease doing it means ceasing to be; and since the requisite doing depends not on themselves alone, but also on the compliance of an environment that can either be granted or denied, the peril of cessation is with the organism from the beginning. Here we have the basic link of life with death, the ground of mortality in its very constitution.

What we have couched so far in the abstract terms of being and doing, the language of ontology, can now be called by its familiar name: *metabolism.* This concretely is the "doing" referred to in our opening remark about entities whose being is their own doing, and metabolism can well serve as the defining property of life: all living things have it, no nonliving thing has it. What it denotes is this: to exist by way of exchanging matter with the environment, transiently incorporate it, use it, excrete it again. The German *Stoffwechsel* expresses it nicely. Let us realize how unusual, nay unique a trait this is in the vast world of matter.

How does an ordinary physical thing—a proton, a molecule, a stone, a planet—endure? Well, just by being there. Its being now is the sufficient reason for its also being later, if perhaps in a different place. This is so because of the constancy of matter, one of the prime laws of nature ever since, soon after the Big Bang, the exploding chaos solidified into discrete, highly durable units. In the universe hence evolving, the single stubborn particle, say a proton, is simply and fixedly what it is, identical with itself over time, and with no need to maintain that identity by anything it does. Its conservation is mere remaining, not a reassertion of being from moment to moment. It is there once and for all. Saying, then, of a composite, macroscopic body—this stone in our collection— that it is the same as yesterday amounts to saying that it still consists of the same elementary parts as before.

Now by this criterion a living organism would have no identity over time. Repeated inspections would find it to consist less and less of the initial components, more and more of new ones of the same kind that have taken their place, until the two compared states have perhaps no components in common anymore. Yet no biologist would take this to mean that he is not dealing with the same organic individual. On the contrary, he would consider any other finding incompatible with the sameness of a living entity *qua* living: if it showed the same inventory of parts after a long enough interval, he would conclude that the body in question has soon after the earlier inspection ceased to live and is in that decisive respect no longer "the same," that is, no longer a "creature," but a corpse. Thus we are faced with the ontological fact of an identity totally different from inert physical identity, yet grounded in transactions among items of that simple identity. We have to ponder this highly intriguing fact.

It presents something of a paradox. On the one hand, the living body is a composite of matter, and at any one time its reality totally coincides with its contemporary stuff—that is, with one definite manifold of individual components. On the other hand, it is not identical with this or any such simultaneous total, as this is forever vanishing downstream in the flow of exchange; in this respect it is different from its stuff and not the sum of it. We have thus the case of a substantial entity enjoying a sort of *freedom* with respect to its own substance, an independence from that same matter of which it nonetheless wholly consists. However, though independent of the sameness of this matter, it is dependent on the exchange of it, on its progressing permanently and sufficiently, and there is no freedom in this. Thus the exercise of the freedom which the living thing enjoys is rather a stern *necessity*. This necessity we call "need," which has a place only where existence is unassured and its own continual task.

With the term *need* we have come upon a property of organic being unique to life and unknown to all the rest of reality. The atom is self-sufficient and would continue to exist if all the world around it were annihilated. By contrast, nonautarky is of the very essence of organism.

Its power to use the world, this unique prerogative of life, has its precise reverse in the necessity of having to use it, on pain of ceasing to be. The dependence here in force is the cost incurred by primeval substance in venturing upon the career of organic—that is, self-constituting—identity instead of merely inert persistence. Thus the need is with it from the beginning and marks the existence gained in this way as a hovering between being and not-being. The "not" lies always in wait and must be averted ever anew. Life, in other words, carries death within itself.

Yet if it is true that with metabolizing existence not-being made its appearance in the world as an alternative embodied in the existence itself, it is equally true that thereby to be first assumes an emphatic sense: intrinsically qualified by the threat of its negative it must affirm itself, and existence affirmed is existence as a *concern*. Being has become a task rather than a given state, a possibility ever to be realized anew in opposition to its ever-present contrary, not-being, which inevitably will engulf it in the end.

With the hint at inevitability, we are ahead of our story. As told so far in these musings of mine, we can sum up the inherent dialectics of life somewhat like this: committed to itself, put at the mercy of its own performance, life must depend on conditions over which it has no control and which may deny themselves at any time. Thus dependent on favor or disfavor of outer reality, life is exposed to the world from which it has set itself off and by means of which it must yet maintain itself. Emancipated from the identity with matter, life is yet in need of it; free, yet under the whip of necessity; separate, yet in indispensable contact; seeking contact, yet in danger of being destroyed by it and threatened no less by its want—imperiled thus from both sides, importunity and aloofness of the world, and balanced on the narrow ridge between the two. In its process, which must not cease, liable to interference; in the straining of its temporality always facing the imminent no-more: thus does the living form carry on its separatist existence in matter—paradoxical, unstable, precarious, finite, and in intimate company with death. The fear of death with which the hazard of this existence is charged is a never-ending comment on the audacity of the original venture upon which substance embarked in turning organic.

But we may well ask at this point, Is it worth the candle? Why all the toil? Why leave the safe shore of self-sufficient permanence for the troubled waters of mortality in the first place? Why venture upon the anxious gamble of self-preservation at all? With the hindsight of billions of years and the present witness of our inwardness, which surely is part of the evidence, we are not without clues for a speculative guess. Let us dare it.

The basic clue is that life says yes to itself. By clinging to itself it declares that it values itself. But one clings only to what can be taken away. From the organism, which has being strictly on loan, it can be taken and will be unless from moment to moment reclaimed. Continued metabolism is such a reclaiming, which ever reasserts the value of Being against its lapsing into nothingness. Indeed to say yes, so it seems, requires the co-presence of the alternative to which to say no. Life has it in the sting of death that perpetually lies in wait, ever again to be staved off, and precisely the challenge of the no stirs and powers the yes. Are we then, perhaps, allowed to say that mortality is the narrow gate through which alone *value*—the addressee of a yes—could enter the otherwise indifferent universe? That the same crack in the massive unconcern of matter that gave value an opening had also to let in the fear of losing it? We shall presently have to say something about the kind of value purchased at this cost. First allow me one further step in this speculation that roams beyond proof. Is it too bold to conjecture that in the cosmically rare opportunity of organismic existence, when at last it was offered on this planet by lucky circumstance, the secret essence of Being, locked in matter, seized the long-awaited chance to affirm itself and in doing so to make itself more and more worth affirming? The fact and course of evolution point that way. Then organisms would be the manner in which universal Being says yes to itself. We have learned that it can do so only by also daring the risk of not-being, with whose possibility it is now paired. Only in confrontation with ever-possible not-being could being come to feel itself, affirm itself, make itself its own purpose. Through negated not-being, "to be" turns into a constant choosing of itself. Thus it is only an apparent paradox that it should be death and holding it off by acts of self-preservation which set the seal upon the self-affirmation of Being.

If this is the burden life was saddled with from the start, what then is its reward? What *is* the value paid for with the coin of mortality? *What* in the outcome was there to affirm? We alluded to it when we said that, in organisms, Being came to "feel" itself. Feeling is the prime condition for anything to be possibly worthwhile. It can be so only as the datum for a feeling and as the feeling of this datum. The presence of feeling as such, whatever its content or mode, is infinitely superior to the total absence of it. Thus the capacity for feeling, which arose in organisms, is the mother-value of all values. With its arising in organic evolution, reality gained a dimension it lacked in the form of bare matter and which also thereafter remains confined to this narrow foothold in biological entities: the dimension of subjective inwardness. Perhaps aspired to since creation, such inwardness found its eventual cradle with the advent of metabolizing life. Where in its advance to higher forms that mysterious dimension actually opened we cannot know. I am inclined to suspect the infinitesimal beginning of it in the earliest self-sustaining and self-replicating cells—a germinal inwardness, the faintest glimmer of diffused subjectivity long before it concentrated in brains as its specialized organs. Be that as it may. Somewhere in the ascent of evolution, at the latest with the twin rise of perception and motility in animals, that invisible inner dimension burst forth into the bloom of ever more conscious, subjective life: inwardness externalizing itself in behavior and shared in communication.

The gain is double edged like every trait of life. Feeling lies open to pain as well as to pleasure, its keenness cutting both ways; lust has its match in anguish, desire in fear; purpose is either attained or thwarted, and the capacity for enjoying the one is the same as that for suffering from the other. In short, the gift of subjectivity only sharpens the yes-no polarity of all life, each side feeding on the strength of the other. Is it, in the balance, still a gain, vindicating the bitter burden of mortality to which the gift is tied, which it makes even more onerous to bear? This is a question of the kind that cannot be answered without an element of personal decision. As part of my pleading for a yes to it, I offer two comments.

The first is about the relation of means and ends in an organism's equipment for living. Biologists are wont to tell us (and, I think, with excellent reasons) that this or that organ or behavior pattern has been "selected" out of chance mutations for the *survival* advantage it bestowed on its possessors. Accordingly, the evolution of consciousness must bespeak its utility in the struggle for survival. Survival as such would be the end, consciousness an incremental means thereto. But that implies its having causal power over behavior, and such a power is—by the canons of natural science—attributable only to the physical events in the brain, not to the subjective phenomena accompanying them; and those brain events in turn must be wholly the consequence of physical antecedents. Causes must be as objective throughout as the effects—so decrees a materialist axiom. In terms of causality, therefore, a nonconscious robot mechanism with the same behavioral output could do as well and would have sufficed for natural selection. In other words, evolutionary mechanics, as understood by its proponents, explains the evolution of brains, but not of consciousness. Nature, then, is credited with throwing in a redundancy, the free gift of consciousness, now debunked as useless and, moreover, as deceptive in its causal pretense.

There is but one escape here from absurdity, and that is to trust the self-testimony of our subjective inwardness, namely, that it is (to a degree) causally effective in governing our behavior, therefore indeed eligible for natural selection as one more *means* of survival. But with the same act of trust, we have also endorsed its inherent claim that, beyond all instrumentality, it is for its own sake and an end in itself. There is a lesson in this about the general relation of means and ends in organic existence.

To secure survival is indeed one end of organic endowment, but when we ask, Survival of what? we must often count the endowment itself among the intrinsic goods it helps to preserve. Faculties of the psychological order are the most telling cases in point. Such "means" of survival as perception and emotion, understanding and will, command of limbs and discrimination of goals are never to be judged as means merely, but also as qualities of the life to be preserved and therefore as aspects of the end. It is the subtle logic of life that it employs means which modify the end and themselves become part of it. The feeling animal strives to preserve itself as a feeling, not just metabolizing creature, that is, it strives to continue the very activity of feeling; the perceiving animal strives to preserve itself as a perceiving creature . . . and so on. Even the sickest of us, if he wants to live on at all, wants to do so thinking and sensing, not merely digesting. Without these subject faculties that emerged in animals, there would be much less to preserve, and this less of what is to be preserved is the same as the less wherewith it is preserved. The self-rewarding experience of the means in action makes the preservation they promote more worthwhile. Whatever the changing contents, whatever the tested utility, awareness as such proclaims its own supreme worth.

But must we assent? This question leads over to my second comment. What if the sum of suffering in the living world forever exceeds the sum of enjoyment? What if, especially in the human world, the sum of misery is so much greater than that of happiness as the record of the ages seems to suggest? I am inclined in this matter to side with the verdict of the pessimists. Most probably the balance sheet, if we could really assemble it, would look bleak. But would that be a valid ground to deny the worth of awareness, that things would be better if it were not in the world at all? There one should listen to the voice of its victims, those least bribed by the tasting of pleasures. The votes of the lucky may be ignored, but those of the suffering unlucky count double in weight and authority. And there we find that almost no amount of misery dims the yes to sentient selfhood. Greatest suffering still clings to it, rarely is the road of suicide taken, never is there a "survival" without feeling wished for. The very record of suffering mankind teaches us that the partisanship of inwardness for itself invincibly withstands the balancing of pains and pleasures and rebuffs our judging it by this standard.

More important still, something in us protests against basing a metaphysical judgment on hedonistic grounds. The presence of any worthwhileness in the universe at all—and we have seen that this is bound to feeling—immeasurably outweighs any cost of suffering it exacts. Since it is in the last resort mortality which levies that cost, but is equally the condition for such to exist that can pay it, and existence of this sort is the sole seat of meaning in the world, the burden of mortality laid on all of us is heavy and meaningful at once.

Up to this point we have been dealing with mortality as the *possibility* of death lurking in all life at all times and countered continually by acts of self-preservation. Ultimate *certainty* of death, intrinsic limitation of individual life spans, is a different matter, and that is the meaning we have mostly in mind when we speak of our own "mortality." We are then speaking of death as the terminal point on the long road of *aging*. That word has so far not appeared in our discourse; and indeed, familiar and seemingly self-evident as the phenomenon is to us, aging—that is, internal organic attrition by the life process itself—is not a universal biological trait, not even in quite complex organisms. It is surprising to learn how many and how diverse species are nonsenescent, for example, in groups such as bony fishes, sea anemones, and bivalve mollusks. Attrition there is left entirely to extrinsic causes of death, which suffice to balance population numbers in the interplay with reproduction and amount to certainty of death for each individual within a time frame typical for the species. However, throughout the higher biological orders, aging at a species-determined rate that ends in dying is the pervasive rule (without exception, for example, in warm-blooded animals) and it must have some adaptive benefits, else evolution would not have let it arise. What these benefits are is a subject of speculation among biologists. On principle, they may derive either directly from the trait itself or from some other traits to which senescence is linked as their necessary price. We will not join in this debate, but rather say a word about the general evolutionary aspect of death and dying in their remorseless actuality, whether from extrinsic or intrinsic necessity. The term *evolution* itself already reveals the *creative* role of individual finitude, which has decreed that whatever lives *must* also die. For what else is natural selection with its survival premium, this main engine of evolution, than the use of death for the promotion of novelty, for the favoring of diversity, and for the singling out of higher forms of life with the blossoming forth of subjectivity? At work to this effect—so we saw—is a mixture of death by extrinsic causes (foremost the merciless feeding of life on life) and the organically programmed dying of parent generations to make room for their offspring. With the advent and ascent of man, the latter kind of mortality, inbuilt numbering of our days, gains increasing importance in incidence and significance, and from here on our discourse will keep to the human context alone and consider in what sense mortality may be a blessing specifically for our own kind.

Reaching ripe old age and dying from mere attrition of the body is, as a common phenomenon, very much an artifact. In the state of nature, so Hobbes put it, human life is nasty, brutish, and short. Civil society, according to him, was founded mainly for protection from violent—and that means premature—death. This is surely too narrow a view of the motives, but one effect of civilization, this comprehensive artifact of human intelligence, is undeniably the progressive taming of the extraneous causes of death for humans. It has also mightily enhanced the powers of their mutual destruction. But the net result is that at least in technologically advanced societies, more and more people reach the natural limit of life. Scientific medicine has a major share in this result, and it is beginning to try to push back that limit itself. At any rate the theoretical prospect seems no longer precluded. This makes it tempting to hitch the further pursuit of our theme to the question of whether it is right to combat not merely premature death but death as such, that is, whether lengthening life indefinitely is a legitimate goal of medicine. We will discuss this on two planes: that of the common good of mankind and that of the individual good for the self.

The common good of mankind is tied to civilization, and this with all its feats and faults would not have come about and not keep moving without the ever-repeated turnover of generations. Here we have come to the point where we can no longer postpone complementing the consideration of death with that of birth, its essential counterpart, to which we have paid no attention so far. It was of course tacitly included in our consideration of individual mortality as a prerequisite of biological evolution. In the incomparably faster, nonbiological evolution the human species enacts within its biological identity through the trans-generational handing-on and accumulation of learning, the interplay of death and birth assumes a very new and profound relevance. "Natality" (to use a coinage of my long-departed friend Hannah Arendt) is as essential an attribute of the human condition as is mortality. It denotes the fact that we all have been born, which means that each of us had a beginning when others already had long been there, and this ensures that there will always be such that see the world for the first time, see things with new eyes, wonder where others are dulled by habit, start out from where they had arrived. Youth with its fumbling and follies, its eagerness and questioning is the eternal hope of mankind. Without its constant arrival, the wellspring of novelty would dry up, for those grown older have found their answers and gotten set in their ways. The ever-renewed beginning, which can only be had at the price of ever-repeated ending, is mankind's safeguard against lapsing into boredom and routine, its chance of retaining the spontaneity of life. There is also this bonus of "natality" that every one of the newcomers is different and unique. Such is the working of sexual reproduction that none of its outcome is, in genetic makeup, the replica of any before and none will ever be replicated thereafter. (This is one reason humans should never be "cloned.")

Now obviously, just as mortality finds its compensation in natality, conversely natality gets its scope from mortality: dying of the old makes place for the young. This rule becomes more stringent as our numbers push or already exceed the limits of environmental tolerance. The specter of overpopulation casts its pall over the access of new life anyway; and the proportion of youth must shrink in a population forced to become static but increasing its average age by the successful fight against premature death. Should we then try to lengthen life further by tinkering with and outwitting the naturally ordained, biological timing of our mortality—thus further narrowing the space of youth in our aging society? I think the common good of mankind bids us answer no. The question was rather academic, for no serious prospect is in sight for breaking the existing barrier. But the dream is taking form in our technological intoxication. The real point of our reflection was the linkage of mortality with creativity in human history. Whoever, therefore, relishes the cultural harvest of the ages in any of its many facets and does not wish to be without it, and most surely the praiser and advocate of progress, should see in mortality a blessing and not a curse.

However, the good of mankind and the good of the individual are not necessarily the same, and someone might say: Granted that mortality is good for mankind as a whole and I am grateful for its bounty paid for by others, for myself I still ardently wish I were exempt from it and could go on interminably to enjoy its fruit—past, present, and future. Of course (so we might imagine him to add) this must be an exception, but why not have a select few equally favored for companions in immortality? For *interminably* you are free to substitute "twice or triple the normal maximum" and qualify *immortality* accordingly.

Would that wish at least stand the test of imagined fulfillment? I know of one attempt to tackle that question: Jonathan Swift's harrowing description in *Gulliver's Travels* of the Struldbrugs or "Immortals," who "sometimes, though very rarely" happen to be born in the kingdom of Luggnagg. When first hearing of them, Gulliver is enraptured by the thought of their good fortune and that of a society harboring such fonts of experience and wisdom. But he learns that theirs is a miserable lot, universally pitied and despised; their unending lives turn into ever more worthless burdens to them and the mortals around them; even the company of their own kind becomes intolerable, so that, for example, marriages are dissolved at a certain age, "for the law thinks . . . that those who are condemned without any fault of their own to a perpetual continuance in the world should not have their misery doubled by the load of a wife"—or a husband, I hasten to add. And so on—one should read Gulliver's vivid description.

For the purposes of our question, Swift's fantasy has one flaw: his immortals are denied death but not spared the infirmities of old age and the indignities of senility—which of course heavily pre-judges the outcome of his thought experiment. Our test of imagined fulfillment must assume that it is not the gift of miraculous chance but of scientific control over the natural causes of death and, therefore, over the aging processes that lead to it, so that the life thus lengthened also retains its bodily vigor. Would the indefinite lengthening then be desirable for the subjects themselves? Let us waive such objections as the resentment of the many against the exception of the few, however obtained, and the ignobility of the wish for it, the breach of solidarity with the common mortal lot. Let us judge on purely egotistical grounds. One of Gulliver's descriptions gives us a valuable hint: "They have no remembrance of anything but of what they learned and observed in their youth and middle age." This touches a point independent of senile decrepitude: we are finite beings and even if our vital functions continued unimpaired, there are limits to what our brains can store and keep adding to. It is the mental side of our being that sooner or later must call a halt even if the magicians of biotechnology invent tricks for keeping the body machine going indefinitely. Old age, in humans, means a long past, which the *mind* must accommodate in its present as the substratum of personal identity. The past in us grows all the time, with its load of knowledge and opinion and emotions and choices and acquired aptitudes and habits and, of course, things upon things remembered or somehow recorded even if forgotten. There is a finite space for all this, and those magicians would also periodically have to clear the mind (like a computer memory) of its old contents to make place for the new.

These are weird fantasies—we use them merely to bring out the mental side of the question concerning mortality and the individual good. The simple truth of our finiteness is that we could, by whatever means, go on interminably only at the price of either *losing* the past and therewith our real identity, or living *only* in the past and therefore without a real present. We cannot seriously wish either and thus not a physical enduring at that price. It would leave us stranded in a world we no longer understand even as spectators, walking anachronisms who have outlived themselves. It is a changing world because of the newcomers who keep arriving and who leave us behind. Trying to keep pace with them is doomed to inglorious failure, especially as the pace has quickened so much. Growing older, we get our warnings, no matter in what physical shape we are. To take, just for once, my own example: a native sensibility for visual and poetic art persists, not much dulled, in my old age; I can still be moved by the works I have learned to love and have grown old with. But the art of our own time is alien to me, I don't understand its language, and in that respect I feel already a stranger in the world. The prospect of unendingly becoming one evermore and in every respect would be frightening, and the certainty that prevents it is reassuring. So we do not need the horror fiction of the wretched Struldbrugs to make us reject the desire for earthly immortality: not even the fountains of youth, which biotechnology may have to offer one day to circumvent the physical penalties of it, can justify the goal of extorting from nature more than its original allowance to our species for the length of our days. On this point, then, the private good does concur with the public good. Herewith I rest my case for mortality as a blessing.

Mind you, this side of it, which is perceived only by thought and not felt in experience, detracts nothing from the burden that the ever present contingency of death lays on all flesh. Also, what we have said about "blessing" for the individual person is true only after a completed life, in the fullness of time. This is a premise far from being realized as a rule, and in all too many populations with a low life expectancy it is the rare exception. It is a duty of civilization to combat premature death among humankind worldwide and in all its causes—hunger, diseases, war, and so on. As to our mortal condition as such, our understanding can have no quarrel about it with creation unless life itself is denied. As to each of us, the knowledge that we are here but briefly and a nonnegotiable limit is set to our expected time may even be necessary as the incentive to number our days and make them count.

10 Death and Dignity: A Case of Individualized Decision Making

Timothy E. Quill, M.D.

Timothy E. Quill, M.D. is in practice at the Genessee Hospital in Rochester, NY.

Diane was feeling tired and had a rash. A common scenario, though there was something subliminally worrisome that prompted me to check her blood count. Her hematocrit was 22, and the white-cell count was 4.3 with some metamyelocytes and unusual white cells. I wanted it to be viral, trying to deny what was staring me in the face. Perhaps in a repeated count it would disappear. I called Diane and told her it might be more serious than I had initially thought—that the test needed to be repeated and that if she felt worse, we might have to move quickly. When she pressed for the possibilities, I reluctantly opened the door to leukemia. Hearing the word seemed to make it exist. "Oh, shit!" she said. "Don't tell me that." Oh, shit! I thought, I wish I didn't have to.

Diane was no ordinary person (although no one I have ever come to know has been really ordinary). She was raised in an alcoholic family and had felt alone for much of her life. She had vaginal cancer as a young woman. Through much of her adult life, she had struggled with depression and her own alcoholism. I had come to know, respect, and admire her over the previous eight years as she confronted these problems and gradually overcame them. She was an incredibly clear, at times brutally honest, thinker and communicator. As she took control of her life, she developed a strong sense of independence and confidence. In the previous 3½ years, her hard work had paid off. She was completely abstinent from alcohol, she had established much deeper connections with her husband, college-age son, and several friends, and her business and her

---

This article first appeared in The New England Journal of Medicine *324 (7 March 1991): 691–694.*

artistic work were blossoming. She felt she was really living fully for the first time.

Not surprisingly, the repeated blood count was abnormal, and detailed examination of the peripheral-blood smear showed myelocytes. I advised her to come into the hospital, explaining that we needed to do a bone marrow biopsy and make some decisions relatively rapidly. She came to the hospital knowing what we would find. She was terrified, angry, and sad. Although we knew the odds, we both clung to the thread of possibility that it might be something else.

The bone marrow confirmed the worst: acute myelomonocytic leukemia. In the face of this tragedy, we looked for signs of hope. This is an area of medicine in which technological intervention has been successful, with cures 25 percent of the time—long-term cures. As I probed the costs of these cures, I heard about induction chemotherapy (three weeks in the hospital, prolonged neutropenia, probable infectious complications, and hair loss; 75 percent of patients respond, 25 percent do not). For the survivors, this is followed by consolidation chemotherapy (with similar side effects; another 25 percent die, for a net survival of 50 percent). Those still alive, to have a reasonable chance of long-term survival, then need bone marrow transplantation (hospitalization for two months and whole-body irradiation, with complete killing of the bone marrow, infectious complications, and the possibility for graft-versus-host disease—with a survival of approximately 50 percent, or 25 percent of the original group). Though hematologists may argue over the exact percentages, they don't argue about the outcome of no treatment—certain death in days, weeks, or at most a few months.

Believing that delay was dangerous, our oncologist broke the news to Diane and began making plans to insert a Hickman catheter and begin induction chemotherapy that afternoon. When I saw her shortly thereafter, she was enraged at his presumption that she would want treatment, and devastated by the finality of the diagnosis. All she wanted to do was go home and be with her family. She had no further questions about treatment and in fact had decided that she wanted none. Together we lamented her tragedy and the unfairness of life. Before she left, I felt the need to be sure that she and her husband understood that there was some risk in delay, that the problem was not going to go away, and that we needed to keep considering the options over the next several days. We agreed to meet in two days.

She returned in two days with her husband and son. They had talked extensively about the problem and the options. She remained very clear about her wish not to undergo chemotherapy and to live whatever time she had left outside the hospital. As we explored her thinking further, it became clear that she was convinced she would die during the period of treatment and would suffer unspeakably in the process (from hospitalization, from lack of control over her body, from the side effects of chemotherapy, and from pain and anguish). Although I could offer support and my best effort to minimize her suffering if she chose treatment, there was no way I could say any of this would not occur. In fact, the last four patients with acute leukemia at our hospital had died very painful deaths in the hospital during various stages of treatment (a fact I did not share with her). Her family wished she would choose treatment but sadly accepted her decision. She articulated very clearly that it was she who would be experiencing all the side effects of treatment and that odds of 25 percent were not good enough for her to undergo so toxic a course of therapy, given her expectations of chemotherapy and hospitalization and the absence of a closely matched bone marrow donor. I had her repeat her understanding of the treatment, the odds, and what to expect if there were no treatment. I clarified a few misunderstandings, but she had a remarkable grasp of the options and implications.

I have been a longtime advocate of active, informed patient choice of treatment or nontreatment, and of a patient's right to die with as much control and dignity as possible. Yet there was something about her giving up a 25 percent chance of long-term survival in favor of almost certain death that disturbed me. I had seen Diane fight and use her considerable inner resources to overcome alcoholism and depression, and I half expected her to change her mind over the next week. Since the window of time in which effective treatment can be initiated is rather narrow, we met several times that week. We obtained a second hematology consultation and talked at length about the meaning and implications of treatment and nontreatment. She talked to a psychologist she had seen in the past. I gradually understood the decision from her perspective and became convinced that it was the right decision for her. We arranged for home hospice care (although at that time Diane felt reasonably well, was active, and looked healthy), left the door open for her to change her mind, and tried to anticipate how to keep her comfortable in the time she had left.

Just as I was adjusting to her decision, she opened up another area that would stretch me profoundly. It was extraordinarily important to Diane to maintain control of herself and her own dignity during the time remaining to her. When this was no longer possible, she clearly wanted to die. As a former director of a hospice program, I know how to use pain medicines to keep patients comfortable and lessen suffering. I explained the philosophy of comfort care, which I strongly believe in. Although Diane understood and appreciated this, she had known of people lingering in what was called relative comfort, and she wanted no part of it.

When the time came, she wanted to take her life in the least painful way possible. Knowing of her desire for independence and her decision to stay in control, I thought this request made perfect sense. I acknowledged and explored this wish but also thought that it was out of the realm of currently accepted medical practice and that it was more than I could offer or promise. In our discussion, it became clear that preoccupation with her fear of a lingering death would interfere with Diane's getting the most out of the time she had left until she found a safe way to ensure her death. I feared the effects of a violent death on her family, the consequences of an ineffective suicide that would leave her lingering in precisely the state she dreaded so much, and the possibility that a family member would be forced to assist her, with all the legal and personal repercussions that would follow. She discussed this at length with her family. They believed that they should respect her choice. With this in mind, I told Diane that information was available from the Hemlock Society that might be helpful to her.

A week later she phoned me with a request for barbiturates for sleep. Since I knew that this was an essential ingredient in a Hemlock Society suicide, I asked her to come to the office to talk things over. She was more than willing to protect me by participating in a superficial conversation about her insomnia, but it was important to me to know how she planned to use the drugs and to be sure that she was not in despair or overwhelmed in a way that might color her judgment. In our discussion, it was apparent that she was having trouble sleeping, but it was also evident that the security of having enough barbiturates available to commit suicide when and if the time came would leave her secure enough to live fully and concentrate on the present. It was clear that she was not despondent and that in fact she was making deep, personal connections with her family and close friends. I made sure that she knew how to use the barbiturates for sleep, and also that she knew the amount needed to commit suicide. We agreed to meet regularly, and she promised to meet with me before taking her life, to ensure that all other avenues had been exhausted. I wrote the prescription with an uneasy feeling about the boundaries I was exploring—spiritual, legal, professional, and personal. Yet I also felt strongly that I was setting her free to get the most out of the time she had left, and to maintain dignity and control on her own terms until her death.

The next several months were very intense and important for Diane. Her son stayed home from college, and they were able to be with one another and say much that had not been said earlier. Her husband did his work at home so that he and Diane could spend more time together. She spent time with her closest friends. I had her come into the hospital for a conference with our residents, at which she illustrated in a most profound and personal way the importance of informed decision making, the right to refuse treatment, and the extraordinarily personal effects of illness and interaction with the medical system. There were emotional and physical hardships as well. She had periods of intense sadness and anger. Several times she became very weak, but she received transfusions as an outpatient and responded with marked improvement of symptoms. She had two serious infections that responded surprisingly well to empirical courses of oral antibiotics. After three tumultuous months, there were two weeks of relative calm and well-being, and fantasies of a miracle began to surface.

Unfortunately, we had no miracle. Bone pain, weakness, fatigue, and fevers began to dominate her life. Although the hospice workers, family members, and I tried our best to minimize the suffering and promote comfort, it was clear that the end was approaching. Diane's immediate future held what she feared the most—increasing discomfort, dependence, and hard choices between pain and sedation. She called up her closest friends and asked them to come over to say goodbye, telling them that she would be leaving soon. As we had agreed, she let me know as well. When we met, it was clear that she knew what she was doing, that she was sad and frightened to be leaving, but that she would be even more terrified to stay and suffer. In our tearful goodbye, she promised a reunion in the future at her favorite spot on the edge of Lake Geneva, with dragons swimming in the sunset.

Two days later her husband called to say that Diane had died. She had said her final goodbyes to her husband and son that morning, and asked them to leave her alone for an hour. After an hour, which must have seemed an eternity, they found her on the couch, lying very still and covered by her favorite shawl. There was no sign of struggle. She seemed to be at peace. They called me for advice about how to proceed. When I arrived at their house, Diane indeed seemed peaceful. Her husband and son were quiet. We talked about what a remarkable person she had been. They seemed to have no doubts about the course she had chosen or about their cooperation, although the unfairness of her illness and the finality of her death were overwhelming to us all.

I called the medical examiner to inform him that a hospice patient had died. When asked about the cause of death, I said, "acute leukemia." He said that was fine and that we should call a funeral director. Although acute leukemia was the truth, it was not the whole story. Yet any mention of suicide would have given rise to a police investigation and probably brought the arrival of an ambulance crew for resuscitation. Diane would have become a "coroner's case," and the decision to perform an autopsy would have been made at the discretion of the medical examiner. The family or I could have been subject to criminal prosecution, and I to professional review, for our roles in support of Diane's choices. Although I truly believe that the family and I gave her the best care possible, allowing her to define her limits and directions as much as possible, I am not sure the law, society, or the medical profession would agree. So I said "acute leukemia" to protect all of us, to protect Diane from an invasion into her past and her body, and to continue to shield society from the knowledge of the degree of suffering that people often undergo in the process of dying. Suffering can be lessened to some extent, but in no way eliminated or made benign, by the careful intervention of a competent, caring physician, given current social constraints.

Diane taught me about the range of help I can provide if I know people well and if I allow them to say what they really want. She taught me about life, death, and honesty and about taking charge and facing tragedy squarely when it strikes. She taught me that I can take small risks for people that I really know and care about. Although I did not assist in her suicide directly, I helped indirectly to make it possible, successful, and relatively painless. Although I know we have measures to help control pain and lessen suffering, to think that people do not suffer in the process of dying is an illusion. Prolonged dying can occasionally be peaceful, but more often the role of the physician and family is limited to lessening but not eliminating severe suffering.

I wonder how many families and physicians secretly help patients over the edge into death in the face of such severe suffering. I wonder how many severely ill or dying patients secretly take their lives, dying alone in despair. I wonder whether the image of Diane's final aloneness will persist in the minds of her family, or if they will remember more the intense, meaningful months they had together before she died. I wonder whether Diane struggled in that last hour, and whether the Hemlock Society's way of death by suicide is the most benign. I wonder why Diane, who gave so much to so many of us, had to be alone for the last hour of her life. I wonder whether I will see Diane again, on the shore of Lake Geneva at sunset, with dragons swimming on the horizon.

11 The PVS Patient and the Forgoing/Withdrawing of Medical Nutrition and Hydration

THOMAS A. SHANNON AND JAMES J. WALTER

Thomas A. Shannon is Professor of Religious and Social Ethics at Worcester Polytechnic Institute in Worcester, Massachusetts. James J. Walter is Professor of Christian Ethics at Loyola University in Chicago, Illinois.

Over the last several decades modern medicine has progressed at a rate that has astonished even its practitioners. Developments in drugs, vaccines, and various technologies have given physicians an incredible amount of success over disease and morbidity, as well as allowing them to make dramatic interventions into the body to repair or replace a problematic system or organ. Yet there are limits we are coming to recognize slowly and only reluctantly. For even many of our best technologies are only halfway technologies, i.e. the technology or intervention compensates for a function but cannot cure the underlying pathology or correct the damaged organ. The respirator is probably the most frequently encountered example of this phenomenon.

Another intervention is our capacity to provide nutrition and hydration to those in a persistent vegetative state (PVS). For long-term feeding of such individuals, a gastrostomy tube is inserted directly into the stomach and the liquid protein diet is delivered in a controlled fashion by a pump. If the individual is reasonably healthy and other reflexes are intact, the life expectancy may be several decades.[1] The PVS will not be cured, and the liquid protein serves to maintain the status quo. The question of how to treat these patients medically is now heavily debated nationally and internationally.

This article first appeared in Theological Studies *49 (December 1988):* 623–647.

In this essay we will examine the issue in several ways: (1) report on a survey of the U.S. hierarchy on bioethics committees in general and on forgoing or withdrawing nutrition and hydration in particular; (2) propose a structured argument which includes a reconceptualization of "quality of life" judgments; and (3) offer suggestions for the future conduct of this debate.

A Survey of the U.S. Hierarchy

General Analysis

In January of 1988 one of the authors (TAS) developed a brief questionnaire which sought information on two broad areas: (1) Were there diocesan bioethics committees and, if so, what was their composition etc.? (2) Did dioceses have specific policies on the issue of nutrition and hydration?[2]

One hundred and sixty-seven questionnaires were sent to the ordinaries of the U.S. dioceses. Seventy-eight ordinaries responded. Of these, 62 indicated that there was no diocesan bioethics committee; 16 indicated the existence of such a committee, and of these, 7 sent in detailed information which will be evaluated separately below.

Of those indicating no diocesan committee, 8 said that there were committees at local Catholic hospitals. Another 8 identified a specific individual within the diocese to whom the ordinary turned for assistance. Another 3 indicated the formation of such a committee, either on a diocesan or on a state level. One respondent stated there was an inoperative committee.

The survey then asked for a description of the membership of the committee, frequency of meetings, its role, whether or not there were guidelines, and how it functioned within the diocese. Committee size ranged from 9 to 23 members, which allowed for a good representation of professions, typically including hospital administrators, physicians, nurses, chaplains, ethicists, lawyers, and other theologians. Six of the committees met monthly, 2 bimonthly, and 1 as needed. Three respondents said their role was to set policy, 2 were to be advisory, and 1 was to be primarily educational. Two respondents had no guidelines, and 9 indicated some form of guidelines ranging from church teachings on medical issues to specific pronouncements of the hierarchy over the past decade.

Part 2 of the survey focused specifically on the moral evaluation of feeding tubes. Of the 78 answering, 17 made no comment on Part 2, 37 made some comments, and 22 respondents reported no cases of PVS patients in their diocese.

Nine respondents reported knowledge of PVS patients within their dioceses. Of those 9, 8 reported figures ranging from 1 to 4–5 per year, and 1 respondent indicated 10 cases in the past year. Eight committees were asked to consider cases and 11 had not been asked. Additionally, 4 respondents reported that they have specific guidelines they follow in such instances and 8 indicated that they have none.

The survey asked if the committee considered feeding tubes to be a medical technology. Six said yes, 4 said no, 8 gave no answer, and 1 said "it depends." The respondents were then asked if they considered the use of such feeding tubes to be routine care. Six said yes, 4 said no, 8 gave no answer, and 1 said "it depends." The next question was whether the removal of a feeding tube from a PVS patient was ordinary or extra-ordinary, or if they had no position. Four responded that the care was ordinary, 4 that it was extraordinary, 1 had no position, 9 gave no ans-wer, and 9 said "it depends." The final question asked whether removal was an act of involuntary euthanasia which is direct and forbidden, or indirect and permitted, or no position. Four responded that removal was direct, 5 that it was indirect, 2 had no position, 4 said "it depends," and 8 had no answer.

Before turning to an analysis of the seven detailed responses (Doc-uments A–G), we would like to make a few general observations about the data so far.

Given the seriousness of contemporary bioethical questions and their pervasiveness within society, it is surprising that so few dioceses have these committees or that so few local Catholic hospitals were indi-cated as having one. While neither seeking to bureaucratize all life nor to reject appropriate patient and family autonomy, nonetheless such com-mittees on a diocesan or state level serve a useful function, minimally by providing workshops or other resources to hospitals or other groups in the diocese. Of those that are in place, the composition is well repre-sented from a disciplinary perspective, and the committees meet with appropriate regularity. The committees appear to be accessible and, while maintaining patient privacy and confidentiality, there is some de-gree of openness in the committees.

Part 2 of the questionnaire provides more interesting data. Nine committees had cases brought to them; taken together, they had a mod-erately large number of cases, about 45. Six committees considered feed-ing tubes to be a medical technology and also routine care, 4 thought they were not a medical technology, and 1 did not consider them routine care. One committee was uncertain in each case. Yet of these committees, only 4 thought that feeding tubes were ordinary means whose removal constituted active euthanasia.

Four committees considered the technology ordinary and 4 judged it to be extraordinary. Four thought their removal to be direct euthanasia, while 5 considered it passive euthanasia. But even more interesting is that 9 committees thought that the placing of the technology into the ordinary/extraordinary categories depended on the individual circumstances of the case, and 8 thought the same thing about the determination of active or passive euthanasia. This suggests substantial ambiguity about the moral status of feeding technologies for PVS patients.

First, there is a difference over whether the procedure is a medical technology. If a technology, its moral evaluation fits conceptually more easily into the traditional format of ordinary/extraordinary means. If not, one might have to structure the argument differently. Most interesting are the differences in perception between whether the therapy is considered ordinary or extraordinary means, on the one hand, and whether its forgoing/withdrawal is morally evaluated as direct or indirect euthanasia, on the other. This interest is compounded when combined with the additional judgment—on the part of 9 and 8 respondents respectively—that such a determination "depends" on the circumstances. Such evaluations suggest room for various analyses of the problem and the possible moral acceptability of several resolutions.

Analysis of Specific Guidelines

Seven respondents sent more detailed information about committee make-up and the bylaws governing these committees. We will discuss each document in some detail, but, to maintain a promised confidentiality, we will simply refer to these documents as A–G.

Document A suggests that the primary locus for decision-making is the local hospital, with the diocesan or proposed state-wide committee serving as a resource. Yet part of the task of the proposed state-wide committee will be to develop guidelines for the local committee. At present, discussions are ongoing among committees but no consensus has been reached.

Document A affirms a presumption in favor of the use of feeding tubes but states that each case must be examined on its own merits. On the other hand, in very exceptional and extraordinary cases the withdrawal of feeding tubes might be passive and therefore permissible euthanasia. Thus, while removal of these tubes is exceptional, their removal is not prohibited. As the document states it, "each case must be considered on its own merits."

Document B represents the responses from three diocesan hospitals, since this diocese has no diocesan committee. B1 indicated that, while there have been cases, the committee did not meet as a committee on them. Rather, individual members of the committee served as resources to the medical staff and the families. This document stated that there is no consensus within the hospital about the issue, and so each case is to be examined on its own merits. The committee understands the practice as passive euthanasia and thus permissible, but also recognizes that there is no consistent position in the hospital.

We detect a problematic area in this document. B1 argues that feeding tubes might be withdrawn on the basis "that continued treatment *will result* in prolonged total dependence, persistent pain, or discomfort, or in a *persistent vegetative state*" (emphasis added). However, one wonders how the withdrawal of feeding tubes causes PVS. This technology is used to *support* patients in this condition; its administration does not *result* in PVS.

Document B2 states that their consultation has been on the placement of such technologies rather than on their withdrawal. Since it has no fixed policy, each case must be dealt with individually. Additionally, this committee considers tube feeding to be a medical technology and can become an extraordinary means in specific cases "which must be individually assessed and reassessed." The decisions are to be considered in "light of the effect of this nutrition and/or the burden to the patient which would be experienced." Again, these decisions cannot be based on a broad application of a policy but must be made according to "case-specific evaluations."

Document B3 comes from an ethicist at a medical center which has no committee. The respondent indicates that conversations about this problem show that many individuals at the medical center have concerns about the issue. Tube feeding, in this individual's judgment, is a technology, but its moral significance resides in "its function in the ongoing treatment of the patient." Thus the central issue is: Does the treatment contribute to restoring life and health, or does it prolong the patient's dying? "If the former, I think it [is] routinely required. If the latter, I judge it foregoable, permissibly not obligatorily foregoable. . . . Tube feeding in some cases is proportionate, hence required, in others, disproportionate, hence not required."

Two other relevant comments were made by this hospital ethicist. First, can feeding tubes ever be withdrawn? If one can

> admit that sometimes tubal feeding need not be *instituted,* then you are already describing conditions which might eventuate *within a case* which justify discontinuing tubal feeding. Put another way, a patient on tubal feeding might become the sort of patient you don't want to begin on tubal feeding. Since you need not start the intervention on the latter patient, why must you stay with it for the former one? (Emphasis in the original.)

Second, never starting or, once begun, removing the tubes is not an intending of death; rather, these decisions indicate that families "recognize and consent to (accept) a dying process which is judged irreversible and imminent."

The two common themes in these three documents from diocesan hospitals are a recognition of the ambiguities in the issue and a strong affirmation of a case-by-case evaluation. The more crucial moral elements are case-specific and determining the usefulness of the technology in relation to the condition of the patient. In addition, the suggestion to use the same criteria for not instituting the therapy and for withdrawing it is a helpful one and could aid in resolving several problems.

Document C is testimony to a state legislature on a natural-death act. At issue is the inclusion of a proviso for withholding feeding tubes in a living will. After a strong affirmation of the dignity, sanctity, and value of all human life, this document states: "The concern to affirm life, however, does not require the maintenance of physiological life by all means. It is recognized that aggressive overtreatment is as ethically unacceptable as is undertreatment. Both lack respect for the dignity and welfare of each person."

This testimony makes four points that lay out several issues very clearly.

1. A clear presumption in favor of life should be established. People who are able to eat, but only with assistance, cannot be discriminated against or be refused appropriate treatment.

2. The law should recognize the right of individuals to be allowed to die in circumstances where medical treatments, including nutrition and hydration, are ineffective or too burdensome for the patient.

3. The law must carefully define useless or ineffective treatment to clearly identify those treatments that offer no benefit of recovery or no relief of pain. The burdens associated with continued medical treatment should be defined in terms of the burdens that an individual experiences in pursuing the goals or ends of life and not defined by a level of invasiveness that may or may not be associated with forced feeding.

4. The clinical setting distinguishes between nutrition and hydration. Although both terms are used as though they are identical, it should be recognized that individuals may not require forced nutrition while still requiring hydration to alleviate

thirst, provide comfort, relieve pain, or provide an open channel for IV medications.

Document C is very nuanced and makes careful distinctions. In particular, the document emphasizes the distinction between basic nutrition
and hydration that requires time and effort on the part of medical personnel to feed the patient orally and the medical procedures that require
total parenteral nutritional support (TPN) or invasive medical techniques to provide nutrition and hydration, e.g. insertion of gastrostomy
tubes.

Document D comes from a research center whose writings and contributions were mentioned by many respondents as a source of guidance
for their committees. Two major points are made. First, forgoing or withdrawing foods and fluids on the rationale of the "assumption that life
itself can be useless or an excessive burden" is morally wrong because it
is euthanasia by omission. This carries out the "proposal, adopted by
choice, to end someone's life because that life itself is judged by others to
be valueless or excessively burdensome." The crucial issues here are the
moral intention of those who would withdraw the means of providing
nutrition, on the one hand, and the justification for the argument adduced to support such a withdrawal, on the other. For this document, the
intention is to end life, and the justification for so acting is that the life
is burdensome or useless. This constitutes direct euthanasia.

Second, the forgoing/withdrawing of medically provided nutrition
and hydration "do not necessarily carry out a proposal to end life."
When certain conditions are met—"if the means employed is judged
either useless or excessively burdensome"—one may forgo or withdraw
treatment.

> Nonetheless, *if it is really useless or excessively burdensome* to pro-
> vide someone with nutrition and hydration, then these means
> may rightly be withheld or withdrawn, *provided* that this omis-
> sion does not carry out a proposal to end the person's life, but
> rather is chosen to avoid the useless effort or the excessive bur-
> den of continuing to provide the food and fluids. (Emphasis in
> the original.)

Two applications follow. If death is imminent, nutrition may become
useless and burdensome, whether administered by tube or otherwise.
On the other hand, if the patients are not dying, feeding provides a great
benefit: "the preservation of their lives and the prevention of their death
through malnutrition and dehydration." Yet even in this instance this
treatment could become useless or futile: "(a) if the person in question is

imminently dying, so that any effort to sustain life is futile, or (b) the person is no longer able to assimilate the nourishment or fluids thus provided."

On the basis of this analysis, Document D concludes:

> We thus conclude that, in the ordinary circumstances of life in our society today, it is not morally right, nor ought it to be legally permissible, to withhold or withdraw nutrition and hydration provided by artificial means to the permanently unconscious or other categories of seriously debilitated but nonterminal persons. Food and fluids are universally needed for the preservation of life, and can generally be provided without the burdens and expense of more aggressive means of supporting life.

This document makes a strong argument in favor of such feeding based on the value of human life, the fact that such feeding can provide benefits to the patient and is not generally burdensome, and that the withdrawal of such technology many times includes the intention to end a person's life. Only when the individual is actually dying and/or cannot assimilate nourishment could the feeding be considered an extraordinary means.

Document E represents an advisory opinion of an archdiocese. This opinion bases its position on Pius XII's teaching on ordinary and extraordinary means, the *Declaration on Euthanasia* of the Congregation for the Doctrine of the Faith, and documents from the Committee for Pro-Life Activities of the National Conference of Catholic Bishops. Document E uses the standards of reasonable hope of success and a determination of excessive burdens as the criteria for decision-making. In addition, it recognizes and accepts the presumption of the use of medically providing nutrition and hydration for individuals.

The advisory opinion makes two statements of importance. The first concerns the decision to forgo or withdraw.

> It can hardly be denied that in certain circumstances artificial hydration and nutrition can be just as burdensome and useless as other means and under these circumstances would not be obligatory. A Catholic in good conscience can come to the conclusion that in a particular set of circumstances such treatment need not be initiated or continued, because it holds no hope that it will be successful in prolonging life or is unduly burdensome for oneself or another.

The second point concerns the intention involved in ending treatment. Document E argues that "even though the omission may shorten life, the intention is not to bring on death but to spare the patient a very burdensome treatment." These actions could constitute direct euthanasia if the intention is to end the life; but if omitted because they are too burdensome or useless in preserving life, "they do not constitute killing any more than any other such omission."

Document E uses the categories of ordinary and extraordinary means and then draws the conclusions that a decision to forgo or withdraw nutrition can be made in good conscience and that people should not be prevented from doing what is morally permissible. While the document does not encourage forgoing or withdrawal, neither does it prohibit such actions.

Document F supports the removal of nutrition and hydration within the context of the Catholic moral tradition that permits withdrawal of all medical technologies either on the basis that a patient has entered the dying phase or that the technologies are nonbeneficial or burdensome. These evaluations are moral as well as medical: "not what will the treatment do . . . , but will the treatment promote human activities and values."

> Merely maintaining biological life is not evaluated as being in and of itself humanly beneficial. Life is something more than biological existence. Life is a conditional value which couples biological existence with social, spiritual and human activities such as loving, praying, remembering, forgiving and experiencing. Life is all these things.

Consequently, when these activities can no longer be realized, there is no moral obligation to continue medical treatment, unless to relieve suffering. The conclusion that treatment can stop "does not mean that the person is worthless, but that the person has activated all human potential." Thus there is "no moral requirement to administer artificial nutrition and hydration. In fact it might be violating the person. . . ." Document F concludes on the interesting note that "people feel intuitively that it is wrong and want to find ways to escape imprisonment by technology."

Finally, Document G discusses this issue within the context of policies of life-sustaining treatment. The general context for thinking about this issue is:

> Prolonging physiological function by itself is not of value if it seems all potential for cognitive functions—mental creativity,

the capacity to know and to love—if all that is irreversibly destroyed. Respect for life is at the heart of medicine, and a person in such a condition must not be put to death, but may be allowed to die.

The document then considers various forms of supportive care following the decision to allow to die. First, when medical procedures that prolong life are to be withheld or withdrawn, other medical procedures not directed to supportive care may also be omitted. These include, e.g., lab work, diagnostic procedures, dialysis, nutritional support by mouth or vein, or transfer to an ICU. Measures not to be omitted are "basic nursing care, including patient hygiene, adequate analgesia, oxygen for comfort, positioning, intake for comfort including intravenous hydration, and nutritional support as tolerated." The document then notes that there may be exceptions to hydration and nutritional support.

Exceptions to the last two care elements do exist, especially when they offer no benefit or comfort to the patient. Intravenous hydration may not be appropriate when it prolongs or increases discomfort. With careful deliberation, nutritional support may be withheld when all three of the following conditions are present, namely: (1) The patient has a terminal condition that is irreversible in the final stages. (2) The patient is comatose and shows no clinical evidence of experiencing hunger or thirst. (3) The patient (or substitute decision-maker) has requested no further treatment. Other situations not meeting the above criteria for withdrawal of nutritional support care will be decided on a case-by-case basis.

Document G concludes that any treatments during this time of dying should aim at maintaining the dignity of the individual and providing compassion and comfort. The guidelines wisely state that the dying are more in need of comfort and company than treatment and diagnostic procedures.

These documents represent a range of opinions, arguments, and conclusions. All are carefully stated, clearly argued, and located squarely within the Catholic tradition. Yet different conclusions are drawn from this common heritage—which indicates that the debate is far from finished. There is strong preference for a case-by-case consideration of the issues and a reluctance to have fixed rules to decide cases. On the other hand, there is a recognition that some consensus needs to be developed. Finally, there is no enthusiasm or joy about the conclusion that forgoing or withdrawing is morally permissible. While the arguments are sound, the conclusion is reached with sadness and reluctance.

In the second part of this paper we turn to our own contribution to the development of a moral consensus by arguing for the permissibility of forgoing or withdrawing medical procedures that provide nutrition and hydration to PVS patients.

ARGUMENT IN SUPPORT OF FORGOING OR WITHDRAWING[3]

The Medical Situation

An important fact about a PVS patient is that he or she is not dying. In these patients the brain stem is intact, with the major damage to the brain occurring in the neocortex and cortex. Thus these patients breathe spontaneously, have their eyes open, have a sleep-wake cycle, their pupils respond to light, and they typically have a normal gag and cough reflex.[4]

With respect to the diagnosis of PVS patients, there is "no set of specific medical criteria with as much clinical detail and certainty as the brain-death criteria. Furthermore, even the generally accepted criteria, when properly applied, are not infallible."[5] Furthermore, "It is not uncommon for patients to survive in this condition for five, ten, and twenty years."[6] Survival is contingent on age, economic, familial, and institutional factors, the natural resistance of the body to disease and infection, and changing moral and social views of this condition.

Of critical importance is knowing whether these patients experience pain and/or suffering. Cranford, following the *amicus curiae* brief of the American Academy of Neurology in the Paul Brophy case, argues that PVS patients "may 'react' to painful and other noxious stimuli, but they do not 'feel' (experience) pain in the sense of conscious discomfort . . . ,"[7] because the centers of the brain required for these experiences are too compromised to be functional. Thus PVS patients are not clinically dying and, if they are otherwise in good health and receive appropriate care, they can have a rather long life-expectancy. We obviously have the medical capacity to provide nutrition and hydration for these individuals, but the ethical difficulty, of course, is whether we must do everything we can to sustain their existence in this clinical condition.

The Value of Life

Clearly the preservation of life is an important goal of the human community in general and of the profession of medicine in particular. Intuitively we know life is valuable and sacred; for were it not, then nothing else would be. Yet, when all is said and done, especially in the

Christian framework, life—even human life—is not of ultimate value. Philosophically and politically, we affirm a variety of values that transcend human life: justice, freedom, charity, the good of the neighbor, etc. On the basis of these values or for their sake, we can qualify our protection of individual human lives. Theologically, only God is of ultimate value; all else, no matter how good or valuable, must take second place. Though heresy trials are one, perhaps unfortunate, example of this priority, we also have the celebrated examples of martyrdom and individual self-sacrifice.

This perspective reminds us, particularly in the health-care context, that while preserving life is a good—and even a great good—biological life is neither the highest value nor a value that holds ultimate claim on us. To make biological life the ultimate value is to forget our real priorities and to create an idol by making a lesser good our ultimate reality.

The Quality of Life

The meaning and validity of quality of life judgments have been debated in the literature for quite some time.[8] One example in recent decades is Joseph Fletcher's criteria of humanhood.[9] Although his criteria establish standards for being human, they also implicitly argued that life without a certain level of rationality was not human and consequently not worth living. Most recently Robert Jay Lifton's examination of Nazi doctors emphasized the role of the concept of *lebenunwertes Leben:* life unworthy of life.[10] Such unworthiness consisted primarily in being Jewish, but also extended to mental illness and retardation, as well as to severe physical handicaps.[11]

Quality of life judgments can serve as a code for a life judged to be worthless or useless. This orientation comes partially from our consumerist society, in which quality is linked with individuals' norms of excellence and is limited only by the horizons of their imagination and desires.[12] This perspective realizes one's worst fears about quality of life judgments, because the removal of any transcendent significance or value to human lives gives the state, institutions, or individuals final control over a person's fate.

The two most crucial levels in the quality of life debate are the evaluative and the normative. At the evaluative level three points need to be made. First, it is necessary to distinguish clearly and consistently between physical or biological life and personal life (personhood). When this important distinction is not made, quality of life judgments can equivocate between the value of biological life and the value of personhood.[13] This possibility must be removed. Second, physical life is indeed a value that is not conditioned on any property or characteristic of the person. Here we disagree with Documents F and G, which appear to imply such a conditional value of physical life, e.g. its rationality.[14] In our view physical life is a *bonum onticum*, a true and real value, though created and therefore limited. By arguing that physical life as such is a *bonum onticum* and not a conditional value, i.e. a *bonum utile*, we can affirm that all physical lives are of equal ontic value and that all persons are of equal moral worth. Third, the issue of the evaluative status of physical life may be misplaced from the start. The word "quality" does not and should not refer to a property or attribute of *life*. Rather, the quality that is at issue is the quality of the *relationship* which exists between the medical condition of the patient, on the one hand, and the patient's ability to pursue life's goals and purposes, understood as the values that transcend physical life, on the other.[15] We maintain that this reconceptualization of quality of life judgments is entirely congruent with the substance of the Catholic tradition.

Normatively, those who oppose quality of life judgments fear that life-and-death decisions will be made solely on the presence or absence of certain qualities or properties that a patient's life possesses. This erodes our duties to protect innocent lives, especially of those most vulnerable in our society.

If one contends that our duties to preserve life are based on a prior judgment of whether a specific quality or property of physical life will result in benefits or good consequences to the patient (personal consequentialism) or to society (social consequentialism), then in our judgment those duties to preserve life are improperly grounded in what the patient earns through social accomplishments or potentialities that his/her life might possess. We reject such a normative position because it denies, at least implicitly, the equal ontic value of all physical lives.

We argue that one derives the prima facie duty to preserve physical life from the ontic value of life and the actual moral obligation to preserve life from a teleological, but not consequentialist, assessment of the relationship between the patient's overall condition and his/her ability to pursue life's goals and purposes. The structure of the actual moral obligation is teleological in that the patient's condition is always viewed in relation to the pursuit of life's purposes, and the grounding of the obligation always involves an evaluative assessment of the qualitative relation which exists between these two components. Because physical life is not an absolute value, even those arguing for the sanctity of life position recognize definite limits to the obligation to support life.[16] We should not reject quality of life judgments, but we should rightly reject any normative derivation of our moral duties from the presence of certain properties of physical or personal life.

Quality of life judgments, which are judgments strictly circumscribed by an assessment of the benefits and burdens of medical treatment considered in itself and/or of those benefits and burdens that will accrue to the patient as a result of treatment, function appropriately as ways of qualifying our duties to preserve life. Thus, as long as the value of both physical life and personhood is assured at the evaluative and normative levels, we not only support the role of quality of life judgments in medicine but also judge them to be indispensable in proper decision-making. In our view, then, quality of life judgments properly supplement and enhance the Christian emphasis on the sanctity of life.[17]

The Technological Imperative

We cannot discuss this debate without including a reference to the technological imperative—"if we can do it, we should (or must) do it"—which infers a moral obligation either from a capacity or from the mere existence of a technology.

In the context of high-tech medicine, such an imperative, even if not explicitly subscribed to, is difficult to resist. The same is true even for low-tech or simple technologies. Some medical technologies that administer nutrition and hydration are relatively simple, e.g. parenteral methods of delivering nutrients. Other methods are more invasive, e.g. gastrostomy tubes, and they carry with them potential iatrogenic dangers, such as infection resulting from the surgical creation of the stoma. Yet they are much less invasive than other procedures and are more risk-free if properly cared for. Furthermore, their use provides a clear and demonstrable benefit: the prolongation of physical life. Indeed, feeding tubes may be unique among all medical technologies in that they almost exceptionlessly deliver on their claims. The technological imperative is augmented by simplicity and predictability of outcome and consequently presents an apparently unassailable case for use. But this very simplicity, ease of use, and ready availability disguises the moral dimension of the technology's use.

One must consider the use with respect to outcome. The outcome, of course, is the preservation of physical life. Prima facie such an outcome is valuable, but it must be considered with respect to other values and/or goods, for physical life is not the only or absolute good. Thus other goods, such as human dignity, ought to be considered. Our point is that, in and of itself, the presence of a technology and the capacity to utilize it constitute at most a prima facie case for its use. One cannot automatically or necessarily infer an actual moral obligation from the mere existence or presence of a technology.[18]

The Ordinary/Extraordinary Means Distinction

This well-used distinction can be dated as early as the 17th century and has been used by popes and theologians in arguments to determine one's moral obligation to preserve human life.[19] Some maintain that the key element in the traditional use of the distinction is the *classification* of technologies, medicines, or procedures. Consequently they are considered apart from the patient on whom they are used. Once classified, the moral question is then essentially resolved. In the feeding-tube example, the late John Connery, S.J., argued that since nutrition and hydration kept individuals alive, the technology fitted the classic definition of ordinary treatment and therefore was morally mandatory.[20]

If one shifts the perspective from an abstract classification of technologies to a *patient-centered* approach[21] which gives moral weight to the autonomy of the patient and looks to the impact of these technologies on the patient's medical and nonmedical condition as a whole, one can establish a different moral argument. Here the expressed wishes of the patient have a legitimate moral claim based on our valuing the dignity of the individual and on our respecting the sacredness of his or her conscience. Second, it is the proportionality or disproportionality of benefits and burdens *to the patient* that makes any medical treatment or procedure, including the medical provision of nutrition and hydration, obligatory or optional. Because the technology can neither ameliorate a PVS patient's general clinical condition nor restore this individual to any state of health where the patient might pursue the values of life, the means are extraordinary and not morally required. Therefore ordinary and extraordinary are determined not by classifying the technology but by considering its impact on the patient and his/her overall condition. Additionally, and following directly from the above, the distinction must adopt a patient-centered perspective to avoid the technological imperative.

The Burdensomeness of Life

The specific issue here is whether the burdensomeness of the life preserved by the offering of nutrition/hydration can or should be part of the overall assessment of burden in the determination of ordinary/ extraordinary as we have just outlined it. Considered only in itself, the medical provision of nutrition and hydration would most often be considered ordinary. Thus for some people any considerations beyond the technology itself would lead to an improper questioning of the value of the patient's life.

We think the concepts of burden and quality of life should be linked. Burden can accrue to the patient precisely through the administration of modern technology and can be a consequence of a life lived merely at the biological level with no hope of restoration or further pursuit of temporal or even eternal goals. In this sense the burden is iatrogenic. For the PVS patient, medicine has reached its limit in bringing this individual to any level of health and wholeness. Again, this patient-centered approach focuses on the conditions under which this valued life is to be lived and seeks to identify what interests of the patient can be achieved. Thus we argue that burden is to be assessed not only from the perspective of the burdensome effects of the technology itself but, like Document C, also from the perspective "of the burdens that an individual experiences in pursuing the goals or ends of life" as a result of the intervention of the medical technology. Although it is doubtful that the PVS patient would experience this burden personally, the burden is real, even if experienced secondhand by the family and/or by those professionals who must care for the patient.[22]

Fear of Being Trapped

The expected benefit of tube feeding is the preservation of life post-trauma or posttreatment so that other important work can go on, e.g. treatment or diagnosis. But there comes a time—sometimes sooner, sometimes later—when one knows that all has been tried and cure is not possible. What was formerly appropriate to do, viz. trying to cure, is now inappropriate, and our efforts must shift to accompanying the patient on his/her final journey.

We agree with Document F that it is precisely here that a family may feel or actually be trapped. Having appropriately initiated medical feeding to preserve life while other tests, procedures, and medications were tried, the family may now be frustrated in its desire to remove the feeding tube. Though such feeding only preserves biological life, attempts to withdraw the feeding may be challenged by medical personnel or by others.

Our fear is that individuals or families may inappropriately refuse to initiate medical procedures for delivering nutrients because of the fear of not being able to withdraw these procedures when that becomes appropriate. Thus individuals who may genuinely benefit from this type of procedure could be deprived of its goods. Such a situation would be tragic beyond belief. But because of the technological imperative, our near absolutizing of biological life, and the fear of taking personal responsibility in medical decision-making, this outcome is almost guaranteed. However, recognizing patient autonomy and shifting to a patient-centered calculation of benefits and burdens in the fashion we have described will counter this unfortunate situation.

Summary

In our judgment, the cumulative effect of our arguments supports the legitimate forgoing or withdrawing of nutrition and hydration to PVS patients. This judgment can properly be reached without supporting any efforts or claims for euthanasia and without making any improper judgments about the worth of a particular life. After carefully considering both the patient's known wishes and the qualitative relation between the patient's medical condition and the pursuit of life's purposes, one may appropriately judge that such a therapy is disproportionate and morally optional. This conclusion seems to be very close to, if not the same as, the judgment contained in Document E.

SUGGESTIONS FOR FUTURE DISCUSSION

Having reviewed the results of the survey, the points raised in the various documents submitted to us, and identified several ethical arguments supporting the removal of medical feeding tubes, we wish to make some suggestions for the future conduct of this debate.

Nomenclature

Here three issues. First, the misuse of "euthanasia" in the debate. In our survey, ordinaries were asked whether the diocesan committee considered the removal of feeding tubes from PVS patients to be an act of involuntary euthanasia. The responses are very interesting. Most answered that they considered the withdrawal of these tubes to be "passive or indirect and therefore permitted." A significant number responded that "it depends," and only four respondents answered that this action was "active or direct and therefore forbidden."

The response from the research center, Document D, states that the withdrawal of feeding tubes from PVS patients, except in very limited cases, is an act of "euthanasia by omission," and in most cases anyone who does this has the moral intention to end a life which is considered valueless or excessively burdensome. Two assumptions, frequently cited among those who consider such actions as euthanasia, seem to underlie this conclusion. The first is that the medical provision of nutrients offers a benefit by preserving the life of the patient. The second is that this nourishment should be considered as ordinary *care,* similar to all other types of care.

The moral characterization of the intention of the one authorizing withdrawal as "ending a life" forces this discussion into the context of euthanasia. In its brief to the New Jersey Supreme Court on the Nancy Ellen Jobes case, the New Jersey Catholic Conference argued that the withdrawal of feeding tubes is "intentional euthanasia."[23] Because we disagree both with the two basic assumptions which underlie this argument and with the description of the moral intention of these acts of withdrawal as killing, we argue that the use of the term "euthanasia" should be avoided in the debate.

A moral analysis of euthanasia necessarily involves an assessment of the intention. Though they may be motivated by humane reasons, morally all acts of euthanasia intend the death of the patient either by commission or by omission, and thus by definition these acts constitute the unjustified killing of a patient. However, we argue that in withdrawing nutrition and hydration the intent is either to end a procedure that no longer benefits the patient or to prevent the person from being entrapped in technology. The patient's death, while foreseen, results from the justified discontinuance of a technology that itself can neither correct the underlying fatal pathology, i.e. the permanent inability to ingest food and fluids orally, nor offer the patient any reasonable hope for what we have defined as quality of life. In our judgment, then, it is inappropriate to characterize the withdrawal of medical nutrition and hydration from PVS patients as euthanasia.

Second, we suggest that in future discussion of this issue the word "forgo" should be used rather than "withhold." The reason is that "withhold" connotes that something is denied to someone who has some entitlement to it. When family members appropriately decide that a medical treatment will not truly benefit the PVS patient, their decision is to refrain from pursuing what is not useful to the loved one, not to deny something for which the patient has a need or a right. Our intent is twofold: to avoid a begging-of the question and to suggest a terminology which allows the argument to come forward and be evaluated on its own merits. The terminology of forgoing and withdrawing, we think, will prevent the argument from becoming confused linguistically and prejudged methodologically.

Third, how describe *nutrition and hydration?* What to call the nourishment administered to a patient introduces a variety of problems, descriptive as well as symbolic. The terms "food and water" conjure up, among other things, a variety of images depending on taste and ethnic background. They also connote a meal in which one actively participates or, if with others, shares. The symbolism associated with food and water is deep, and rightly so. For they symbolize membership and participation in a community, and to deny these common but significant realities to someone is more than depriving that individual of nourishment; it is cutting him/her off from the community.

The symbolic level of food and water is what inclines several individuals to argue against the removal of nourishment from the PVS patient.[24] The forgoing or the removal of nutrition says that the individual has been marked and put outside the community, outside society. This further signifies the valuelessness of the person and his/her uselessness to the community. Therefore one must continue to provide this nourishment precisely as a symbol of inclusion.

However, one must also recognize the limits of this symbolism, particularly in the case of PVS patients. To begin with, we have a situation in which the patient is fed and does not eat; the experience is entirely passive. Orderlies or nurses do not deny trays of food to patients nor do they forcibly remove these from the hands of patients. Nutrition and hydration are administered to the patient and the body absorbs them; the feeding process is completely involuntary. Second, the symbolism of the meal is utterly absent, even if others are there. There is no meal, only a medical feeding. Though nourishing, it is difficult to consider such a liquid protein diet as food. For food, in addition to having a certain biological reality, is also a human construct and is more than the sum of its nutritional value. It is the color, texture, aroma, taste, and company in which it is shared. For the PVS patient, all of this is absent. To call this nourishment food is to invest it with more meaning than the reality of the situation can bear.

Also, these patients do not consciously hunger or thirst. But even if these states were experienced, medical procedures for supplying nutrition and hydration might not relieve the feelings.[25] "Medical nutrition and hydration" seems an appropriate phrase for this form of nourishment, because it captures in a nonjudgmental fashion the medical provision of the nourishment as well as the passivity of the experience. The patient is fed and consequently the body is nourished, but he/she certainly does not participate in a meal and clearly does not share table fellowship. This terminology also describes the procedure without begging the moral question of whether one ought to provide it, and it avoids the intrusion of inappropriate symbolism. This terminology will keep us from making more of the situation than is there, but it will also keep us from making less of it.

Ordinary and Extraordinary Treatment

Here are three considerations. First, as noted above, there is a difference in how these traditional terms can be used. For some, the terms are the basis on which the procedure or technology is classified. Once classified, the correct action is relatively clear. If ordinary, the procedure or technology is morally obligatory; if extraordinary, it is morally optional. This schema encounters significant problems when the pace of technological change increases. In addition, the term "ordinary" in its moral or normative sense has been used to declare a certain technology routine or customary in a medical or descriptive sense. The descriptive use of "ordinary" generally refers to what is usually done, but this involves little or no moral analysis of what ought to be done.

These equivocations have precipitated a re-thinking of the terminology that now aims at the evaluation of the benefit-burden ratio for the patient.[26] Consequently a procedure is judged ordinary in a normative sense if its effects on the patient provide proportionately more benefits than burdens. On the other hand, a treatment is extraordinary in a moral sense if the evaluation produces the contrary conclusion. Thus these terms are now seen as the conclusion of a process of evaluation rather than as a classification of a procedure. It is not unusual that a Jehovah's Witness would judge a clinically routine blood transfusion morally extraordinary because of the disproportionate consequences for his or her eternal salvation. Similarly, a person on long-term dialysis might conclude in some circumstances that use of this technology is extraordinary because of its impact on diet and life style.

Understanding ordinary and extraordinary as conclusions of an evaluative process rather than as a classification schema permits a much more appropriate use of the terms in the practice of contemporary medicine. Furthermore, the danger of equivocation is now removed and the meaning of the terms is moral, not descriptive.

Second, autonomy. Though the concept has undergone some criticism in the last few years because it has been taken to an extreme by functioning independently of or to the exclusion of other values, nonetheless we might do well to remember the old adage that abuse does not take away use. Autonomy is an important value, and the proper starting point for these discussions is the expressed wishes of the competent patient. To begin at this point is to respect the dignity of patients and their conscientious decisions. Statements that individuals make about their death or the circumstances of their dying are extremely important. Minimally, they form the foundation of any and all discussion about the initiation or withdrawal of therapy. These statements, which need to be discussed and evaluated in light of the clinical situation and other relevant moral values, always constitute a core element in the final decision about treatment.

Third, quality of life considerations and the goal of medicine. As we have noted, quality of life judgments should not be construed as judgments about the worth of either physical or personal life. They are not concerned with assessing qualities or properties that, when present, make life itself valuable. Rather, these judgments are evaluative and normative claims or assessments about the relation between the patient's overall condition and his/her ability to pursue material, moral, and spiritual values which transcend physical life but do not give that life its very meaning and worth. Consequently quality of life judgments help specify concretely the meaning of the terms "benefits," "burdens," and "best interests" of a patient, as well as the limits of medical interventions within a given historical and cultural situation.

Whereas all physical life is of equal ontic worth and all personal life is of equal moral value, the quality of the relation between these lives and the pursuit of values is not equal. Due to multiple factors, some of which have to do with individual genetic endowment and the ways in which we live our lives and some of which are dependent on the nurturing and accessibility of values in a given culture, a large portion of the population is fortunate enough to attain a high quality of life. Other individuals, regrettably, are not as fortunate, and they must live most of their lives pursuing life's purposes at a less than optimal level. But some have no discernible or such a minimal qualitative relation between their overall condition and the pursuit of values that we would argue that those in this last category have no moral obligation to prolong their physical lives. In these cases all treatment can be withdrawn from them. Not long ago all PVS patients' lives would have been mercifully ended by their inability to ingest food orally, but the intervention of modern technology today has not been as merciful.

No doubt, one of the principal factors that has provoked this debate has been the ambiguity about the central goal of medicine itself. Medicine rightfully seeks to prevent death, especially an untimely death, to alleviate pain and physical suffering, and to promote health as far as possible. Indeed, these are important goals. However, we argue that all these goals are really subordinate to the more encompassing goal of serving the purposefulness of personal existence.[27] In other words, the central and overarching goal of clinical medicine is to enhance the qualitative relation between the patient's condition and the pursuit of life's goods. Thus, other things being equal, when medicine can intervene to ameliorate the quality of the relation between the patient's condition and the pursuit of life's goals, then such an intervention can be considered a benefit to the patient and is in his/her best interests. On the other hand, because of the overall condition of the patient, when a proposed intervention cannot offer the patient any reasonable hope of pursuing life's purposes at all or can only offer the patient a condition where the pursuit of life's purposes will be filled with profound frustration or with utter neglect of these purposes because of the energy needed merely to sustain physical life, then any medical intervention (1) can only offer burden to the life treated, (2) is contrary to the best interests of the patient, (3) can cause iatrogenic harm or the risk of such harm, and (4) has reached its limit based on medicine's own principal reason for existence, and thus treatment should not be given except to palliate or to comfort.[28]

Responsibility in Decision-Making

When the biotechnological revolution began in earnest and humans discovered new powers and capacities, one of the first slogans to describe this new state of affairs was "playing God." This phrase denoted the power humans now wielded over previously untamed and uncontrolled natural realities. But we detect a shift emerging. Rather than humans "playing God," it is now technology that is "playing God." Our machines seem to have developed a life and power of their own. How, for example, does someone with an artificial heart die? How does someone on a respirator stop breathing? How does someone with a feeding tube refuse to be nourished? Very often, once in place, there seems to be no way, short of a cosmic power failure, to end the domination of the machine. We are, clearly, much better about removing machines now than we were initially, but many are still very reluctant to intervene in the activities of the machinery. Often enough, court intervention is the only recourse the family or guardian has to stop a machine.[29]

Have we surrendered our decision-making powers to machines? Do they "play God" by exercising their untiring, endless vigilance over us and our loved ones? We have not improved our situation much if indeed we have turned our appropriate decision-making responsibilities over to machines. Although such decisions are dangerous and difficult at times, humans have a legitimate level of responsibility for deciding about the forgoing or withdrawing of treatment. Surrendering that responsibility because a machine is in place is truly the worship of a false god.

The family typically plays an important role in these decisions, because often the individual most affected by a decision cannot participate directly. Such involvement is proper, because generally the family has a relationship with the patient and knows his/her wishes. The family is normally in the best position to discern the patient's wishes or desires. Thus it can either relate what the patient actually wanted or, failing that, relate its best judgment of what the patient would have wanted. If the family has no direct knowledge of the patient's wishes, it is still the appropriate decision-maker. The family has a socially recognized relation to the patient and can be presumed to have the best interests of the patient in mind.

Should conflicts arise which simply cannot be resolved at the local level with the assistance of the physicians, an ethics committee, a patient's rights advocate, the clergy, or other resources, then—and only then in our judgment—is it appropriate to think of turning to the courts for a resolution of the issue.

CONCLUSION

On both practical and theoretical levels, the question of forgoing or withdrawing medical nutrition and hydration from PVS patients appears to have reached no clear consensus inside or outside the Catholic community, although our sense is that many, if not most, people are uncomfortable with continuing this technology when there is no reasonable hope of an improvement in the patient's prognosis. This is not to say that there is an atmosphere of joy about the situation or a zeal to begin a withdrawal procedure. Rather, there is a sense of reluctance, a very great sense of caution and care, and a most careful focusing on the moral arguments.

Finally, we wish to highlight two aspects of the debate that we think are particularly crucial. First, the moral intention to forgo or withdraw medical nutrition and hydration is not identical with the intention in euthanasia. This conclusion is confirmed by our own work and in most of the literature. People who advocate the forgoing or the withdrawal of feeding tubes are not advocating any kind of euthanasia policy. The clear intent is to end a procedure that is not proportionately benefiting the person or to release the person from entrapment in technology. Thus, while forgoing or withdrawing feeding tubes is not "medical killing," maintaining them may well produce "involuntary medical living." Second, forgoing or withdrawing this technology is argued as a moral option, not as a mandatory practice. Therefore the conclusion we share with most authors is either that forgoing or withdrawal is not prohibited or it is within the permitted range of moral activities. We also agree with Document E that individuals who conclude that such a practice is morally appropriate should not be prohibited from acting on that conclusion.

We expect that the debate will continue and that different aspects of it will be further examined. Our hope is that this report and presentation of an argument will help structure that process and assist in its resolution.[30]

NOTES

1. The longest case of coma is that of Elaine Esposito, who died 37 years and 111 days after falling into coma. See The President's Commission for the Study of Ethical Problems in Medicine and Biomedical and Behavioral Research, *Deciding to Forego Life-Sustaining Treatment: A Report on the Ethical, Medical, and Legal Issues in Treatment Decisions* (Washington, D.C.: U.S. Government Printing Office, 1983) 177 n. 16.

2. Some dioceses may not have received a survey either because the see was vacant or because of error on TAS's part. Additionally, not every respondent answered every question. Thus, in terms of data analysis there is no constant "n"; yet an overall impression can be gained from the data.

3. Throughout the remainder of this essay we have adopted the terminology used by the Hastings Center in describing the technique by which nutrition and hydration are provided to the PVS patient. As defined by the Hastings Center, "medical procedures for supplying nutrition and hydration are medical enteral procedures and parenteral nutritional procedures. . . ." "Medical enteral procedures are procedures in which nutritional formulas and water are introduced into the patient's stomach or intestine by means of a tube, such as

a gastrostomy tube or nasogastric tube." "Parenteral nutritional procedures are procedures in which nutritional formulas and water are introduced into the patient's body by means other than the gastrointestinal tract. Such procedures include total parenteral nutritional support (TPN), in which a formula capable of maintaining the patient for prolonged periods is infused into a vein—usually a large, central vein in the patient's chest—and intravenous procedures in which water and/or a formula supplying limited nutritional support is introduced into a peripheral vein" (Hastings Center, *Guidelines on the Termination of Life-Sustaining Treatment and the Care of the Dying* [Briarcliff Manor, N.Y.: Hastings Center, 1987] 140–41).

4. For a more detailed discussion of the condition of a patient in persistent vegetative state, see Ronald E. Cranford, "The Persistent Vegetative State: The Medical Reality (Getting the Facts Straight)," *Hastings Center Report* 18 (February/March, 1988) 27–32. Also, the President's Report, *Deciding to Forego Life-Sustaining Treatment* 174–81.

5. Cranford, "The Persistent Vegetative State" 29.

6. Ibid. 31.

7. Ibid. In addition, see the recent "Position of the American Academy of Neurology on Certain Aspects of the Care and Management of the Persistent Vegetative State Patient," reprinted in *Medical Ethics Advisor* 4 (August 1988) 111–13.

8. E.g., see George J. Annas, "Quality of Life in the Courts: Earle Spring in Fantasyland," *Hastings Center Report* 10 (August 1980) 9–10; Daniel Callahan, *Setting Limits* (New York: Simon & Schuster, 1987) 187–93; John R. Connery, S.J., "Quality of Life," *Linacre Quarterly* 53 (February 1986) 26–33; Brian V. Johnstone, C.SS.R., "The Sanctity of Life, the Quality of Life and the New 'Baby Doe' Law," ibid. 52 (August 1985) 258–70; Edward W. Keyserlingk, *Sanctity of Life or Quality of Life in the Context of Ethics, Medicine and Law* [a study written for the Law Reform Commission of Canada] (Ottawa: Minister of Supply and Services Canada, 1979) 49–72, 75–105, 185–90; Richard A. McCormick, S.J., "A Proposal for 'Quality of Life' Criteria for Sustaining Life," *Hospital Progress* 59 (1975) 76–79; idem, "The Quality of Life, the Sanctity of Life," *Hastings Center Report* 8 (February 1978) 30–36; Warren T. Reich, "Quality of Life," in *Encyclopedia of Bioethics* 2 (New York: Free Press, 1978) 829–40; idem, "Quality of Life and Defective Newborn Children: An Ethical Analysis," in *Decision Making and the Defective Newborn: Proceedings of a Conference on Spina Bifida and Ethics,* ed. Chester A. Swinyard (Springfield, Ill.: Charles C. Thomas, 1978) 489–511.

9. Joseph Fletcher, "Indicators of Humanhood: A Tentative Profile of Man," *Hastings Center Report* 2 (November 1972) 1–4.

10. Robert Jay Lifton, *The Nazi Doctors: Medical Killing and the Psychology of Genocide* (New York: Basic Books, 1986) 21.

11. For an interesting contrast between the Nazi interpretation of "quality of life" and what contemporary authors tend to mean by this criterion, see Cynthia B. Cohen, " 'Quality of Life' and the Analogy with the Nazis," *Journal of Medicine and Philosophy* 8 (1983) 113–35.

12. Albert R. Jonsen, "Purposefulness in Human Life," *Western Journal of Medicine* 125 (July 1976) 5.

13. E.g., Warren Reich's theological position grounds both the value and the equality of "human life" in the belief that "all men are created as persons in the image of God" ("Quality of Life and Defective Newborn Children" 504). His use of the phrase "human life" is ambiguous here and therefore misleading. The context of his argument is a critique

of what he believes to be Richard A. McCormick's position on the value of *physical life*, yet Reich completes his argument by referring to *persons* and their nature and value as images of God.

14. In fact, several contemporary Catholics have given the impression that the value of physical life is dependent on some inherent property or attribute which, when present, gives physical life its value. It is possible that this way of phrasing the value of physical life is due to the lack of a terminology in the contemporary discussion that can mediate between the two traditional categories of value, viz. *bonum honestum* and *bonum utile*. E.g., see Kevin D. O'Rourke, O.P., and Dennis Brodeur, *Medical Ethics: Common Ground for Understanding* (St. Louis: Catholic Health Association of the U.S., 1986) 213; Richard A. McCormick, *How Brave a New World? Dilemmas in Bioethics* (Washington, D.C.: Georgetown University, 1981) 405–7; David Thomasma et al., "Continuance of Nutritional Care in the Terminally Ill Patient." *Critical Care Clinics* 2 (January 1986) 66.

15. See James J. Walter, "The Meaning and Validity of Quality of Life Judgments in Contemporary Roman Catholic Medical Ethics," *Louvain Studies* 13 (fall 1988) 195–208, esp. 201.

16. E.g., see John R. Connery, S.J., "Prolonging Life: The Duty and Its Limits," *Linacre Quarterly* 47 (May 1980) 151–65; Johnstone, "The Sanctity of Life, the Quality of Life," esp. 265–69; Reich, "Quality of Life and Defective Newborn Children," esp. 505–9.

17. Keyserlingk also argues a similar position in his report for the Law Reform Commission of Canada. See his *Sanctity of Life or Quality of Life*, esp. 49–72.

18. We agree with the report from the Hastings Center that "All invasive procedures for supplying nutrition and hydration—all enteral and parenteral techniques—should be considered procedures that require the patient's or surrogate's consent . . ." (*Guidelines on the Termination of Life-Sustaining Treatment* 61).

19. See Gerald Kelly, S.J., *Medico-Moral Problems* (St. Louis: Catholic Hospital Association, 1958) 128–41.

20. John R. Connery, S.J., "The Clarence Herbert Case: Was Withdrawal of Treatment Justified?" *Hospital Progress* 65 (February 1984) 32–35 and 70.

21. Recently several authors have argued for a patient-centered approach in clinical decision-making: e.g., see Robert M. Veatch, *Death, Dying, and the Biological Revolution: Our Last Quest for Responsibility* (New Haven: Yale University, 1976); James J. Walter, "Food & Water: An Ethical Burden," *Commonweal* 113 (Nov. 21, 1986) 616–19.

22. Though we have refrained from making any judgment about the financial burden either on society or on insurance companies in providing funds for PVS patients, the fact that there are approximately 10,000 of these patients in the U.S. strongly inclines us to agree with Daniel Callahan that "It is hard to see how a debate on that reimbursement issue can be forestalled much longer." See Callahan's "Vital Distinction, Mortal Questions: Debating Euthanasia & Health-Care Costs," *Commonweal* 115 (July 15, 1988) 404. It is important to note here that the *Declaration on Euthanasia* and Document E, both following Pius XII, do permit one to assess the burden on the family or on the community in judging whether a treatment is disproportionate. See the *Declaration on Euthanasia* in *Origins* 10 (Aug. 10, 1980) 16.

23. New Jersey State Catholic Conference Brief, "Providing Food and Fluids to Severely Brain Damaged Patients," in *Origins* 16 (Jan. 22, 1987) 583. The Conference was following the Lutheran theologian Gilbert Meilaender in his "On Removing Food and Water: Against the Stream," *Hastings Center Report* 14 (December 1984) 11–13. An oppos-

198   THOMAS A. SHANNON, JAMES J. WALTER

ing position was taken by Bishop Louis Gelineau of Providence, R.I., in the Marcia Gray court case. See his statement in *Origins* 17 (Jan. 21, 1988) 546–57.

24. E.g., see Daniel Callahan, "On Feeding the Dying," *Hastings Center Report* 13 (October 1983) 22.

25. Hastings Center, *Guidelines on the Termination of Life-Sustaining Treatment* 59.

26. See the *Declaration on Euthanasia*, where the terminology has shifted to a discussion of proportionality between the benefits and the burdens.

27. Jonsen, "Purposefulness in Human Life" 6.

28. Walter, "The Meaning and Validity of Quality of Life Judgments" 207.

29. There have been several court cases recently involving patients in a persistent vegetative state. Two of the more notable cases are Paul Brophy and Nancy Ellen Jobes.

30. Support for the survey was provided by the Research Development Council of Worcester Polytechnic Institute, and the authors acknowledge their gratitude for this assistance.

12 *Unsuccessful Emergency Medical Resuscitation: Are Continued Efforts in the Emergency Department Justified?*

WILLIAM A. GRAY, M.D., ROBERT J. CAPONE, M.D., AND ALBERT S. MOST, M.D.

Dr. William Gray is in the Division of Cardiology, Rhode Island Hospital. Dr. Robert Capone is with the Brown University Program in Medicine, Providence, R.I. Dr. Albert Most is in the Division of Cardiology, University of Rochester Medical Center, Rochester, N.Y.

Cardiopulmonary resuscitation has been implemented extensively in hospitals throughout the United States in the 30 years since its inception.[1] Originally used for victims of acute but reversible insult,[2] its application has grown to include attempts to resuscitate some patients in whom the prognosis is extremely poor. Studies have demonstrated that the usefulness of resuscitation in hospitalized patients is limited, especially in elderly persons[3-5] and in patients with renal failure,[3,6] pneumonia,[6] cancer,[4,6] or sepsis.[4] Recognizing that sometimes it is more appropriate to withhold this therapy from certain patients, most U.S. hospitals have adopted do-not-resuscitate policies to preempt efforts at resuscitation in hospitalized patients with a poor prognosis.

In addition to the widespread use of in-hospital resuscitation, emergency medical systems have been implemented throughout the United States to deliver care rapidly when arrests occur outside the hospital. The majority of such arrests result from cardiac events, usually ventricular fi-

---

This article first appeared in The New England Journal of Medicine *325 (14 November 1991): 1393–1398.*

brillation, in patients with coronary artery disease.[7-9] Several factors have been shown to improve outcome in cardiac arrests occurring outside the hospital: the presence of witnesses,[10,11] the administration of cardiopulmonary resuscitation by a bystander,[11-18] an initial cardiac rhythm of ventricular tachycardia or fibrillation,[13,14,17,19] and early defibrillation.[12-15,19,20] In the Seattle area, where an extensive, tiered response system is in place and lay education in techniques of cardiopulmonary resuscitation has been emphasized, the overall rates of survival until hospital discharge of patients with cardiac arrest occurring outside the hospital and due to ventricular fibrillation have reached approximately 30 percent.[14]

Although much is known about the outcomes in patients who have cardiac arrests in the inpatient and outpatient settings, little information is available about the relation between the two systems in the case of patients who have arrests outside the hospital, who undergo unsuccessful attempts at resuscitation by the emergency medical system, and who are then transported to the hospital for continued, and usually more extensive, resuscitation. To assess the efficacy and cost effectiveness of this practice, we reviewed the case histories of 185 patients with such arrests who lacked vital signs when they were transported to our emergency department by ambulance.

METHODS

Rhode Island Hospital is a 719-bed university teaching hospital located in Providence, the state's largest city. It functions as a community hospital for the greater Providence area and serves as the principal tertiary care referral center and designated trauma center for patients in southeastern New England.

A review of the patient logs of the Rhode Island Hospital emergency department between October 1, 1985, and June 30, 1987, identified patients for inclusion in this study. Only patients who came to the emergency department by ambulance without spontaneous pulse or respirations (i.e., without vital signs) after an arrest outside the hospital and in whom initial resuscitative efforts were unsuccessful but ongoing were included for analysis. Patients were excluded from the study if their arrests were due to trauma or drowning or if they were under 16 years old. All other patients were included, regardless of the primary cause of their arrests (e.g., cardiac, respiratory, or resulting from an overdose).

In the state of Rhode Island, it is standard for resuscitation to be initiated by the emergency medical system in all patients found without a pulse, regardless of their initial cardiac rhythm, except patients in whom prolonged arrest is evident (i.e., cases of rigor mortis). Once begun, resuscitation is continued until the emergency medical unit transfers the care of the patient to the staff of the emergency department. In the case of emergency medical units capable of advanced cardiac life support,[21] full and aggressive implementation of the cardiac-arrest protocol is undertaken at the scene, with subsequent transport to the emergency department only after these initial attempts at resuscitation. Alternatively, in basic cardiac life-support units,[22] immediate transport of the patient is the primary directive.

One hundred eight-five patients met the criteria for entry into the study. Prehospital resuscitation factors were ascertained, including an estimate of the time from the arrest to the arrival of the ambulance, the initial cardiac rhythm recorded by the ambulance personnel, and the extent of resuscitative efforts in the field—either basic cardiac life support, defined as resuscitation limited to chest compression and assisted ventilation, or advanced cardiac life support, defined as the basic treatments plus defibrillation, intravenous medication, and esophageal obturator airway or endotracheal intubation. The time required for resuscitation (both at the scene and during transport to the emergency department) was noted, and the distance traveled by the emergency medical unit was estimated on the basis of the patient's township of origin. Accounts of witnessed as compared with unwitnessed arrests and of the initiation of cardiopulmonary resuscitation by bystanders could not be obtained reliably in a majority of cases and are not included in our data.

All patients presenting to the emergency department received resuscitation according to the advanced cardiac life-support protocol,[21] including chest compression, intubation, the use of vasopressors and antiarrhythmic agents, direct-current cardioversion, the placement of a central venous catheter or pacemaker, and pericardiocentesis, as deemed necessary by the attending physician. The emergency department records of those cases were reviewed, and the patient's outcome (death or resuscitation) was determined. Demographic data were recorded, including age, sex, race, and previous medical history. Information was obtained about resuscitation efforts in the emergency department, such as the time of admission, the duration of resuscitation (to the pronouncement of death or the first evidence of a pulse), cumulative recorded nursing time, cardiac rhythm on arrival in the emergency department, arterial blood gas levels, and serum potassium levels. The cumulative time spent by physicians was estimated, with the assumption that at least two physicians were present for the duration of the resuscitation or longer. The cause of the arrest was determined from the circumstances surrounding the event or from postmortem examination, if available.

In the case of patients who were successfully revived in the emergency department and admitted to the hospital, information on their subsequent course was gathered from a review of hospital charts. Information about the following was obtained: hospital outcome (death or survival until discharge), neurologic status at the time of death or discharge, time in the intensive care unit and total duration of hospital stay, in-hospital cause of death, and outpatient course.

The costs of hospitalization for the patients admitted to the hospital were estimated from the charges accrued in the various departments (i.e., pharmacy, laboratory, radiology, and the like) and the charges related to the patients' stay in the intensive care unit and elsewhere in the hospital, as well as the cost of any procedures they may have undergone. Once these figures were determined, cost-to-charge ratios for each department were used to calculate the total hospital cost for each patient. These figures were then adjusted to reflect 1991 dollars. Professional fees were not included in cost determinations.

To assess differences between the characteristics of survivors and those of the patients who died, a statistical analysis using the chi-square test (or Fisher's exact test, as appropriate) for categorical variables or Student's t-test (unpaired and two-tailed) for continuous data was performed.

RESULTS

Characteristics of Patients and Resuscitations

During the 21-month study period, a total of 185 patients who lacked vital signs were brought to the emergency department for further care after an arrest outside the hospital with initially unsuccessful, but continuing, resuscitation by the emergency medical system. The mean ($\pm$SD) age was 67 ± 15 years. Patients who died of other than cardiac causes (16 of 185, or 9 percent) tended to be younger than the other patients (mean age, 47 ± 21 vs. 68 ± 13 years, $P<0.01$), and most had respiratory arrests. One hundred twenty-three patients (66 percent) were men, and 148 (80 percent) were white. Most of the patients (94 percent) were ambulatory at the time of their arrest. Coronary artery disease was the most common preexisting medical condition reported (in 34 percent), followed by congestive heart failure (16 percent), hypertension (15 percent), and diabetes mellitus (15 percent).

Most of the emergency medical units arrived at the scene of the arrest (61 of 82, or 74 percent) within five minutes of receiving the call for help. Approximately two thirds of all the patients (114 of 185, or 62 percent) received advanced cardiac life support from the responding emergency medical unit, and one third of all patients (68 of 185, or 37 percent) had defibrillation according to protocol for ventricular tachycardia or ventricular fibrillation. The initial cardiac rhythm that the emergency medical units reported finding most often at the scene was ventricular tachycardia or ventricular fibrillation, seen in 60 percent (68 of 114) of the electrocardiographically monitored patients (i.e., those treated by emergency medical units capable of advanced cardiac life support). For the same group of patients, however, ventricular tachycardia and ventricular fibrillation represented only 32 percent (36 of 114) of the rhythms seen in the emergency department.

The cases were divided into tertiles—<5, 5 to 8, and >8 km (<3, 3 to 5, and >5 miles)—according to the distance traveled by the emergency medical units from the scene of the arrest to the emergency department. The time required for the initial resuscitation and transport of the patient to the emergency department was more than 15 minutes in two thirds of the cases (128 of 185, or 69 percent).

The mean resuscitation time in the emergency department was 22.4 minutes, and the cumulative nursing time averaged 116 minutes. The estimated time spent by physicians during these resuscitation efforts was 45 minutes.

Outcomes

Sixteen patients (9 percent) were successfully resuscitated in the emergency department and admitted to the hospital (Table 1). There were no significant differences in age, race, or cause of arrest between these surviving patients and those who died. There was, however, a significant predominance of women among the survivors, and this finding was independent of age and cause of arrest. Improved survival was also noted in patients who had a history of congestive heart failure.

The shorter the distance from the scene of the arrest to the hospital (i.e., the more urban the setting), the more likely the patient was to receive advanced cardiac life support from the responding emergency medical unit ($P = 0.0001$ for distances ≤8 km [5 miles] vs. >8 km). However, the extent of resuscitation by emergency-medical-system personnel (advanced cardiac life support vs. basic cardiac life support) did not affect survival in the emergency department, and there was no association between the use of defibrillation and hospital admission (Table 2). Although ventricular tachycardia and ventricular fibrillation constituted the majority of the rhythms noted by the emergency medical units at the scene of the arrest, there was a significant decline in their prevalence in the emergency department. There were no differences, however, in survival in the emergency department according to cardiac rhythm, in either the field or the emergency department. Improved survival in the emergency department was observed when less than 15 minutes was required for initial emergency-medical-system field resuscitation and transport to the emergency department; this improvement

**Table 1.   Characteristics of Patients and Outcomes in the
Emergency Department**

Characteristic	Outcome	
	Death (N = 169)	Resuscitation (N = 16)
Age (yr)	67±15	70±13
	no. (% of total)	
Sex		
Male	119 (70)	4 (25)*
Female	50 (30)	12 (75)*
Racial or ethnic group		
White	135 (80)	13 (81)
Black	9 (5)	1 (6)
Hispanic	25 (15)	2 (13)
Medical history		
Coronary artery disease	56 (33)	6 (38)
Congestive heart failure	22 (13)	7 (44) †
Hypertension	28 (17)	0 (0)
Diabetes mellitus	26 (15)	2 (13)
Chronic obstructive pulmonary disease	14 (8)	1 (6)
Cancer	11 (7)	1 (6)
Cerebrovascular disease	9 (5)	0 (0)
End-stage renal disease	6 (3)	1 (6)
Other (e.g., arrhythmias, hypothyroidism)	14 (8)	1 (6)
None reported	46 (27)	2 (13)
Cause of arrest		
Cardiac	154 (91)	15 (94)
Other	15 (9)	1 (6)

*P<0.001 for the comparison between men and women with respect to the proportion who were successfully resuscitated (chi-square test with one degree of freedom and a continuity correction).

†P<0.005 by Fisher's exact test for the comparison between the patients who died and those who were resuscitated.

Table 2. Characteristics of Attempts at Resuscitation and Outcomes in the Emergency Department

Characteristic*	Outcome		P Value†
	Death	Successful Resuscitation	
	no. (%) of patients		
Time to arrival of EMS (min) (n = 82)			
<5	57 (76)	4 (57)	
5–10	5 (7)	3 (43)	
>10	13 (17)	0 (0)	
Cardiac rhythm (n = 114)			
At the scene			
VT or VF	64 (61)	4 (44)	
EMD or asystole	41 (39)	5 (56)	
In the ED			<0.0001‡ §
VT or VF	34 (32)	2 (22)	
EMD or asystole	71 (68)	7 (78)	
Resuscitation efforts by EMS (n = 185)			
BCLS	64 (38)	7 (44)	
ACLS	105 (62)	9 (56)	
Defibrillation	64 (38)	4 (25)	
No. of miles from scene to ED¶			
<3	65 (38)	6 (38)	
3–5	50 (30)	8 (50)	0.10‖
>5	54 (32)	2 (13)	
Time required (min)			
<15	46 (27)	11 (69)	<0.001‡
≥15	123 (73)	5 (31)	
Resuscitation efforts in ED			
Duration (min)—mean±SD	22.6±17.9	18.7±11.6	
Cumulative staff time (min)			
Nurses—mean±SD	105±56	231±169	NA (see text)
Physicians (estimated)	45	38	NA (see text)

*EMS denotes emergency medical system, VT ventricular tachycardia, VF ventricular fibrillation, EMD electromechanical dissociation, ED emergency department, BCLS basic cardiac life support, ACLS advanced cardiac life support, and NA not applicable.

†P values refer to the comparison between patients who died and those who were resuscitated; only values ≤0.10 are shown.

‡By the chi-square test with one degree of freedom and a continuity correction.

§For the comparison of patients treated at the scene with ventricular tachycardia or ventricular fibrillation vs. those treated in the emergency department.

¶To convert miles to kilometers, multiply by 1.609.

‖For the comparison of >5 miles vs. ≤5 miles (Fisher's exact test).

was independent of the extent of emergency-medical-system resuscitation. Although differences in the time it took for the emergency medical unit to arrive at the scene did not result in a statistically significant difference in emergency department outcome, it should be noted that no patient was revived with subsequent resuscitative efforts when it took more than 10 minutes for the emergency medical unit to arrive. Similarly, when the distance traveled by the emergency medical unit from the scene to the emergency department was more than 8 km, there was a decline in survival in the emergency department, albeit not a statistically significant one.

Analysis of the duration of resuscitation in the emergency department for each group revealed that it did not predict survival. The cumulative nursing time was not statistically compared in the two groups; significant differences would have been expected because of the additional time needed to prepare the survivors for admission and transport to their inpatient beds, and not necessarily by any intrinsic differences between the groups.

Hospital Course and Medical Costs in Resuscitated Patients

Of the 16 patients admitted to the hospital after successful resuscitation in the emergency department, none lived to be discharged. The mean stay was 12.6 days (range, 1 to 132), with an average stay in the intensive care unit of 2.3 days (range, 1 to 11). Only one of the patients resuscitated regained consciousness (but remained intubated) before her death on the first hospital day; the others were comatose until death. One patient's prehospital arrest was due to a subarachnoid hemorrhage, whereas the remainder had apparently primary cardiac events. In about half the patients, the cause of hospital death was refractory hypotension (in 7 of 16 patients, or 44 percent); recurrent arrhythmias (in 5 of 16 patients, or 31 percent) and neurologic causes (in 4 of 16 patients, or 25 percent), including the discontinuation of life-support measures (e.g., ventilation and dialysis) after persistent coma, accounted for the rest of the deaths. The total cost of hospitalization for these 16 patients was $180,908, with an average cost per patient of $11,307 (range, $1,984 to $95,144).

DISCUSSION

This study was undertaken to evaluate the outcomes and costs of continued hospital resuscitation in patients after a cardiac or respiratory arrest outside the hospital, when initial efforts at resuscitation proved unsuccessful. With approximately 350,000[21] cardiac arrests in the United States every year, at least two thirds of which take place outside hospital settings,[9] there are undoubtedly many patients similar to those we studied. Patients who had other forms of arrest, including but not limited to victims of hypothermia, trauma, and drowning, were excluded from this study.

We believe that the care given to our patients by the emergency medical system and the emergency department and the resulting outcomes are representative of those in many urban and suburban centers. During the period of our study, a review of the records from 3 emergency medical services that contributed more than half the patients to this study (in which 25 services participated) disclosed that the rate of successful resuscitation by the emergency medical system after cardiopulmonary arrest was approximately 20 percent. A telephone survey of emergency medical systems in major New England cities revealed similar success rates, ranging from 12 to 20 percent. A retrospective design was chosen, because a prospective study might have influenced the length and intensity of hospital resuscitation and perhaps the outcome in the emergency department.

Of the patients transported to our emergency department after an unsuccessful attempt at resuscitation, only 9 percent were revived by further efforts and admitted. No patient lived to be discharged from the hospital, however, and all but one were comatose at the time of death, having had profound and irreversible anoxia and brain injury as a result of prolonged arrest. For the average patient, the total time spent undergoing resuscitation efforts before reaching the hospital and being treated in the emergency department was more than 35 minutes. Although the mean stay was just over 12 days, one comatose patient lived for more than 4 months before dying. The poor outcomes and lack of survival in the hospital in these patients who have undergone prolonged resuscitation are not surprising, since studies of survival after cardiac arrest occurring either in the hospital or before the patient reaches it have established that for an arrest to last more than 12 to 15 minutes is an independent predictor of death.[4,17]

Subgroup analysis of the patients who survived resuscitation efforts in the emergency department has limited value because all patients died before discharge, but two features of this group are worth noting. First, the predominant cardiac rhythms noted in the field were ventricular tachycardia and ventricular fibrillation, whereas electromechanical dissociation and asystole were the primary rhythms noted in the emergency department. These data, along with those of previous studies,[14,23] suggest that electromechanical dissociation and asystole represent terminal rhythms, probably the result of the deterioration, with prolonged arrest, of the ventricular tachycardia or ventricular fibrillation that had precipitated the event. Most important, for both the patients who had an arrest in the hospital and those with a prehospital arrest, dramatic differences in the rates of successful outcome have been demonstrated to be associated with cardiac rhythm, with only occasional survival noted once electromechanical dissociation or asystole is present.[3,4,14,16,24] Second, the only characteristic of treatment by the emergency medical system that was predictive of improved outcome in the emergency department was a total resuscitation time of less than 15 minutes—confirmation of the ineffectiveness of prolonged resuscitation.

Previous studies of unsuccessful resuscitation in medical patients before they reach the hospital have also documented extremely poor outcomes. In a review of the records of 281 consecutive patients arriving in the emergency department after failed attempts at resuscitation by the emergency medical system, Kellermann et al.[25] reported that only 4 patients survived until hospital discharge. Two who were reported to be neurologically intact had their arrests shortly before their arrival in the emergency department, whereas the other two required nursing home care because of severe neurologic deficits. The results of our study also closely parallel what has been observed in both pediatric patients and trauma patients—populations in which the causes of arrest are largely non-cardiac. In a review by Shimazu and Shatney[26] of 267 trauma patients without vital signs who were treated in the emergency department, only 2.6 percent survived and only 1.5 percent were considered functional. The results were just as grim when O'Rourke[27] reviewed 34 pediatric patients brought to the emergency department with apnea and without a pulse; 7 (21 percent) survived, but all were discharged to a chronic care facility, and most were in a persistent vegetative state.

Our study raises important questions about the need for continued resuscitative measures and their advisability once patients reach the hospital, given our observations of the apparent futility of such efforts and their consumption of health care resources. For all the patients we studied, cumulative nursing time in the emergency department averaged almost 2 hours, and estimated physicians' time approximately 45 minutes. The patients who survived to be admitted to the hospital had a mean stay in the intensive care unit of more than two days and a mean hospital stay of almost two weeks, and they required complete care until their deaths. This represented a considerable allocation of beds in the intensive care unit and elsewhere in the hospital, equipment, respiratory therapy, and nursing and physicians' time, all of which are scarce commodities. Given the uniformly fatal outcome, it is difficult to justify the use of the facilities and personnel required for this care.

Furthermore, these efforts resulted in a cost to the hospital of

$180,908 for the 16 patients surviving until hospital admission. Additional costs, conservatively estimated at between $100,000 and $150,000, were incurred for the 169 patients who underwent unsuccessful attempts at resuscitation in the emergency department. When one considers the magnitude of the problem presented by sudden death in this country and the fact that our data represent only one hospital's experience, the implication is that there are considerable nationwide outlays for seemingly little benefit, and perhaps at the expense of more productive practices.

Provided that expert advanced cardiac life support is administered before the patient reaches the hospital, it seems reasonable to establish emergency-medical-system protocols to stop prolonged, unsuccessful resuscitation at the scene, perhaps after consultation with the physician in the emergency department, and this concept should be supported by appropriate legislation in all states. This would eliminate much of the current need to use the resources of the emergency department to treat these patients. In addition, the members of the emergency department team should temper their efforts when a patient arrives after undergoing prolonged resuscitation, since such patients have as dire an outlook as any identifiable group of patients who have had an arrest. Several authors and commissions have proposed[28-32] that the physician is under no obligation to perform procedures when there is little or no expectation of medical benefit, and the population of patients certainly has little hope of meaningful recovery as a result of continued resuscitative efforts.

An occasional patient who has had an arrest outside the hospital can be resuscitated successfully in the emergency department. Physicians caring for these hospitalized patients can advise relatives about the prognosis and considerations for further therapy and resuscitation on the basis of the uniformly poor outcomes noted in this study, as well as the individual patient's condition at the time of admission.

In a broader context, emphasis should be placed on prehospital care for the patient with cardiopulmonary arrest, since it is clear that patients treated in this setting have the greatest chance of successful resuscitation. Specifically, measures should be taken to increase the number and responsiveness of emergency medical units capable of defibrillation, performed either by trained paramedics or with automatic external defibrillators (for which efficacy at lower cost has been demonstrated even with minimally trained personnel),[33] and to provide widespread instruction for lay people in techniques of cardiopulmonary resuscitation, since these are the two modifiable determinants of survival. Many experts have strongly endorsed these proposals in the past to improve the outcome after an arrest occurring outside the hospital,[12-15,17,20,34-36] but their

210   WILLIAM A. GRAY, ROBERT J. CAPONE, ALBERT S. MOST

recommendations take on even greater importance given the lack of survival after subsequent attempts at resuscitation in the emergency department, since the only real opportunity to rescue such patients appears to be in the field.

We are indebted to Mrs. Dawn Oliveira and Mrs. Arlene Grant for assistance in the preparation of the manuscript and to Patricia O'Sullivan, Ph.D., for assistance with the statistical analysis.

REFERENCES

1. Kouwenhoven WB, Jude JR, Knickerbocker GG. Closed-chest cardiac massage. JAMA 1960;173:1064–7.

2. Talbott JH. Introduction. In: Jude JR, Elam JO, eds. Fundamentals of cardiopulmonary resuscitation. Philadelphia: F.A. Davis, 1965:1–3.

3. Murphy DJ, Murray AM, Robinson BE, Campion EW. Outcomes of cardiopulmonary resuscitation in the elderly. Ann Intern Med 1989;111:199–205.

4. Taffet GE, Teasdale TA, Luchi RJ. In-hospital cardiopulmonary resuscitation. JAMA 1988;260:2069–72.

5. Saphir R. External cardiac massage. Medicine (Baltimore) 1968;47:73–87.

6. Bedell DE, Delbanco TL, Cook EF, Epstein FH. Survival after cardiopulmonary resuscitation in the hospital. N Engl J Med 1983;309:569–76.

7. Weaver WD, Lorch GS, Alvarez HA, Cobb LA. Angiographic findings and prognostic indicators in patients resuscitated from sudden death. Circulation 1976;54:895–900.

8. Tresch DD, Grove JR, Siegal R, Keelan MH, Brooks HL. Survivors of prehospitalization sudden death: characteristic clinical and angiographic features. Arch Intern Med 1981;141:1154–7.

9. Cobb LA, Werner JA, Trobaugh GB. Sudden cardiac death. I. A decade's experience with out-of-hospital resuscitation. Mod Concepts Cardiovasc Dis 1980;49:31–6.

10. Bachman JW, McDonald GS, O'Brien PC. A study of out-of-hospital cardiac arrests in northeastern Minnesota. JAMA 1986;256:477–83.

11. Einarsson O, Jacobsson F, Sigurdsson G. Advanced cardiac life support in the prehospital setting: the Reykjavik experience. J Intern Med 1989;225:129–35.

12. Weaver WD, Copass MK, Bufi D, Ray R, Hallstrom AP, Cobb LA. Impaired neurologic recovery and survival after early defibrillation. Circulation 1984;69:943–8.

13. Roth R, Stewart RD, Rogers K, Cannon GM. Out-of-hospital cardiac arrest: factors associated with survival. Ann Emerg Med 1984;13:237–43.

14. Weaver WD, Cobb LA, Hallstrom AP, et al. Considerations for improving surviving from out-of-hospital cardiac arrest. Ann Emerg Med 1986;15:1181–6.

15. Eisenberg M, Bergner L, Hallstrom A. Paramedic programs and out-of-hospital cardiac arrest. I. Factors associated with successful resuscitation. Am J Public Health 1979; 69:30–8.

16. Myerburg RJ, Conde CA, Sung RJ, et al. Clinical, electrophysiologic and hemodynamic profile of patients resuscitated from prehospital cardiac arrest. Am J Med 1980;68: 568–76.

17. Cummins RO, Eisenberg MS, Hallstrom AP, Litwin PE. Survival of out-of-hospital cardiac arrest with early initiation of cardiopulmonary resuscitation. Am J Emerg Med 1985;3:114–9.

18. Hallstrom AP, Cobb LA, Swain M, Mensinger K. Predictors of hospital mortality after out-of-hospital cardiopulmonary resuscitation. Crit Care Med 1985;13:927–9.

19. Aprahamian C, Thompson BM, Gruchow HW, et al. Decision making in prehospital sudden cardiac arrest. Ann Emerg Med 1986;15:445–9.

20. Stults KR, Brown DD, Schug VL, Bean JA. Prehospital defibrillation performed by emergency medical technicians in rural communities. N Engl J Med 1984;310:219–23.

21. McIntyre KM, Lewis AJ, eds. Textbook of advanced cardiac life support. Dallas: American Heart Association, 1983.

22. Standards and guidelines for cardiopulmonary resuscitation (CPR) and emergency cardiac care (ECC). JAMA 1980;24:453–509.

23. Hallstrom AP, Eisenberg MS, Bergner L. The persistence of ventricular fibrillation and its implication for evaluating EMS. Emerg Health Serv Q 1983;1:41–9.

24. Myerburg RJ, Kessler KM, Zaman L, Conde CA, Castellanos A. Survivors of prehospital cardiac arrest. JAMA 1982;247:1485–90.

25. Kellermann AL, Staves DR, Hackman BB. In-hospital resuscitation following unsuccessful prehospital advanced cardiac life support: 'Heroic efforts' or an exercise in futility? Ann Emerg Med 1988;17:589–94.

26. Shimazu S, Shatney CH. Outcomes of trauma patients with no vital signs on hospital admission. J Trauma 1983;23:213–6.

27. O'Rourke PP. Outcome of children who are apneic and pulseless in the emergency room. Crit Care Med 1986;14:466–8.

28. Brett AS, McCullough LB. When patients request specific interventions: defining the limits of the physician's obligation. N Engl J Med 1986;315:1347–51.

29. Blackhall LJ. Must we always use CPR? N Engl J Med 1987;317:1281–5.

30. Law Reform Commission of Canada. Euthanasia, aiding suicide, and cessation of treatment. Ottawa, Ont.: Law Reform Commission of Canada, 1983. (Report 20.)

31. Tomlinson T, Brody H. Ethics and communication in do-not-resuscitate orders. N Engl J Med 1988;318:43–6.

32. Schneiderman LJ, Jecker NS, Jonsen AR. Medical futility: its meaning and ethical implications. Ann Intern Med 1990;112:949–54.

33. Weaver WD, Hill D, Fahrenbruch CE, et al. Use of the automatic external defibrillator in the management of out-of-hospital cardiac arrest. N Engl J Med 1988;319:661–6.

34. Tweed WA, Wilson E. Is CPR on the right track? Can Med Assoc J 1984;131:429–33.

35. Thompson RG, Hallstrom AP, Cobb LA. Bystander-initiated cardiopulmonary resuscitation in the management of ventricular fibrillation. Ann Intern Med 1979;90:437–40.

36. Cummins RO, Eisenberg MS. Prehospital cardiopulmonary resuscitation: is it effective? JAMA 1985;253:2408–12.

13 Friend-of-the-Court Brief for Larry James McAfee

Georgia Man Asks to Turn Off Life-Supporting Ventilator

THE ATLANTA ARCHDIOCESE

At the court's request, the Most Reverend Eugene A. Marino, on behalf of the Roman Catholic Archdiocese of Atlanta (hereinafter the "archdiocese"), hereby submits this amicus brief relating to petitioner's request for declaratory relief. This brief will address both the legal and ecclesiastical positions relevant to the petitioner's request.

BACKGROUND

In his petition, Larry James McAfee informed the court that he is a quadriplegic patient being sustained on a ventilator who, as a result, has "no control over his person and receives no enjoyment out of life" (Petition, Para. 2). He suffered a motorcycle accident on May 5, 1985, and has since been paralyzed from the neck down. His lungs no longer function on their own, and he cannot care for himself. He has petitioned the court for an order allowing him to "turn off his own ventilator by means of a mechanical device operated on a timer, that he be provided with a sedative before turning off said ventilator and, thereafter, that said ventilator not be restarted even though such is a life-sustaining medical treatment" (Petition, Para. 3).

Mr. McAfee contends that he is competent to decide as to his medical treatment, that his living relatives all consent to his request for relief, that he has no dependents, that his condition is irreversible and that "the continued treatment by ventilator merely prolongs petitioner's emotional pain and suffering" (Petition, Para. 9).

This friend-of-the-court brief was reprinted in Origins 19 *(28 September 1989): 273, 275–279.*

On Aug. 16, 1989, the court conducted a bedside hearing with Mr. McAfee, along with attorneys for the Fulton-DeKalb Authority and Grady Hospital, and therein received testimony that confirmed the allegations contained in the petition. Thus, the material facts of this case appear not to be contested.

The sole question before the court appears to be whether Mr. McAfee, a competent adult, has the right to refuse extraordinary medical treatment, without interference from third parties, even though such refusal will likely result in his immediate death. Recognizing the unsettling nature of this question, the archdiocese neither opposes nor advocates Mr. McAfee's petition, but is of the opinion that granting his request would not be assisting in suicide or undermining the state's and the Roman Catholic Church's interest in preserving life. This amicus brief will present and discuss both legal and ecclesiastical authorities on the issue.

I. LEGAL AUTHORITIES

It has been said that "(t)he law always lags behind the most advanced thinking in every area. It must wait until the theologians and the moral leaders and events have created some common ground, some consensus" (Burger, "The Law and Medical Advances," 67 Annals Internal Med. Supp. 7, 15, 17 (1967), quoted in *Superintendent of Belchertown State School vs. Saikewicz*, 373 Mass. 728, 370 N.E. 2d 417, 423 (Mass. 1977). This case represents a morally troubling issue for this court and for society in general. As to this situation, however, the law, the theologians, moral leaders and events have apparently arrived at "some common ground, some consensus."

A. The Constitutional Right to Privacy

As pointed out in Mr. McAfee's brief, virtually every court that has addressed this issue in recent years has found that competent adult patients have the right, both under common law and constitutional bases, to choose to receive either active, aggressive medical treatment, something less than that or no treatment at all. This right includes the right to choose an early death rather than a later one, but does not include taking direct steps to terminate life. *Griswold vs. State of Connecticut*, 381 U.S. 479, 85 S. Ct. 1678 (1965); *Zant vs. Prevatte*, 248 Ga. 832, 286 S.E. 2d 715 (1982); *Kirby vs. Spivey*, 167 Ga. App. 751, 307 S.E. 2d 538 (1983); *Bartling vs. Superior Court*, 163 Cal. App. 3d 186, 209 Cal. Rptr. 220 (1984); *Lane vs. Candura*, 6 Mass. App. 377, 376 N.E. 2d 1232 (1978); *In re: Gardner*, 534 A.2d 947 (Me. 1987); *Satz vs. Perlmutter*, 379 So. 2d 359 (Fla. 1980); *Tune vs. Walter Reed Hospital*, 602 F. Supp. 1452 (D.C. 1985); *In re Farrell*, 108 N.J. 335, 529 A. 2d 404 (1987).

In the landmark case of *Griswold vs. State of Connecticut,* 381 U.S. 479, 85 S. Ct. 1678 (1965), the U.S. Supreme Court expressly recognized a constitutional "penumbral" guarantee of privacy inherent within the Bill of Rights. Specifically, in holding that a Connecticut law forbidding the use of contraceptives unconstitutionally intruded upon the right of marital privacy, the court recognized that the various guarantees inherent in the First, Third, Fourth and Fifth Amendments to the U.S. Constitution created "zones of privacy" (*id.* at 1681), and that this inherent right of privacy and repose is "no less important than any other right carefully and particularly reserved to the people." *Id.* at 1682.

B. Georgia Authorities

Relying on this constitutional right of privacy, Georgia courts have consistently upheld the right of competent individuals to refuse medical care or food, even if such refusal resulted in death. For example, in *Zant vs. Prevatte,* 248 Ga. 832, 286 S.E. 2d 715 (1982), the superintendent of the Georgia Diagnostic and Classification Center in Butts County petitioned the court for an order authorizing him to impose medical examinations upon a prison inmate against his will "and, if necessary, to force-feed Prevatte to prevent his death." *Id.* at 832. The court found that Mr. Prevatte was sane and rational and that "without food, Prevatte would die within three weeks, sooner if no liquid is taken." *Id.* at 833. It nevertheless concluded that "the state has no right to monitor this man's physical condition against his will; neither does it have the right to feed him to prevent his death from starvation if that is his wish." *Id.* at 834.

Later, in *Kirby vs. Spivey,* 167 Ga. App. 751, 307 S.E. 2d 538 (1983), the heirs of a decedent, Mr. Echols, sued a nursing home and the attending physician, Dr. Spivey, claiming that Mr. Echols' death resulted from Dr. Spivey's malpractice in failing "to diagnose and treat Mr. Echols for renal failure and cancer of the prostate, the conditions alleged to have ultimately led to his death." *Id.* at 751. Prior to his death, Mr. Echols was lucid and, in Dr. Spivey's opinion, "entirely capable of making a rational decision to decline treatment." *Id.* He had no wife or children, and his other relatives never visited him. According to Dr. Spivey, Mr. Echols, upon learning of his illness, refused to authorize further diagnostic testing and treatment and eventually died. The court first turned to the language of O.C.G.A., Sec. 31-9-7, which provides that a person 18 years of age or over has a right "to refuse to consent to medical and surgical treatment as to his own person." It then concluded as a matter of law that "a lucid adult has the right to withhold his consent to suggested and recommended medical procedures" and that "a patient, by virtue of his right of privacy, can refuse to allow intrusion on his person, even though calculated to preserve his life." *Id.* at 753.

The case of *In re L.H.R.*, 253 Ga. 439, 321 S.E. 2d 716 (1984), involved a petition for declaratory relief as to whether life-support systems could be removed from a terminally ill infant. In again upholding an individual's right to decline treatment, the court first noted that "in Georgia, as elsewhere, a competent adult patient has the right to refuse medical treatment in the absence of conflicting state interest." *Id.* at 722. It then went on to address the "narrow question" as to "who may exercise this right on behalf of a terminally ill infant who is in a chronic vegetative state with no reasonable possibility of attaining cognitive function." *Id.* The court concluded that "the decision whether to end the dying process is a personal decision for family members or those who bear a legal responsibility for the patient." *Id.* at 723.

Effective July 1, 1984, the Georgia General Assembly enacted the Living Wills Act, O.C.G.A. Sec. 31-32-1 *et seq.*, in which it expressly recognized "the right of a competent adult person to make a written directive, known as a living will, instructing his physician to withhold or withdraw life-sustaining procedures in the event of a terminal condition." Although confined to patients who are certified by two physicians as having a "terminal condition" (defined as those having "no reasonable expectation for improvement" and facing imminent death), the statute expressly recognizes "the dignity and privacy which patients have a right to expect" O.C.G.A. Sec. 31-32-1(d). Thus, Georgia law and Georgia courts recognize the personal right of a lucid adult to refuse medical treatment, even if he is not terminally ill and even if such refusal will result in his death.

C. Authorities From Other Jurisdictions

As pointed out in the petitioner's brief, other jurisdictions have likewise upheld the right of non-terminally ill competent adults to refuse medical treatment. In *Bartling vs. Superior Court*, 163 Cal. App. 3d 186, 209 Cal. Rptr. 220 (1984), the California Court of Appeals upheld the right of a non-terminally ill patient to disconnect his ventilator, a situation virtually identical to this:

"In short, the law recognizes the individual interest in preserving the inviolability of the person. . . . The constitutional right of privacy guarantees to the individual the freedom to choose to reject, or refuse to consent to, intrusions of his bodily integrity." *Id.* at 225.

Likewise, in *Lane vs. Candura*, 6 Mass. App. 377, 376 N.E. 2d 1232 (1978), the court, in upholding the right of a patient to refuse amputation of a gangrenous leg, stated:

"The constitutional right to privacy, as we conceive it, is an expression of the sanctity of individual free choice and self-determination as fundamental constituents of life. The value of life as so perceived is lessened not by a decision to refuse treatment, but by the failure to allow a competent human being the right of choice." *Id.* at 1233.

D. Medical Authorities

Finally, experts on medical ethics appear to have arrived at a consensus as to a competent patient's right to decline medical treatment under virtually all situations. A 1983 report from the President's Commission for the Study of Ethical Problems in Medicine and Biomedical and Behavior Research concluded, in part:

"(T)he voluntary choice of a competent and informed patient should determine whether or not life-sustaining therapy will be undertaken, just as such choices provide the bases for other decisions about medical treatment. . . . Healthcare professionals serve patients best by maintaining a presumption in favor of sustaining life, while recognizing that competent patients are entitled to choose to forgo any treatments, including those that sustain life." *Deciding to Forgo Life-Sustaining Treatment,* at pp. 3, 5 (U.S. Govt. Printing Office, 1983).

Likewise, the American Hospital Association policy and statement of patients' choices of treatment options, approved by the AHA in 1985, provided in pertinent part: "Whenever possible, however, the authority to determine the course of treatment, if any, should rest with the patient," and "the right to choose treatment includes the right to refuse a specific treatment or all treatment."

Finally, the Council on Ethical and Judicial Affairs of the American Medical Association adopted a statement on March 15, 1986, titled "Withholding or Withdrawing Life-Prolonging Medical Treatment" that provided in relevant part that "the social commitment of the physician is to sustain life and relieve suffering. Where the performance of one duty conflicts with the other, the choice of the patient, or his family or legal representative, if the patient is incompetent to act on his own behalf, should prevail."

E. Countervailing State Interests

The legal right to refuse medical treatment is not absolute, however, and can in certain circumstances be limited by one of several countervailing state interests. These overriding interests can include: 1) the preservation of life in general (discussed in *Superintendent of Belchertown State School vs. Saikewicz,* 373 Mass. 728, 370 N.E. 2d 417, 423–427 (Mass. 1977); 2) the prevention of suicide (See *Erickson vs. Dilgard,* 44 Misc. 2d. 27, 252 N.Y.S. 2d 705 [N.Y. Sup. Ct. 1962]); 3) the protection of innocent third persons, such as dependent children (See *Holmes vs. Silver Cross Hosp. of Joliet, Ill.,* 340 F. Supp. 125 (N.D. Ill. 1972); and 4) the preservation of the medical profession's integrity. See Ezekiel J. Emanuel, "A

Review of the Ethical and Legal Aspects of Terminating Medical Care," 84 Am. J. Med. 291 (1988). In this case, however, none of these counter-vailing state interests appears to be applicable or overriding.

In *Jefferson vs. Griffin-Spaulding County Hospital Authority*, 247 Ga. 86, 274 S.E. 2d 457 (1981), the Georgia Supreme Court found that "an expectant mother in the last weeks of pregnancy lacks the right to refuse necessary life-saving surgery and medical treatment where the life of the unborn child is at stake." *Id.* at 90. Thus, in that case, the state's interest in the life of the unborn child outweighed the mother's right to refuse life-sustaining medical treatment. Here, however, Mr. McAfee has no dependent children and, as noted by Justice Hill, "a competent adult does have the right to refuse necessary life-saving surgery and medical treatment (i.e., has the right to die) where no state interest other than saving the life of the patient is involved." *Id.* at 89–90.

F. Refusing Treatment vs. Suicide

Neither the U.S. Constitution nor common law provides an individual with the right to commit suicide, and no court, to date, has authorized anyone or any entity to take direct steps to terminate life. As a matter of civil law, however, several states have held that "declining life-sustaining medical treatment may not properly be viewed as an attempt to commit suicide." *Brophy vs. New England Sinai Hospital Inc.*, 398 Mass. 417, 439, 497 N.E. 2d 626, 638 (1986). Rather: "Refusing medical intervention merely allows the disease to take its natural course; if death were eventually to occur, it would be the result, primarily, of the underlying disease and not the result of self-inflicted injury." *Id.*

In *Brophy*, the petitioning patient was not terminally ill, although he was rendered incompetent as a result of a ruptured aneurysm. Acting on Mr. Brophy's behalf, his wife requested that the hospital stop feeding her husband by way of gastronomy tube. *Id.* at 422, 497 N.E. 2d at 628. The court found that removing the feeding tube merely allowed the patient's body to follow its natural course, *id.* at 439, 497 N.E. 2d at 638, and rejected the state's argument that the discontinuance of medical treatment constituted suicide.

Similarly, in *Bartling vs. Superior Court*, 163 Cal. App. 3d 186, 209 Cal. Rptr. 220 (1984), the California Court of Appeals found that disconnecting a ventilator on a patient did not assist him in committing suicide, but "merely have hastened his inevitable death by natural causes" 163 Cal. App. 3d 196, 209 Cal. Rptr. 225 (1984). Finally, in the case of *In re Gardner*, 534 A.2d 947 (Me. 1987), the court found that in allowing a patient's ventilator to be disconnected, "the cause of his death will not be his refusal of care but rather his accident and his resulting medical condition, including his inability to (breathe on his own)." *Id.* at 956.

Thus, the legal and medical authorities seem to be in agreement that:

1) Competent adult patients have the right to refuse medical treatment or intrusions on their persons, even if such refusal will likely result in death.

2) This right exists whether the patient is terminally ill or not; and

3) If death occurs, it results from the underlying disease or injury and not from the refusal of care.

II. Ecclesiastical Authorities

This brief will focus on the basic principles which underlie Roman Catholic tradition relative to the artificial prolongation of life. On June 26, 1980, the Vatican Congregation for the Doctrine of the Faith issued a declaration on euthanasia which was approved by His Holiness Pope John Paul II and which represents the official position of the church. The declaration, which is a definitive statement, represents a compilation based on writings and opinions from theological ethicists of the Roman Catholic faith over many centuries and therefore effectively presents what might be described as a universal ecclesiastical consensus on the subject.

A. The Sanctity of Life

The Roman Catholic Church views life as "a gift of God's love, which (believers) are called upon to preserve and make fruitful." "Declaration on Euthanasia," p. 3. In light of this view, "intentionally causing one's own death or suicide is therefore equally as wrong as murder; such an action on the part of a person is to be considered as a rejection of God's sovereignty and loving plan." Id.

Nevertheless, one must clearly distinguish suicide from the sacrifice of one's life whereby for a higher cause, such as God's glory, the salvation of souls or the service of one's brethren, a person offers his or her own life and puts it in danger. Id. In this case, it does not appear that Mr. McAfee seeks to commit suicide.

B. The Physician's Obligation to His Patient

The obligation to preserve or prolong life ultimately resides with the patient. If a mentally competent patient decides not to prolong his life, however, a conflict may arise between the patient and his physician. In such a case:

"The obligation of the physician, therefore, is to do nothing to the patient without first informing the patient of what he thinks should be done, with the significant alternatives (including doing nothing), and the probable risks and benefits of each. . . . The doctor's right and responsibility extends only to informing the patient truthfully about his or her terminal condition and the possible ways in which this can be handled medically. The choice among these is the patient's, although this choice cannot be made prudently without honest and substantially complete medical information." *Moral Responsibility in Prolonging Life Decisions,* Pope John Center, St. Louis, 1981, p. 120.

In making his decision, it is essential that the patient be fully informed and understand the consequences of his decision:

"In numerous cases, the complexity of the situation can be such as to cause doubts about the way ethical principles should be applied. In the final analysis, it pertains to the conscience either of the sick person, or those qualified to speak in the sick person's name, or the doctor's to decide in the light of moral obligations and of the various aspects of the case." "Declaration on Euthanasia," Congregation for the Doctrine of the Faith, June 26, 1980, p. 8.

C. Ordinary vs. Extraordinary Treatment

From the perspective of moral theology, there are two major categories of treatment: ordinary and extraordinary. A patient is obligated to accept the former, but may decline the latter if he, in his informed capacity, so chooses. The competent patient (mentally, emotionally and psychologically) is the one to decide whether a medical treatment is ordinary or extraordinary, and his informed, subjective decision should not be subject to interference or criticism.

The two categories are not specifically defined in the "Declaration on Euthanasia," but moral theologians have compiled their own definitions which are helpful. Thus, *ordinary* means of preserving life "are those means commonly used in given circumstances, which this individual in his present physical, psychological and economic condition can reasonably employ with definite hope of proportionate benefit." Cronin, Daniel, "The Moral Law in Regard to the Ordinary and Extraordinary Means of Conserving Life" (dissertation, Pontifical Gregorian University), Rome, 1958, pp. 127–28. On the other hand, *extraordinary* means of preserving life are "those not commonly used in given circumstances, or those means in common use which this individual in his present physical, psychological and economic condition cannot reasonably employ, or if he can, will not give him hope of proportionate benefit." *Id.* at 128.

Thus, the category in which a particular treatment falls is necessarily judged by subjective criteria on a case-by-case basis. A means of preserving life may be deemed ordinary for one patient, but extraordinary for another, depending on the patient's particular physical, psychological or economic condition at the time of his perception of the "hope of proportionate benefit" resulting from the treatment.

In making his decision, the patient must focus on a number of questions:

1. What sort of treatment is proposed/ongoing?
2. What degree of complexity or risk is involved?
3. What is the cost and availability of the treatment?
4. Taking into account the state of the patient, including his physical, psychological and economic resources, what result can be hoped for by employing the proposed/ongoing treatment?

D. Ecclesiastical Guidelines

The "Declaration on Euthanasia" provides the following clarifications when reviewing these difficult questions:

> If there are no other sufficient remedies, it is permitted, with the patient's consent, to have recourse to the means provided by the most advanced medical techniques, even if these means are still at the experimental stage and are not without a certain risk. By accepting them, the patient can even show generosity in the service of humanity.
>
> It is also permitted, with the patient's consent, to interrupt these means where the results fall short of expectations. But for such a decision to be made, account will have to be taken of the reasonable wishes of the patient's family, as also of the advice of the doctors who are specially competent in the matter. The latter may in particular judge that the investment in instruments and personnel is disproportionate to the results foreseen; they may also judge that the techniques applied impose on the patient strain or suffering out of proportion with the benefits which he or she may gain from such techniques.
>
> It is also permissible to make do with the normal means that medicine can offer. Therefore one cannot impose on anyone the obligation to have recourse to a technique which is already in use, but which carries a risk or is burdensome. Such refusal is not the equivalent of suicide; on the contrary, it should be considered as an acceptance of the human condition or a wish to avoid the application of a medical procedure disproportionate to the results that can be expected or a desire not to impose excessive expense on the family or the community.
>
> When inevitable death is imminent in spite of the means used, it is permitted in conscience to take the decision to refuse forms of treatment that would only secure a precarious and burdensome prolongation of life, so long as the normal care due to the sick person in similar cases is not interrupted. In

such circumstances, the doctor has no reason to reproach himself with failing to help the person in danger.

"Declaration on Euthanasia," pp. 9–10.

In its conclusion, the "Declaration on Euthanasia" states that "life is
a gift of God, and on the other hand, death is unavoidable; it is necessary
therefore that we, without in any way hastening the hour of death,
should be able to accept it with full responsibility and dignity." *Id.* at 11.

Here, Mr. McAfee has testified that as a result of his present condition and his treatment he "receives no enjoyment out of life" (Petition,
Para. 2), his "continued treatment by ventilator merely prolongs (his)
emotional pain and suffering (Petition, Para. 9), he is currently without
economic resources and is being maintained by public funds (Transcript,
pp. 10–11); he has discussed his wishes with his family, who consent to
his request (Transcript pp. 21–23), he is "still in a lot of pain" (Transcript,
p. 18), his condition is irreversible (Transcript, p. 29), and "there is
nothing to look forward to" (Transcript p. 18). Applying the subjective
criteria presented by (Bishop) Daniel Cronin to Mr. McAfee's situation,
the ventilator, as applied to Mr. McAfee to prolong his life, clearly constitutes an "extraordinary means of preserving life."

Based on the facts as set forth above as well as the basic principles
which outline Catholic tradition relative to the artificial prolongation of
life, it is the position of the Archdiocese of Atlanta that the patient, Mr.
McAfee, has the right under ecclesiastical law either to continue his present treatment or to interrupt that treatment even though such interrup-
tion will end in death.

E. Use of Painkillers When Refusing Medical Treatment

Mr. McAfee has requested that he be given a sedative before he
activates a timer which will turn off his ventilator. In the opinion of the
archdiocese, this request is irrelevant to Mr. McAfee's and this court's
decision in this case. The Roman Catholic Church recognizes that while
physical suffering is an unavoidable element of the human condition, "it
often exceeds its own biological usefulness and so can become so severe
as to cause the desire to remove it at any cost." "Declaration on Euthanasia," p. 6.

The Roman Catholic Church teaches:

"(I)t would be imprudent to impose a heroic way of acting as a general rule. On the contrary, human and Christian prudence suggest for
the majority of sick people the use of medicines capable of alleviating
or suppressing pain, even though these may cause as a secondary effect
semiconsciousness and reduced lucidity." *Id.* at 7.

Thus, Mr. McAfee's request for sedation is not offensive to the Roman Catholic Church.

CONCLUSION

The archdiocese is submitting this brief to be used as guidance for addressing a difficult and unsettling issue. The archdiocese takes no official position as to whether the relief requested by Mr. McAfee should or should not be granted. The consensus of legal, theological and moralistic authorities, however, supports Mr. McAfee's right to refuse further treatment by ventilator, and such refusal in this case would not be the equivalent of suicide. Rather, it can be considered as Mr. McAfee's acceptance of his condition, his wish to avoid the application of a medical procedure disproportionate to the expected results and his desire not to impose excessive expense on his family and the community at large.

14 *Living Wills: Past, Present, and Future*

EZEKIEL J. EMANUEL, M.D. AND LINDA L. EMANUEL, M.D.

Ezekiel Emanuel, M.D. is an oncologist and medical ethicist at Harvard Medical School. Linda Emanuel, M.D. is the Assistant Director of Medical Ethics and is in the Department of Medicine at Harvard Medical School.

The living will was first proposed more than 20 years ago. In the first decade after proposal, it was not adopted by any state. However, in the years following the *Quinlan* decision,[1] the living will was widely endorsed as the model document for advance care and the solution to the medical-ethical problems of terminating life-sustaining interventions. During these same years, deficiencies in the living will became apparent. Yet there were few attempts either to revise the living will or to replace it with a more useful advance care document. Recently, efforts have shifted from criticism to substantive reform; new approaches to remedy the problems of living wills are likely to produce a more useful advance care document.

In this article, we aim to review the current state of advance care documents. First, we will distinguish between advance care documents and living wills. Second, we will review the history of living wills. Third, we will examine the deficiencies of existing living wills. Fourth, we will consider recent revisions and replacements for living wills. Finally, we will consider the future of advance care documents and propose areas for additional inquiry.

DEFINITIONS

Until recently, living wills and advance care documents were thought to be one and the same, terms to be used interchangeably. Some use *living will* as a "generic term."[2] Living wills and advance care documents are,

---

This article first appeared in The Journal of Clinical Ethics 1 *(Spring 1990): 9–19.*

however, distinct concepts. To avoid confusion and errors, it is best to distinguish between the two.

Advance care document is the generic term for a general category of documents. Advance care documents are general statements of a patient's preferences regarding the medical interventions to be implemented if he or she becomes incompetent. Consequently, these documents request particular types of interventions while refusing others. There are many kinds of advance care documents; some may refer to specific conditions, such as persistent vegetative state; some may appoint a proxy decision maker; others may be general declarations of values without reference to specific medical interventions; still others may be requests that everything possible be done. Advance care documents need *not* be restricted to statements concerning life-sustaining procedures and they need not pertain only to the person who is dying. In this sense, advance care documents are not necessarily "natural death statements" or requests for a "right to die." Conversely, living wills are restricted to rejecting life-sustaining medical interventions, usually, although not exclusively, when a person is terminally ill.[3] For this reason, living wills might be called a "rejectionist" advance care document.

Advance care documents and living wills have been considered synonymous by historical accident: Living wills were the first type of advance care document to gain widespread public support. But other types of advance care documents have been proposed, for instance, the Directive for Maximum Care.[4] And recently the authors have published the Medical Directive,[5] an advance care document that is not a living will. As we shall see, the progress in statements of patient preferences regarding medical interventions has been characterized by a shift from living wills to other types of advance care documents. In the next sections, we recount the history of living wills and the deficiencies that have stimulated creation of other types of advance care documents.

THE HISTORY OF THE LIVING WILL

The historical record shows that the widespread enactment of living will laws has been a very recent phenomenon. While living will laws have been proposed for more than two decades, and while the first one was passed more than 13 years ago, 75 percent of the laws have been adopted since 1982 and almost 50 percent in the past four years.

In 1967, at a Euthanasia Society of America meeting (the forerunner of the Society for the Right to Die and Concern for Dying), the living will was proposed as an advance care document by which an individual could specify his or her wish to terminate life-sustaining medical interventions. The next year, Walter Sackett, a Florida physician and state

Table 1.   History of the Enactment of Living Will Laws

Years	No. of States Enacting Laws This Year	Cumulative
1976	1	1
1977	7	8
1979–1981	3	11
1982–1984	12	23
1985–1986	16	39
1987–1989	2	41

legislator, introduced legislation to recognize the living will.[6] Like similar efforts in other states, Dr. Sackett's legislation failed.

Not until 1976 did the fate of living will legislation change. The difference was the *Quinlan* case.[1] Publicity surrounding this case alerted the general public to the possibility that physicians could prolong the lives of patients who lack—and have no hope of regaining—higher mental functioning. This realization led to a strong consensus in favor of permitting individuals to specify their wishes regarding life-sustaining medical interventions before they became comatose. Consequently, California passed the first natural death act in September 1976, recognizing living wills. In 1977, living will laws were introduced in 42 states and enacted in seven (see Table 1).[2]

In 1978, however, momentum for living will laws waned and the rate of enactment slowed. Between 1982 and 1984, interest in living wills was rekindled by two events. The first was the push to permit the termination of artificial nutrition and hydration[7,8] and the second was the landmark *Conroy* decision,[9] which legalized the termination of artificial nutrition and hydration under some circumstances. As Table 1 demonstrates, there ensued a rush of states enacting living will legislation between 1982 and 1986. In addition, six other states revised or replaced living will laws that had been enacted before 1980.[2] Since 1986, two more states have adopted living will laws. And in some states that lack legislatively enacted living will laws, such as New Jersey, the courts have ruled that living wills are legally binding expressions of patient preferences and must be respected.

EXISTING LIVING WILLS

Not all living wills are the same. Each state's law codifies a slightly different text, and individuals have modified the actual text of standard forms. Nevertheless, during the past two decades, several living wills have served as models for either public distribution or legislative enact-ment. To understand the deficiencies of living wills, it is important to consider the actual text of three influential living wills (see Figure 1).

The original document from Concern for Dying has been distrib-uted to almost 10 million people and is probably the single most recog-nized and available living will. The original California Natural Death Act, adopted in September 1976, has been important because of its precedent value as the first living will law adopted. The third prominent living will comes from the 1985 National Conference of Commissioners on Uni-form State Laws, which drafted a model living will law, the Uniform Rights of the Terminally Ill Act. This uniform act has been adopted *in toto* or in part by at least seven states.

Each living will contains two operative clauses: 1) the condition of the patient that determines when medical interventions should be with-drawn and 2) the types of medical interventions that can be withdrawn. These are emphasized in Figure 1.

Concern for Dying
If at such a time the situation should arise in which there is *no reasonable expectation of my recovery from extreme physical or mental disability,* I direct that I be allowed to die and not be kept alive by *medications, artificial means or "heroic measures."*

California Natural Death Act
If at any time I should have *an incurable injury, disease, or illness cer-tified to be a terminal condition* by two physicians, and where the application of life-sustaining procedures would serve only to arti-ficially prolong the moment of my death and where my physician determines that my death is imminent whether or not *life sustaining procedures* are utilized, I direct that such procedures be withheld or withdrawn and that I be permitted to die naturally.

Uniform Rights of the Terminally Ill Act
If I should have *an incurable or irreversible condition that will cause my death within a relatively short time,* and I am no longer able to make decisions regarding my medical treatment, I direct my attending physician, pursuant to the Uniform Rights of the Terminally Ill Act of this State, to withhold or withdraw *treatment that only prolongs the process of dying and is not necessary to my comfort or to alleviate pain.*

Figure 1.   Prominent Living Wills

DEFICIENCIES OF EXISTING LIVING WILLS

Examination of the prominent living wills presented in Figure 1 suggests four important deficiencies of living wills: 1) They pertain only to the termination of medical treatments; 2) they tend to apply to terminally ill patients; 3) they are vague in defining the patient's condition; and 4) they are vague in delineating interventions to be withheld.

First, existing living wills concentrate on *terminating* medical interventions. Living wills profess to permit "adult person[s] to control decisions regarding administration of life-sustaining treatment."[10] Unfortunately, the only control living wills facilitate is a rejection of medical treatments; they contain no suggestion that patients specify medical treatments they might want maintained.

Second, existing living wills tend to apply only to terminally ill patients. Clearly the living will statements contained in both the California Natural Death Act and the Uniform Rights of the Terminally Ill Act apply only to terminally ill patients (see Figure 1). While the language of the Concern for Dying living will does not require the patient to be terminally ill, Concern for Dying's explanation of living wills states that "a Living Will is a signed, dated and witnessed document which allows you to state *in advance* your wishes regarding the use of life-sustaining procedures when you are dying."[3]

More importantly, the living will laws adopted by at least 35 states require medical certification of a patient's terminal condition before the document can be executed. The living wills enacted by most states contain language concerning the patient's condition that is identical or similar to the California Natural Death Act. States define *terminal* differently. Some states, such as Arkansas, have qualified the terminal condition requirement to include permanently unconscious patients; however, other states, such as Connecticut, Missouri, Oklahoma, Tennessee, and Texas, maintain that a terminal patient must have "an incurable condition . . . which within reasonable medical judgment would produce death regardless of the application of life-sustaining procedures."[11]

The requirement that a patient be dying *regardless* of the application of medical interventions before the living will becomes effective has prompted some to ask whether living wills are more "help or hindrance."[12] The terminally ill requirement also limits the utility of living wills by limiting the number of eligible patients. For example, Karen Quinlan was not terminally ill when her father requested withdrawal of her respirator. As some commentators have noted, Quinlan, and most patients in a persistent vegetative state or with other permanent medical deficits, do not suffer from a disease that will lead to their death regardless of medical interventions. A physician from Idaho vividly documented how this requirement prevented him from removing the ventilator from an 84-year-old woman who became semicomatose after an operation.[13]

Quinlan and most incompetent patients are *hopelessly* ill; they do not suffer from a disease process that will kill them and they are not necessarily dependent upon medical interventions. Instead, they may require few and minor interventions and may require these interventions only episodically. Nevertheless, they are hopelessly ill because medical interventions cannot reverse their mental disabilities but can only maintain their biological existence.[14] Many believe it should be permissible for patients to request termination of medical interventions when they are hopelessly ill, even if they are not terminally ill.

The third deficiency of living wills is that they are vague in characterizing the state the patient must be in before the living will can be implemented. For instance, in the Concern for Dying living will, care is to be stopped when "there is no reasonable expectation of recovery from extreme physical or mental disability." Obviously, this phrase is open to a multitude of interpretations. The New York case of *Evans v. Bellevue Hospital*[15] illustrates this point well. A patient with acquired immunodeficiency syndrome-related complex (ARC) who developed toxoplasmosis and became stuporous had a living will that stated the following:

> I direct that life-sustaining procedures should be withheld or withdrawn if I have an illness, disease or experience mental deterioration such that there is no reasonable expectation of recovering or regaining a meaningful quality-of-life.[15]

There arose a conflict between the Bellevue Hospital administration and the patient's friend about whether his condition—ARC with toxoplasmosis and stupor—constituted irreversible mental deterioration with no reasonable expectation of recovering a meaningful quality of life. Some observers believed the patient could recover a meaningful quality of life since with treatment for the toxoplasmosis he would probably regain full consciousness even if he were not cured of ARC. Others argued that the patient's ARC ruled out the possibility of his ever regaining a meaningful quality of life. Unfortunately, the vagueness of the living will engenders such conflicting interpretations.

A fourth shortcoming of living wills is that they are vague in delineating the types of medical interventions to be terminated. The Concern for Dying living will requests that "medications, artificial means, or 'heroic measures'" be terminated. The President's Commission[16] and many state supreme courts[9] have long maintained that concepts such as "artificial means" and "heroic measures" have "too many conflicting meanings" to offer physicians, patients, and others suitable guidance in terminating life-sustaining medical treatments.

Other living wills request the termination of "life-sustaining procedures" or "treatments that only prolong the process of dying." These phrases are no more specific. Indeed, it has taken many legal battles just to clarify whether or not nutrition and hydration through intravenous lines or gastrostomy tubes constitute life-sustaining procedures. While most states have included these under the heading of life-sustaining treatments, others have not. Clearly, these terms are vague and open to a wide range of interpretations, making it difficult to apply living wills.

These four deficiencies of living wills—their restriction to the termination of care, their restriction to terminal patients, their vagueness regarding the patient's condition, and their vagueness regarding interventions to be withheld—have limited their usefulness. Despite the widespread support for living wills, they are hardly ever used in clinical practice. Indeed, most practicing physicians have rarely encountered them.[17]

REPLACEMENT AND REVISION OF LIVING WILLS

The recognition of these deficiencies has prompted two types of responses: the replacement and the revision of existing living wills.

The first response has been to supplant living wills and advance care documents with proxy decision makers. Many physicians feel, for instance, that written living wills were too vague and imprecise to guide their judgments for incompetent patients in particular cases, and they have urged the use of proxies instead. A 1979 *New England Journal of Medicine* editorial[18] called legislation to permit the appointment of proxies a "sensible living will" because it replaced abstract, rigid, and imprecise documents with people who are cognizant of the nuances of each individual case and can thus make informed choices.

Many states have followed this view in recent years. More than 10 states have attached proxy decision-maker clauses or sections to their living will laws. Twenty-one other states have specifically authorized the use of the durable power-of-attorney for the termination of life-sustaining medical treatments.[19] All other states have general durable power-of-attorney laws. Recently, the New Jersey Supreme Court upheld the use of such laws to appoint a proxy for terminating medical interventions.[20] Rulings in other state supreme courts seem to concur with this view.[21] Finally, a year ago, Concern for Dying issued a revised version of its living will that included a section for a durable power-of-attorney for health care decisions to supplement the standard document.

Using proxy decision makers, either with existing living wills or without any specific indications of the incompetent person's wishes, does not resolve the difficulties associated with living wills but is in fact likely to compound them. In particular, although a proxy decision maker may be related to the patient, he or she may never have discussed terminal care decisions with the patient. And even when proxy decision makers have had such discussions, they are likely to be expressed in the same vague terms that plague the living will.[22] The consequence of such proxy decision making is less likely to be an expression of the patient's preferences than an expression of the proxy's preferences for the patient. Indeed, an empirical study of elderly patients, their spouses, and physicians and nurses revealed that these potential proxies had a strikingly poor ability to predict correctly the patient's wishes regarding resuscitation.[23] Finally, there are no data to suggest that proxies either reflect the patient's views or are even willing to accept responsibility for choosing to withdraw, withhold, or continue life-sustaining medical interventions for incompetent patients. In fact, a general survey[24] indicated that people are less willing to terminate medical interventions for their relatives than for themselves. Proxies have been advocated less because of their proven usefulness than because of the deficiencies of living wills. Yet there is little reason to think that proxy decision makers will solve the problems of existing living wills.

A second response has been to revise existing living wills, especially by specifying the types of interventions to be terminated. Even before a single living will law had been enacted, Sissela Bok suggested that the living will proposed by Concern for Dying was "vague in such a way that real risks of misinterpretation arise."[25] A main focus of her remedy was to specify the medical interventions to be terminated: surgery, resuscitation, mechanical ventilation, intensive care services, antibiotics, blood products, and other life-prolonging procedures. Bok's revision was an improvement over the Concern for Dying living will because it specified the types of interventions to be withheld. It thus reduced much of the vagueness related to the interventions to be terminated. Nevertheless, it perpetuated many of the other deficiencies of the living will. First, it remained a "rejectionist" advance care document. All interventions were lumped together and rejected; no space was granted for specifying interventions to be requested or tried. Second, the list of interventions was incomplete because dialysis and artificial nutrition and hydration were not mentioned.

Within the past few months, Concern for Dying has devised a more specific version of its living will.[26] The operative section of the document reads as follows:

*If I am permanently unconscious or there is no reasonable expectation
of my recovery from a seriously incapacitating or lethal illness or condition, I do not wish to be kept alive by artificial means.* I request that
I be given all care necessary to keep me comfortable and free of
pain, even if pain-relieving medications may hasten my death,
and I direct that no life-sustaining treatment be provided except as I or my surrogate specifically authorize.

Many of the criticisms of the original living will apply to this revised one.
However, the patient is informed that "optional specific provisions" may
be added to increase the specificity of the document, especially by listing
particular interventions to be rejected. On an overlay are the following
instructions:

You may wish to add specific statements to the Living Will in
the space provided for that purpose. Such statements might
concern:
  • Cardiopulmonary resuscitation
  • Artificial or invasive measures for providing
    nutrition and hydration
  • Kidney dialysis
  • Mechanical or artificial respiration
  • Blood transfusions
  • Surgery (such as amputation)
  • Antibiotics

This list of specific interventions is clearly an improvement. Unfortunately, it does not appear in the document itself, and thus many people
who use the living will are unlikely to specify the interventions they do
not want. Furthermore, it can be anticipated that placing the specific
interventions on an overlay to be completed by the patient will probably
create a whole new set of problems in implementing the patient's
wishes. For instance, we can imagine a patient particularly concerned
about resuscitation and dialysis because he or she has a relative who
endured these interventions. The patient might specify preferences
against these interventions but not against others. When the living will is
to be implemented, what is the significance of the failure to list specific
interventions? Does the absence of antibiotics on a list of rejected interventions mean that the patient actually desires such an intervention? Are
physicians and others to consider patient silence an error, an oversight,
or intentional?

As noted, most attempts at reforming existing living wills have concentrated on eliminating the vagueness surrounding the types of inter-

ventions to be terminated. Unfortunately, the other deficiencies of living wills—their rejectionist character and their vagueness regarding the patient's condition—have not been corrected.

THE MEDICAL DIRECTIVE

To remedy the four major deficiencies of existing living wills and thereby to create a more comprehensive and useful advance care document, we recently proposed the Medical Directive (see the appendix).[5] We can delineate how the Medical Directive overcomes each of the deficiencies.

First, the Medical Directive is not a living will because it is not rejectionist. Instead, as the introduction declares, "the Medical Directive states a person's wishes for or against types of medical interventions." This position is put into practice in the Medical Directive because there is not just a "do not want" option attached to each intervention, but patients are also able to choose whether they "want," "do not want," "want a trial," or are "undecided" about a particular intervention. Furthermore, the Medical Directive recognizes that patient preferences may vary depending upon clinical circumstances. Consequently, patients are asked to indicate their preferences in four different scenarios, and the preferences for treatment need not be the same for each one. These choices allow patients to control—not just to reject—decisions regarding medical interventions.

Second, the Medical Directive does not only apply to terminally ill patients. The Medical Directive is organized with four paradigmatic scenarios describing a patient's condition. In only one of the scenarios (Situation C) is the patient described as terminally ill. The other three scenarios describe hopelessly ill patients who have varying degrees of mental deficits, from persistent vegetative state to significant dementia, but no illness or disease that will bring about death within a short time regardless of medical interventions.

Third, the Medical Directive characterizes the patient's condition in specific language. Rather than "extreme physical or mental disability," the Medical Directive outlines four different scenarios: 1) a patient in a persistent vegetative state, 2) a comatose patient with a small but uncertain chance of recovery, 3) a terminally ill, significantly demented patient lacking the capacity to recognize people or speak understandably, and 4) a significantly demented patient without a terminal illness. These scenarios are the most relevant to the physician because they encompass the spectrum of mental incompetence and also the principal circumstances that confront physicians and have prompted court battles.

Of course, these scenarios are not unambiguous; there can never be absolute clarity. There is what might be called medical vagueness, the uncertainty inherent in the practice of medicine. The accumulated knowledge of the medical profession rarely permits precise predictions for any individual about the course of his or her disease. When physicians state that a patient has a "small and uncertain chance" of recovery from a coma, they are not being evasive or cautious; medical knowledge simply does not permit any more specific statement. Such uncertainty is often annoying to physicians, patients, and families. Nevertheless, it is irreducible and forms the setting of medical practice and the human condition. The Medical Directive cannot eliminate this medical vagueness but does clarify the linguistic vagueness that plagues other living wills.

Fourth, the Medical Directive eliminates the vagueness regarding medical interventions. The document lists 12 interventions and asks patients to indicate their preferences regarding these interventions in each of the four paradigmatic scenarios. The list aims to be comprehensive by eliciting preferences concerning the medical interventions likely to be administered to incompetent patients as well as those interventions that have provoked legal conflicts. In this way the Medical Directive replaces "artificial means and heroic measures," providing a more comprehensive list of interventions than previous reforms, which listed only five or seven specific interventions.[27] Furthermore, unlike previous advance care documents, the Medical Directive provides a brief explanation of each intervention to ensure that patients understand what they are being asked.

The Medical Directive also aims to be a more comprehensive advance care document. To this end, it combines into one document a durable power-of-attorney section and the section for eliciting patient preferences. It also recognizes that there may be conflicts between proxy decisions and the patient's stated preferences and requests that the patient indicate which will have final authority. In addition, the Medical Directive recognizes that many patients' views about the end of life go beyond specifying what interventions they might want; for example, a patient may wish to specify that his or her organs not be made available for donation. Again, by eliciting preferences on organ donation, the Medical Directive aims at providing patients with the opportunity to control their fate at the end of life. Also, the Medical Directive's introduction informs patients that the decisions to be made are of a "personal, philosophical, and religious" nature. It suggests that the patient consider the types of medical conditions that would make life intolerable and discuss these terminal care issues with his or her "family, friends, and religious mentor." These suggestions are combined with a section in which the patient may make a personal statement.

Finally, and most importantly, the Medical Directive attempts to incorporate the issues related to the termination of medical interventions into the physician-patient relationship. Previous living wills have been developed and propagated by right to die advocacy groups, lawyers, and legislators. Often, the pivotal role of the physician has been completely ignored. The Medical Directive is designed to be discussed and completed by a physician and a patient; it should foster an understanding by the physician, the ultimate clinical authority, of the patient's preferences.

Therefore, the Medical Directive represents a new type of advance care document. It is designed to eliminate the problems of previous living wills and to incorporate positive attempts at reforming these living wills. It is also a simple but comprehensive document through which patients can express their preferences for care at the end of life in a way that will guide their physicians in clinical decision making.

FUTURE DIRECTIONS FOR ADVANCE CARE DOCUMENTS

Progress in developing useful advance care documents cannot stop with the Medical Directive. The Medical Directive is certainly not the ultimate or final advance care document, overcoming all of the deficiencies of existing living wills. Indeed, it may be necessary to revise the four scenarios, the list of specific interventions, or other sections. Therefore, the authors hope that publication of the Medical Directive will not prompt complacency but will herald a period of critical evaluation of advance care documents and the development of new ideas. While there are many avenues for future work, emphasis should be placed on two particular areas: empirical studies and better means of exploring patient values.

The single most important area for future efforts is empirical research. For more than 20 years, major organizations have published living wills, a majority of states have enacted living will laws, many ethicists have endorsed these documents, and yet we hardly know anything about their utility in the clinical setting. Living wills have been the subject of few empirical evaluations. There have been fewer than a dozen empirical research publications on living wills, and most of these are assessments of physician attitudes toward living wills.[28,29] Similarly, there have been few empirical studies of proxy decision makers. Indeed, most arguments concerning the utility of living wills or proxies have been based on unsubstantiated analogies to other practices, such as soliciting organ donations.[30]

If we are to have more useful advance care documents, then this ignorance of the facts must change. Four areas of empirical research suggest themselves: 1) patient attitudes and understanding of advance care documents, 2) the best format and setting for discussing advance care documents, 3) the effect of advance care documents on the physician-patient relationship, and 4) the effect of advance care documents on clinical care.

First, we must study patient attitudes toward and understanding of advance care documents. Preliminary research among elderly patients[31,32] suggests that most want to discuss cardiopulmonary resuscitation with their physicians prior to hospitalization. Such studies should be extended to all adults and to all types of critical care interventions. Indeed, we need to determine what types of interventions patients want to discuss with their physicians and whether they prefer to fill out advance care documents or to appoint proxies. We must also try to understand what factors impede patient use of advance care documents and how these can be overcome. Are patients unaware of the existence of advance care documents? Are patients afraid to mention critical care issues to their physicians? Do patients think terminal care planning is not relevant to them in their current state of health? Are patients waiting for physicians to introduce the issue of terminal care planning? In addition, we need to discover the level of patient understanding of advance care documents and terminal care planning. Do patients understand the different types of interventions? Do they understand the difference between persistent vegetative state and mild dementia? Are patient choices about particular critical care interventions consistent with their expressed views?

Second, we should explore the proper format and setting for presenting advance care documents to patients. Until now, living wills have been distributed by national organizations and through lawyers specializing in estate planning. Unfortunately, the medical profession generally, and most physicians in particular, have not taken an active role in discussing advance care documents with patients. In this regard, we need to study whether such documents can be discussed in the outpatient setting or whether they should be introduced during hospitalization. We must determine how much time it takes to fill out an advance care document, whether a patient should fill out an advance care document with a physician during an office visit, and whether an entire document can be discussed during one office visit. We must also examine whether preferences expressed once are durable over time. How often should advance care documents be re-discussed to be sure that patient preferences are durable? Are patient preferences expressed in the outpatient setting consistent with their preferences when they become ill and are hospitalized?

Third, we must understand how advance care documents affect the physician-patient relationship. Existing research[32,33] suggests that many physicians have not discussed and do not understand their patients' terminal care preferences. The purpose of advance care documents is to permit patients to control the type of medical interventions they receive if they become incompetent. If this goal is to be realized, then we must determine whether the use of such documents enhances the physician's understanding of a patient's critical care preferences. When physicians and patients discuss an advance care document, is the physician's ability to predict patient preferences in common clinical circumstances increased? Are physicians and patients more trusting of each other and more satisfied with their relationship after discussing an advance care document? Or do they find discussions of terminal care issues to be too speculative, frustrating, or a waste of time?

Finally, we must examine how advance care documents affect clinical practice. At one level, we need to determine how patient preferences are implemented. Are advance care documents available during hospitalizations? Do physicians and nurses know a patient's advance care document preferences? In appropriate situations, are the patient's expressed preferences respected or ignored? Do patient preferences expressed in advance care documents provide suitable and specific guidance for actual clinical decisions? Or do advance care documents create more confusion than clarity for clinical decisions? On another level, we should understand how the use of advance care documents affects patient outcomes and hospital costs. Does the use of such documents change the causes of death among patients? Does the use of advance care documents affect patient longevity? What is the effect of advance care documents on medical care costs at the end of life?

Empirical research into each of these four areas has yet to be undertaken. If we are to develop better advance care documents and if advance care documents are to be effectively implemented, then such research is imperative.

The second area for future work is the assessment of patient values. Some argue that the best way of permitting patients to control their terminal care is through more general assessments of values. According to these commentators, advance care documents are too specific and inflexible, and proxies are often uninformed about patient preferences. And so a third alternative should be devised: an assessment of general patient values from which preferences about specific interventions can be deduced.

Within the past year or so, the development of such "value assessments" has begun. The Center for Health Law and Ethics at the University of New Mexico has launched a pilot study of a form they call a Values History.[34] This form includes 10 sections with 45 open-ended questions to assess patient views. The "value areas" range from religious beliefs to overall attitude toward life to living environment. Similarly, Doukas et al.[35] have devised another assessment scheme, also called a Values History, to be used with geriatric patients. In their values history, elderly patients are asked to choose between two "basic life values," stating whether they prefer to live as long as possible or to preserve a high quality of life. In a subsequent section, the patients are to define quality of life by selecting three "most important" values from among 15 value statements that include being treated with respect, being treated in accord with one's religious beliefs, and avoiding unnecessary pain and suffering.

Such value assessments seem liable to the same defects as the original living wills, especially since the original living wills were more statements of general values than documents regarding specific interventions. First, these value assessments are designed to elicit a patient's general health care-related values. Consequently, the responses are likely to be characterized in general and therefore vague language. For instance, the Values History of Doukas et al. suggests a stark dichotomy between quantity and quality of life values. Naturally, the relationship between these two values is much too complex to be stated as a simple choice. Furthermore, the 15 value statements used to define quality of life more clearly are themselves fairly vague. What is *unnecessary* pain and suffering? What does it mean to be treated with respect? These general and noncontroversial statements have a multitude of meanings that will differ among individuals.

A second deficiency of value assessments is that there is no guarantee that knowing a patient's general values will be a suitable guide in deducing a patient's views on specific interventions. Does a patient who values quality of life want to be given medical interventions if he or she is "pleasantly senile" and not suffering any pain? Or does being pleasantly senile, even without pain, already entail a poor quality of life? Indeed, some philosophers maintain that ethical reasoning is inductive, beginning from examples. This is true because it is easier to gain a mutual understanding of specific ethical decisions than of general values, and an agreement on general values does not ensure agreement on specific ethical decisions.[36] Empirical studies support this skeptical attitude toward deducing specific interventions from general values. As mentioned above, one study[23] has indicated that a patient's spouse, who should know the patient's values, is unable to predict the patient's preferences on a single intervention, cardiopulmonary resuscitation.

Value assessments also do not take into consideration that people rarely develop completely consistent value systems. Indeed, people espouse certain general values but also express particular ethical judgments that conflict with these values. They also may espouse two different values that conflict in particular situations and lack any clear resolution for such conflicts. These value conflicts may be quite common when it comes to critical care issues, and yet they are not elicited by value histories.

Finally, physicians may be very reluctant to discuss general values without reference to specific clinical situations and interventions. They may perceive such general discussions as too open ended and time consuming to be worthwhile.

Despite these defects, there may be some role for value assessments. It might be possible to combine value assessments with advance care documents, such as the Medical Directive, that delineate preferences concerning specific scenarios and interventions. Linking general values with specific preferences may help to illuminate the patient's specific choices, especially in guiding physicians when patients express uncertainty over a particular intervention or when they desire an intervention only for a trial period. These values may also be helpful when the actual clinical situation departs in important ways from the standard scenario outlined in the advance care documents.

But if value assessments are to supplement specific advance care documents, then the type of values explored and the way in which they are explored will have to be altered. First, the values elicited will have to be both more specific and more relevant to actual clinical practice. It is no use asking if a person wants to be treated with respect or in accordance with his or her religious beliefs. Physicians must know whether or how much a patient values being able to talk, to walk independently, to live at home, etc. Second, it is not clear that in critical care situations patients make their choices on the basis of what they value. Indeed, many critical choices are motivated by attempts to avoid highly undesirable situations. John Rawls calls this reasoning by the "maximum rule."[37] Hence, value assessments should elicit the patient's views on goods he or she finds desirable as well as on situations he or she hopes to avoid. Finally, a value assessment should ask patients to both rate and rank values. A value assessment that fits these criteria is presented in Figure 2.

Combining value assessments with specific advance care documents and the value assessment offered here are only suggestions. Their worthiness cannot be determined apart from actual use in clinical circumstances. Like all aspects of advance care documents, value assessments must be subjected to empirical study before we can assess their ultimate utility. Indeed, as with proxies, we may find that value assessments, while appearing to be a good idea, do not help us to realize the

Figure 2.   A Proposed Value Assessment Scheme

Desirable States	Rank 3 Most Important Values (1, not valuable; 5, very valuable)
1 2 3 4 5	Being pain free.
1 2 3 4 5	Being able to talk to my family and friends and being able to understand what they say to me.
1 2 3 4 5	Being able to express my emotions and feelings even if I cannot communicate with words and being able to feel the emotional expressions of others even if I cannot understand their words.
1 2 3 4 5	Being mentally alert enough to be aware of what I am doing and saying and to understand the significance of what I am doing and saying, as well as what others are doing and saying to me.
1 2 3 4 5	Living with my spouse, friends, or family.
1 2 3 4 5	Living in my own apartment or house, not in a nursing home or other long-term care facility.
1 2 3 4 5	Being independent in bodily care activities so that another person does not have to take me to the bathroom, wash me up, brush my teeth, comb my hair, etc.
1 2 3 4 5	Being able to walk without assistance so that I am not bed bound or in a wheelchair.
1 2 3 4 5	Having my bodily integrity so that there are not tubes or needles or other things stuck into my body and having none of my limbs amputated.
1 2 3 4 5	Being physically and mentally fit to continue my work, hobbies, and other leisure activities.
1 2 3 4 5	Living as long as possible using the available medical technologies.
1 2 3 4 5	Contributing to the good of other people by whatever means I can.
1 2 3 4 5	Being financially independent so that I do not have to rely on my parents, brothers, sisters, or children to support my living.
1 2 3 4 5	Living long enough for a personal or family milestone such as the birth of a grandchild or the college graduation or marriage of a child.

Figure 2.   A Proposed Value Assessment Scheme   (*continued*)

Undesirable States	Rank 3 Worst Situations (1, tolerable; 5, intolerable)
1 2 3 4 5	Being paralyzed. You are unable to walk but can move around in a wheelchair. You can talk and interact with other people.
1 2 3 4 5	Being unable to speak meaningfully. You are unable to speak or write to others. You can walk on your own, feed yourself, and take care of daily needs such as bathing and dressing yourself.
1 2 3 4 5	Being unable to care for yourself. You are paralyzed and bed bound, and unable to wash, feed, or dress yourself. You are totally cared for by others.
1 2 3 4 5	Being in pain. You are in severe bodily pain that cannot be totally controlled or completely eliminated by medications.
1 2 3 4 5	Being pain free but not completely awake. You have pain that can be controlled by medications but are unconscious or very sleepy or confused most of the time because of the pain medications.
1 2 3 4 5	Being mildly demented. You can neither remember things, such as where you are, nor reason clearly. You are not aware that you have these mental impairments. You are capable of speaking with others, although you are not capable of remembering the conversations; you are capable of washing, feeding, and dressing yourself and are experiencing no chronic pain. These mental impairments cannot be reversed.
1 2 3 4 5	Being severely demented. You have suffered brain damage and can neither remember things, such as where you are, nor reason clearly, nor are you able to initiate very many actions. You are awake and alert but have a very limited awareness of your environment. You can withdraw from pain and have limited actions, such as smiling or scratching. You are not capable of speaking, washing, feeding, or dressing yourself and are totally cared for by others. These mental impairments cannot be reversed.

Figure 2.   A Proposed Value Assessment Scheme   *(continued)*

Undesirable States	Rank 3 Worst Situations (1, tolerable; 5, intolerable)
1 2 3 4 5	Being in a coma or persistent vegetative state. You have suffered brain damage and are not conscious and are not aware of your environment in any way. You cannot even feel pain. You are totally cared for by others. These mental impairments cannot be reversed.
1 2 3 4 5	Being in a coma temporarily. You are not conscious and are not aware of your environment in any way. You are totally cared for by others. This state of unconsciousness is temporary. In a short time you will probably regain your normal mental and physical function.
1 2 3 4 5	Being financially dependent. You require frequent nursing or medical care that is not covered by insurance, Medicare, or your own savings and is being paid for by your family.
1 2 3 4 5	Being a financial burden. You require frequent nursing or medical care that is very expensive and is being paid for by your family. The cost is a large amount of your family's income and is making it hard for them to do things they want to do.

goal of permitting patients to control their terminal care, but divert us from this goal in actual practice.

CONCLUSION

Living wills were introduced more than 20 years ago. They have been endorsed by ethicists and the courts and propagated by many groups and individuals. Over the past decade, the deficiencies of living wills have become obvious. Until publication of the Medical Directive, however, there had not been any substantive attempt to overcome the deficiencies of living wills and to create a specific and comprehensive advance care document. In this sense, the introduction of the Medical Directive has marked an end to a past that was concerned with rejecting life-sustaining interventions and has created a present focused on developing new advance care documents to elicit patient preferences over a comprehensive range of medical interventions. The future will usher in the first real empirical studies on the use of advance care documents in clinical settings.

ACKNOWLEDGMENT
The authors would like to thank Dr. Robert A. Pearlman for insightful comments.

NOTES

1. *In re Quinlan,* 70 NJ 10 (1976).

2. Society for the Right to Die, *Handbook of Living Will Laws,* New York, Society for the Right to Die, 1987.

3. Concern for Dying, *Questions and Answers About the Living Will,* New York, Concern for Dying, 1984.

4. M. B. Kapp, "Response to the Living Will Furor: Directive for Maximum Care," *American Journal of Medicine* 72 (1982): 855–859.

5. L. L. Emanuel and E. J. Emanuel, "The Medical Directive: A New Comprehensive Advance Care Document," *Journal of the American Medical Association* 261 (1989): 3288–3293.

6. Society for the Right to Die, *The First Fifty Years: 1938–1988,* New York, Society for the Right to Die, 1988. Concern for Dying offers a somewhat different history, stating that the living will was developed in 1968 from five letters.

7. C. Strong, "Can Fluids and Electrolytes Be 'Extraordinary Treatment'?" *Journal of Medical Ethics* 7 (1981): 83–85.

8. J. Lynn and J. F. Childress, "Must Patients Always Be Given Food and Water?" *Hastings Center Report* 13 (October 1983): 17–21.

9. *In re Conroy,* 98 NJ 321 (1988).

10. Uniform Rights of the Terminally Ill Act, Section 1–18, 9A U.L.A. 456 (Supp. 1986).

11. Oklahoma Natural Death Act, *Okla. Stat. Ann.,* tit. 63 section 3102.

12. S. J. Eisendrath and A. R. Jonsen, "The Living Will: Help or Hindrance?" *Journal of the American Medical Association* 249 (1983): 2054–2058.

13. E. R. W. Fox, "Nora's Living Will," *Western Journal of Medicine* 146 (1987): 118.

14. E. J. Emanuel, "A Review of the Ethical and Legal Aspects of Terminating Medical Care," *American Journal of Medicine* 84 (1988): 291–301.

15. *Evans v. Bellevue Hospital,* No. 16536/87 (N.Y. Sup. Ct., N.Y. County, July 27, 1987).

16. President's Commission for the Study of Ethical Problems in Medicine and Biomedical and Behavioral Research, *Deciding to Forgo Life-Sustaining Treatment*, Washington, DC, US Government Printing Office, 1983.

17. T. A. Brennan, "Ethics Committees and Decisions to Limit Care: The Experience at the Massachusetts General Hospital," *Journal of the American Medical Association* 260 (1988): 803–807.

18. A. S. Relman, "Michigan's Sensible 'Living Will'," *New England Journal of Medicine* 300 (1979): 1270–1272.

19. R. Steinbrook and B. Lo, "Decision Making for Incompetent Patients by Designated Proxy: California's New Law," *New England Journal of Medicine* 310 (1984): 1598–1601.

20. *In re Peter*, 108 N.J. 365 (1987).

21. *Rasmussen v. Fleming*, 741 P.2d 674 (1987).

22. L. J. Schneiderman and J. D. Arras, "Counseling Patients to Counsel Physicians on Future Care in the Event of Patient Incompetence," *Annals of Internal Medicine* 102 (1985): 693–698.

23. R. F. Uhlmann, R. A. Pearlman, and K. C. Cain, "Physicians and Spouses' Prediction of Elderly Patients' Resuscitation Preferences," *Journal of Gerontology* 43 (1988): M115–M121.

24. S. R. Steiber, "Right to Die: Public Balks at Deciding for Others," *Hospitals* 61 (1987): 72.

25. S. Bok, "Personal Directions for Care at the End of Life," *New England Journal of Medicine* 295 (1976): 367–369.

26. Concern for Dying, *A Living Will and Appointment of a Surrogate Decision Maker*, New York, Concern for Dying, 1989.

27. US Office of Technology Assessment, *Life-Sustaining Technologies and the Elderly*, Washington, DC, US Government Printing Office, July 1987.

28. D. L. Redleaf, S. B. Schmitt, and W. C. Thompson, "The California Natural Death Act: An Empirical Study of Physicians' Practices," *Stanford Law Review* 31 (1979): 913–945.

29. R. S. Shapiro, F. Tavill, G. Rivkin, and H. Gruchow, "Living Will in Wisconsin," *Wisconsin Medical Journal* 85 (1986): 17–23.

30. A. L. Caplan, "Living Wills and the Lessons of Organ Donations," *New Physician* 34 (September 1985): 7, 19.

31. A. Wagner, "Cardiopulmonary Resuscitation in the Aged: A Prospective Survey," *New England Journal of Medicine* 310 (1984): 1129–1130.

32. R. H. Shmerling, S. E. Bedell, A. Lilienfeld, and T. L. Delbanco, "Discussing Cardiopulmonary Resuscitation: A Study of Elderly Outpatients," *Journal of General Internal Medicine* 3 (1988): 317–321.

33. S. E. Bedell and T. L. Delbanco, "Choices About Cardiopulmonary Resuscitation in the Hospital: When Do Physicians Talk with Patients?" *New England Journal of Medicine* 310 (1984): 1089–1093.

34. Personal communication with Joan McIver Gibson, University of New Mexico, Albuquerque.

35. D. J. Doukas, S. Lipson, and L. B. McCullough, "Value History," in *Clinical Aspects of Aging*, 3rd ed. (W. Reichel, ed.), Baltimore, Williams and Wilkens, 1989.

36. J. Rawls, "Justice as Fairness: Political Not Metaphysical," *Philosophy and Public Affairs* 14 (1985): 223–251.

37. J. Rawls, *A Theory of Justice*, Cambridge, MA, Harvard University Press, 1971.

Appendix

The Medical Directive: An Introduction

As part of a person's right to self determination every adult has the freedom to accept or refuse any recommended medical treatment. This is relatively easy when people are well and can communicate. Unfortunately, during severe illness, people are often unable to communicate their wishes at the time that many critical decisions about medical interventions need to be made.

The Medical Directive states a person's wishes for or against types of medical interventions in several key situations, so that the person's wishes can be respected even when he or she cannot communicate.

A Medical Directive only comes into effect if a person becomes incompetent or unable to make decisions or to express his or her wishes. It can be changed at any time up until then. Decisions not involving incompetence should be discussed directly with the physician.

The Medical Directive also allows for appointing someone to make medical decisions for a person should he or she become unable to make his or her own; this is a proxy or durable power of attorney. The Medical Directive also allows for a statement of wishes concerning organ donation.

A copy of the completed Medical Directive should be given to a person's regular physician and to his or her family or friends to ensure that it is available when necessary.

Medical Directives should be seen not only as legal protection for personal rights but also as a guide to a person's physician. Discussion of Medical Directives with the physician can help in making plans for health care that suit a person's values.

Reprinted with permission from the *Journal of the American Medical Association* 261 (1989): 3288–3293.

A person's wishes usually reflect personal, philosophical, and religious views, so one may wish to discuss the issues with his or her family, friends, and religious mentor as well.

Before recording a personal statement in the Medical Directive it may be helpful to consider the following questions. What kind of medical condition, if any, would make life hard enough that attempts to prolong life would be undesirable? Some may say none. For others the answer may be intractable pain. For other people the limit may be permanent dependence on others, or irreversible mental damage, or inability to exchange affection.

Under such circumstances as these the goal of medical treatment may be to secure comfort only, or it may be to use ordinary treatments while avoiding heroic ones, or to use treatments that offer improved function (palliation), or to use all appropriate interventions to prolong life independent of quality. These points may help to clarify a person's thoughts and wishes.

Durable Power of Attorney

I understand that my wishes expressed in these four cases may not cover all possible aspects of my care if I become incompetent. I also may be undecided about whether I want a particular treatment or not. Consequently there may be a need for someone to accept or refuse medical interventions for me in consultation with my physicians. I authorize:

_____

_____

_____

_____

as my proxy(s) to make the decision for me whenever my wishes expressed in this document are insufficient or undecided.

Should there be any disagreement between the wishes I have indicated in this document and the decisions favored by my above named proxy(s), I wish my proxy(s) to have authority over my medical directive /I wish my medical directive to have authority over my proxy(s). (Please delete as necessary.)

Should there be any disagreement between the wishes of my

proxies, _____

_____

_____ shall have final authority.

Organ Donation

   I hereby make this anatomical gift to take effect upon my death.
   I give: ☐ my body;   ☐ any needed organs or parts;
☐ the following organs or parts

_____

_____

_____

☐ to the following person or institution;   ☐ the physician in attendance at my death;   ☐ the hospital in which I die;   ☐ the following
named physician, hospital, storage bank or other medical institution

_____

_____

_____

for the following purposes: ☐ any purpose authorized by law;
☐ transplantation;   ☐ therapy;   ☐ research;
☐ medical education.

   My Personal Statement (use another page if necessary.)

_____

_____

_____

_____

_____

_____

Signed _____

Date _____

Witness _____

Date _____

Witness _____

Date _____

My Medical Directive

This Medical Directive expresses, and shall stand for, my wishes regarding medical treatments in the event that illness should make me unable to communicate them directly. I make this Directive, being 18 years or more of age, of sound mind and appreciating the consequences of my decisions.

Situation (A)

If I am in a coma or in a persistent vegetative state, and in the opinion of my physician and several consultants have no known hope of regaining awareness and higher mental function no matter what is done, then my wishes regarding use of the following, if considered medically reasonable, would be:

I WANT	I DO NOT WANT	I AM UNDECIDED	I WANT A TRIAL: IF NO CLEAR IMPROVEMENT STOP TREATMENT	
			X	1. **Cardiopulmonary Resuscitation**—if on the point of dying the use of drugs and electric shock to start the heart beating, and artificial breathing.
				2. **Mechanical Breathing**—breathing by a machine.
				3. **Artificial Nutrition and Hydration**—nutrition and fluid given through a tube in the veins, nose, or stomach.
			X	4. **Major Surgery**—such as removing the gall bladder or part of the intestines.
				5. **Kidney Dialysis**—cleaning the blood by machine or by fluid passed through the belly.
				6. **Chemotherapy**—drugs to fight cancer.
			X	7. **Minor Surgery**—such as removing some tissue from an infected toe.
			X	8. **Invasive Diagnostic Tests**—such as using a flexible tube to look into the stomach.
				9. **Blood or Blood Products.**
				10. **Antibiotics**—drugs to fight infection.
			X	11. **Simple Diagnostic Tests**—such as blood tests or x-rays.
			X	12. **Pain Medications,** even if they dull consciousness and indirectly shorten my life.

My Medical Directive (*continued*)

Situation (B)

If I am in a coma, and I have a small likelihood of recovering fully, a slightly larger likelihood of surviving with permanent brain damage, and a much larger likelihood of dying, then my wishes regarding the use of the following, if considered medically reasonable, would be:

I WANT	I DO NOT WANT	I AM UNDECIDED	I WANT A TRIAL; IF NO CLEAR IMPROVEMENT STOP TREATMENT	
			X	1. **Cardiopulmonary Resuscitation**—if on the point of dying the use of drugs and electric shock to start the heart beating, and artificial breathing.
				2. **Mechanical Breathing**—breathing by a machine.
				3. **Artificial Nutrition and Hydration**—nutrition and fluid given through a tube in the veins, nose, or stomach.
			X	4. **Major Surgery**—such as removing the gall bladder or part of the intestines.
				5. **Kidney Dialysis**—cleaning the blood by machine or by fluid passed through the belly.
				6. **Chemotherapy**—drugs to fight cancer.
			X	7. **Minor Surgery**—such as removing some tissue from an infected toe.
			X	8. **Invasive Diagnostic Tests**—such as using a flexible tube to look into the stomach.
				9. **Blood or Blood Products.**
				10. **Antibiotics**—drugs to fight infection.
			X	11. **Simple Diagnostic Tests**—such as blood tests or x-rays.
			X	12. **Pain Medications,** even if they dull consciousness and indirectly shorten my life.

My Medical Directive (*continued*)

Situation (C)

If have brain damage or some brain disease which cannot be reversed and which makes me unable to recognize people, or to speak understandably, *and I also have a terminal illness,* such as incurable cancer which will likely be the cause of my death, then my wishes regarding use of the following, if considered medically reasonable, would be:

I WANT	I DO NOT WANT	I AM UNDECIDED	I WANT A TRIAL: IF NO CLEAR IMPROVEMENT STOP TREATMENT	
			X	1. **Cardiopulmonary Resuscitation**—if on the point of dying the use of drugs and electric shock to start the heart beating, and artificial breathing.
				2. **Mechanical Breathing**—breathing by a machine.
				3. **Artificial Nutrition and Hydration**—nutrition and fluid given through a tube in the veins, nose, or stomach.
			X	4. **Major Surgery**—such as removing the gall bladder or part of the intestines.
				5. **Kidney Dialysis**—cleaning the blood by machine or by fluid passed through the belly.
				6. **Chemotherapy**—drugs to fight cancer.
			X	7. **Minor Surgery**—such as removing some tissue from an infected toe.
			X	8. **Invasive Diagnostic Tests**—such as using a flexible tube to look into the stomach.
				9. **Blood or Blood Products.**
				10. **Antibiotics**—drugs to fight infection.
			X	11. **Simple Diagnostic Tests**—such as blood tests or x-rays.
			X	12. **Pain Medications,** even if they dull consciousness and indirectly shorten my life.

My Medical Directive (*continued*)

Situation (D)

If have brain damage or some brain disease which cannot be reversed and which makes me unable to recognize people, or to speak understandably, *but I have no terminal illness,* and I can live in this condition for a long time, then my wishes regarding use of the following, if considered medically reasonable, would be:

I WANT	I DO NOT WANT	I AM UNDECIDED	I WANT A TRIAL; IF NO CLEAR IMPROVEMENT STOP TREATMENT	
			X	1. **Cardiopulmonary Resuscitation**—if on the point of dying the use of drugs and electric shock to start the heart beating, and artificial breathing.
				2. **Mechanical Breathing**—breathing by a machine.
				3. **Artificial Nutrition and Hydration**—nutrition and fluid given through a tube in the veins, nose, or stomach.
			X	4. **Major Surgery**—such as removing the gall bladder or part of the intestines.
				5. **Kidney Dialysis**—cleaning the blood by machine or by fluid passed through the belly.
				6. **Chemotherapy**—drugs to fight cancer.
			X	7. **Minor Surgery**—such as removing some tissue from an infected toe.
			X	8. **Invasive Diagnostic Tests**—such as using a flexible tube to look into the stomach.
				9. **Blood or Blood Products.**
				10. **Antibiotics**—drugs to fight infection.
			X	11. **Simple Diagnostic Tests**—such as blood tests or x-rays.
				12. **Pain Medications,** even if they dull consciousness and indirectly shorten my life.

15 Initiative 119: What Is at Stake?

ALBERT R. JONSEN

Albert Jonsen is Professor and Chair of the Department of Medical History and Ethics at the University of Washington, Seattle.

The state of Washington is a place of serene and majestic beauty. Wide expanses of water, towering forests, broad plains, and splendid mountains surround its 5 million inhabitants in the northwest corner of the "lower forty-eight," as our Alaska neighbors say. In the midst of this beauty lies peril. One of its peaks, Mt. St. Helens, erupted ten years ago, devastating the landscape and, only a few weeks ago, geologists announced that our risk of major earthquake was much greater than had previously been assumed. The Pacific Plate could slip beneath our lovely landscape and busy cities and tear our state to pieces.

The state of Washington is also on the edge of a moral cataclysm. On November 5, 1991, the citizens of this state will vote on Initiative 119. This ballot provision would allow a competent, terminally-ill patient to request of his or her physician "aid-in-dying." These innocuous, indeed benign words, refer to what its proponents describe as "a new medical service." This service consists in the administration or provision of a lethal drug to effect the immediate death of the patient. The benign phrase, "aid-in-dying," like the deceptively beautiful slopes of Mt. St. Helens, conceals the potential for cataclysm. If our citizens approve Initiative 119, we will make our state the first American jurisdiction, indeed, the first jurisdiction in the world, to legalize active euthanasia.

Some persons, particularly its proponents, would see this not as a moral cataclysm, but as moral enlightenment. At last, they say, a government has listened to the voices of those philosophers who construct rational arguments justifying euthanasia and to the pleas of suffering patients requesting a humane and dignified death. Obviously, I take a

This article first appeared in Commonweal *118 (9 August 1991): 466–468.*

different view. I am opposed to Initiative 119 and to any policy permitting active euthanasia. However, I rely on others in this issue to put forth extended arguments against the proposition. I will explain what Initiative 119 is and how Washington came to be the site for this historic public decision.

The state of Washington has a history of reasonable public policy about death and dying. California passed the first Natural Death Act in 1976; Washington was the second state to do so, enacting a bill substantially similar to California's in 1979. Its Natural Death Act permits persons to prepare an advance directive authorizing their physician to withhold or withdraw life-sustaining procedures when death is imminent. The legislature subsequently passed a Durable Power of Attorney for Health Care law and amended the state statutes to include a list of authorized surrogate decision makers for incompetent patients. Several Supreme Court decisions in the early 1980s endorsed the concepts of total brain death, of forgoing life support of the patient in a persistent vegetative state, and of the right to refuse life-sustaining care. Only on the issue of withdrawal of nutrition and hydration has Washington's Supreme Court maintained a conservative position, at least for mentally incapacitated persons. That decision, *In the Matter of Grant,* is a legal chimera: the majority opinion presents an eloquent argument justifying withdrawal, while the majority vote rejects withdrawal, a judicial oddity resulting from one justice who changed her vote on reconsideration after the opinion was published!

The state, then, has a legal climate open to liberal opinions about issues of death and dying. Its judicial and legislative policies reflect the wide agreement among bioethics scholars and national advisory groups on most issues. This climate might be a favorable one in which to introduce the next question: Should the law tolerate active euthanasia? The Hemlock Society has been seeking an opportunity to put this question before the public. California, Oregon, and Washington are among the few states that have an initiative and referendum process; Washington's dates back to 1911. The process is the heritage of the strong populism that reigned in the Western states at the turn of the century. Citizens can circulate a petition for signatures and, if enough are obtained, place their proposition on the ballot at a general election. A legislative system such as this is ideal for the debate and resolution of broad issues of public concern, although it can place severe restraints on policymakers on such issues as taxation and education.

The Hemlock Society chose to bring the issue of the legality of active euthanasia before the people of California in 1988. The society had its first chapter in Southern California and had developed an organizational base in the state. The group began to gather signatures on an initiative that would exempt from prosecution under the homicide statutes any physician who caused the death of a patient voluntarily requesting such assistance. Because only 137,000 of the requisite 378,000 signatures had been obtained by the deadline, the initiative failed to reach the ballot. Hemlock officials believe that the failure to obtain sufficient signatures was due not so much to opposition to their proposal as to the large number of signatures needed. Given the size of California's electorate, paid signature-gatherers are necessary and Hemlock did not have the funds to organize such an extensive activity. Next, an attempt to mount an initiative in Oregon failed to qualify for signature gathering because of a successful challenge to the ballot title.

Washington was the next target of opportunity. In many ways it was more ideal than California. Its population is much smaller and thus only 150,000 signatures were needed. In addition to the progressive legislation and judicial climate about death, Washington has a liberal ethos. The state has a heritage of progressive, even radical, politics. (In the 1930s, one of Roosevelt's cabinet officers raised a toast to "the forty-seven states and the Soviet of Washington!") Perhaps most significant, the attitude of Washington inhabitants is strongly live-and-let-live (or, in this case, let die). Respect for autonomy and privacy is a cherished social value in the Great Northwest. Also, religious opposition, which could be expected to be strong, would not be as powerful in Washington as elsewhere. A recent survey showed Washington as one of the most unchurched states in the nation: at 14 percent, it is surpassed only by its neighbor Oregon (17 percent) in the number of persons who claim no religious affiliation (the national average is 8 percent). Thus, Hemlock's message would be received with tolerance in such a political and moral climate.

Initiative 119 was circulated with the official ballot title, "Shall adult patients who are in a medically terminal condition be permitted to request and receive from a physician aid-in-dying?" The official summary of the initiative read:

> This initiative expands the right of adult persons with terminal conditions to have their wishes, expressed in a written directive, regarding life respected. It amends current law to: Expand the definition of terminal condition to include irreversible coma and persistent vegetative state or condition which will result in death within six months; Specify which life-sustaining procedures may be withdrawn; Permit adult persons with terminal conditions to request and receive aid-in-dying from their physicians, facilitating death.

The current law which these provisions will expand is the 1979 Natural Death Act. This legislation, following the California model, has been criticized for its overly cautious definition of "terminal condition" and for its omission of explicit reference to nutrition and hydration as life-sustaining measures that may be forgone. The initiative amends the act to correct these deficiencies. This aspect of the initiative has generally been welcomed (although defining persistent vegetative state as a "terminal condition" seems a semantic sleight of hand). The final provision, permitting "aid-in-dying," is the radical departure from prevailing law and medical ethics.

The Natural Death Act would be amended to define "aid-in-dying" as "aid in the form of a medical service, provided in person by a physician, that will end the life of a conscious and mentally competent qualified patient in a dignified, painless, and humane manner, when requested voluntarily by the patient through a written directive . . . at the time the medical service is to be provided." The directive is to be witnessed by two unrelated and impartial persons and the patient must be declared "in a terminal condition" by two physicians. While it is odd to find this mention of an active, voluntary request in a document otherwise devoted to advance directives to be carried out on behalf of incompetent patients, the idea of amending the extant Natural Death Act was politically and psychologically astute. It makes this radical change seem less radical by incorporating it into accepted legislation. It associates it with useful and broadly approved amendments. It fits the radical provision within the relatively conservative safeguards of the extant act.

These safeguards are, however, only relatively conservative. Like most Natural Death legislation, they require witnesses unrelated by family or financial interest and the written declaration by two physicians that the patient is in a terminal condition, that is, the reasonable medical judgment that death will result within six months. However, there is no mention of presence or evaluation of pain and suffering, no reference to stability of the patient's request over time, no requirement for psychological evaluation (safeguards that are mentioned in reports of the Dutch tolerance of active euthanasia). The patient must simply be diagnosed as being in a terminal condition and make an uncoerced request for aid-in-dying. Most important (and most different from the Dutch practice), Initiative 119 appears to remove the aid-in-dying decision and execution from all legal oversight. The failure of the California initiative, which directly called for exemption from the homicide statutes, was instructive. Proposition 119 buries this feature in the text, mingling it with the previous exemption from criminal liability for physicians who forgo life sustaining treatments in accord with a Directive to Physicians (a very different issue, legally and ethically!).

The public response to the initiative was quite positive. Washington Citizens for Death with Dignity, supported by the Hemlock Society, was able to gather 223,000 signatures. Fortuitously, two cases that received media exposure occurred during the signature gathering: the U.S. Supreme Court's decision in the matter of Nancy Cruzan, which stimulated interest in advance directives, and the "mercy killing" of Janet Adkins by means of Dr. Jack Kervorkian's "suicide machine." Ironically, neither case would fit under the provision of the amended act, since Ms. Cruzan was incapable of making a voluntary request and Mrs. Adkins was not suffering from a "terminal condition." Still, the exposure in the media must have stimulated interest and spurred the signature campaign. The evidence of public acceptance is not out of line with the results of recent national opinion polls that show slight majorities in favor, when asked clear questions about the permissibility of active euthanasia.

Washington's initiative and referendum law allows an approved initiative to go before the state legislature for action. If the legislature fails to enact the initiative, it is to go on the ballot at the next general election. The legislature decided not to consider the initiative. Astute politicians judged that a ballot measure would split the vote in such a way that Initiative 119 would be assured of victory.

Reaction within the medical community has been hard to interpret. The Washington State Medical Association (WSMA) found itself in a quandary. It had previously endorsed the AMA Ethics and Judicial Council statement that forbids physicians to participate in active euthanasia. At the annual meeting in 1990, the WSMA House of Delegates voted by an overwhelming majority to oppose Initiative 119. However, by March 1991, WSMA members seemed nearly evenly split over the issue. An informal poll of 2,000 members (50 percent responding) indicated a shift in attitude: 49 percent favored WSMA support of Initiative 119, while 51 percent opposed it. The same poll, however, showed that only 28 percent of respondents thought that it should be legal for a physician to give a lethal injection to knowingly hasten death and 30 percent stated that they would personally be willing to aid in a patient's death. In April, the WSMA board of trustees, without rescinding the earlier House of Delegates vote, decided not to recognize officially the private group, Washington Physicians Against 119, which was formed to mount a campaign against passage of the initiative. The WSMA spokesperson stated that since the membership was divided, "there were other ways to oppose it without getting directly involved." The Washington State Hospital Association takes an opposed position and, while it will not actively campaign, will assist its member institutions to do so. The Washington State Nurses Association at first opposed the initiative and then, after intense lobbying, withdrew its statement of opposition in favor of "no position."

As of this writing, opposition efforts have been modest. Most media coverage has tended to present the initiative in a favorable light, since the appealing stories relate tragic instances of terminal care. It appears to many observers that the public continues to confuse the problem of forgoing life-support with the problem of active euthanasia. The ambiguity of the phrase "aid-in-dying" contributes to that confusion. Most of the anecdotes tell of overuse of life-sustaining technologies rather than of unrelieved pain and suffering. An informal and unpublished survey taken by some opponents suggests that public approval of Initiative 119 diminishes somewhat when people are informed of the difference and when terms such as lethal injection are used rather than aid-in-dying. Still, a recent poll showed that if the vote were held today, 119 would pass. Whether opposition can effect a change in public understanding and sympathy between now and November remains to be seen.

This article began with the dire prediction of a moral cataclysm. This may seem an extreme judgment. Yet to become the first jurisdiction in the world to authorize by formal legal enactment active euthanasia has, in my view, cataclysmic implications. The term literally means a deluge. There will be a flood of persons seeking aid-in-dying, coming from all over the United States and Canada, since only in Washington will their desire to end their lives be honored without fear of prosecution. Hospitals will have to decide not only what stance they will take, but how to inform patients of their position (in accord with the new patient self-determination provisions of Medicare) and even how the new law will affect their admissions and credentialing policies. Physicians will have to form their consciences and, if they choose to provide aid-in-dying, learn how to do it (as a new "medical service" it will, like all others, require standards and training: it is not so easy to effect a "dignified and humane" death). Professional groups will be faced with the task of establishing appropriate self-discipline and surveillance, since, like other medical services, aid-in-dying falls within professional self-regulation. Third-party payers will have to decide whether aid-in-dying is a covered and reimbursable medical service. Legal authorities, since they seem to have no jurisdiction, will have to determine how they deal with suspicious cases and allegations of abuse. Above all—and this is the properly "moral" aspect of the cataclysm—all persons will be presented with the opportunity to relieve themselves and their families and the society of the burdens of their own final illnesses. This is not, I think, an unambiguous opportunity: its implications go far beyond the beneficent promotion of autonomy and the relief of pain and suffering. The considerations, private and public, that must surround it will constitute a social order that, as the dictionary defines cataclysm, sweeps away the old order of things.

PART THREE

CONSENT, THERAPY, AND RESEARCH

Andrew W. McThenia
Steven H. Miles, M.D.
Terrence F. Ackerman
Carol Levine, M.A.
Nancy Neveloff Dubler, LL.B.
Robert J. Levine, M.D.
Giles R. Scofield
Dorothy C. Wertz, Ph.D.
John C. Fletcher, Ph.D.

16 *Deciding for Others: Issues of Consent*

Andrew W. McThenia

Andrew McThenia is Professor of Law at Washington and Lee University in Lexington, Virginia.

> Every human being of adult years and sound mind has a right to determine what shall be done with his own body, and a surgeon who performs an operation without his patient's consent commits an assault for which he is liable in damages.
> —*Scholendorff v. Society of New York Hospitals* (1914)

That often quoted statement of Judge Benjamin Cardozo states the premises underlying the current "patients' rights" movement in American law. The 1970s were a time of ferment about questions of consent—whether consent was required, what exceptions to the doctrine of informed consent existed, who could give consent, and what standards would be required of surrogate decision makers. Many courts struggled to give some coherent shape to the doctrine of informed consent, while legislatures generally sought to limit the expansion of that doctrine.

We have in recent years extended Cardozo's dictum to say that one has not only the right to choose a particular treatment but also the right to refuse treatment—the right to die. Numerous natural death acts have been passed, so that a competent adult can, with legislative approval in perhaps a majority of the states, choose to "die with dignity." More recently questions have centered on the refusal of treatment for those who cannot, when treatment decisions are required, speak for themselves. But for the concept of the "right to die" to make any sense at all, it must at least incorporate the notion that one's right to die should not be determined by another's needs. As the concept has been worked out in cases involving incapacitated patients, there is cause to worry.

This article first appeared in Second Opinion 5 *(1987): 76–99.*

How, even in the relatively simple case where the patient is in the eyes of the law fully competent, can we be so sure that we are honoring his or her request for autonomy in allowing the patient to die, and not succumbing to our own darker desire to remove the sufferer from our presence? As we move further from the case of a rational adult exercising his or her own choice, what happens to our model for decision making? What if the patient, formerly competent, is no longer of sound mind but is comatose and kept alive only by a respirator—a Karen Quinlan? What if the patient is an elderly nursing home resident suffering from serious and permanent mental and physical impairments who will likely die within a year even with medical treatment and from whom it is proposed that food and water be withheld—a Claire Conroy? And what if the patient is a terminally ill adult, severely retarded since birth, who never had the mental capacity to make decisions and who without chemotherapy will soon die—a Joseph Saikewicz?[1] And what about the severely handicapped newborn—Baby Doe? We could continue the litany. Even if we confine ourselves to the cases involving adults, we can see how weak is the notion of patient autonomy for deciding these cases.

The task of this article is first to examine two questions: (1) who speaks for the silent patient; and (2) what standards guide the decision maker? The courts in Massachusetts and New Jersey have had extensive experience with termination of treatment decisions, and they provide contrasting models of decision making for our consideration. Two cases in particular, *Superintendent of Belchertown State School v. Saikewicz* and *In re Conroy* highlight the contrasts. In addition, a proposed legislative approach, the Model Health-Care Consent Act, merits attention because it encourages coming to grips with some of the issues of death and dying in advance of a courtroom drama. But I would like to conclude by attempting the more formidable task of critiquing the law's response to the problem from the vantage of the Judeo-Christian tradition—a tradition which knows how to care for people as they die.

THE LAW'S RESPONSE

When a patient cannot make treatment decisions, who decides and under what standards? For a long time both questions remained unanswered, at least in any formal sense. Generally physicians, sometimes in consultation with family members and sometimes acting alone, decided whether to withhold treatment. For all sorts of reasons, that system is no longer workable; for better or worse those questions have been dumped into the lap of the law. Since an estimated 80 percent of all deaths now occur in institutional settings—nursing homes or hospitals—it is not surprising that we have turned to the social institution of the law to sort out these issues (see President's Commission 1983:17–18). The law is in many ways a poor substitute for the family "deathbed," but it seems to be all we have.

The normal way of making decisions in American law is rigidly to separate the act of interpreting what ought to be done from the act of carrying out what is to be done. The institution of the law doesn't know when it is "time to assemble the family." It must await a formal request for an assembly from someone who must first ask a court to designate him as a person (a guardian) who can officially assemble others. If that is accomplished and if there is a conversation, it does not take place around the deathbed; it is not about living and dying in communities but about medical techniques and rights. If the decision is to terminate treatment, it is not finally a shared decision. It is the judge's decision.

Judges in American law don't pull the switch or the plug. They are insulated from the consummation of their decisions by layers of hierarchy and bureaucracy. The judge who orders that treatment be terminated doesn't have to see the patient die. Nor does the judge who refuses a request to withhold treatment have to watch the suffering that his order might occasion. Those who have been assembled don't experience the same mystery in a courtroom that they would share in the presence of the dying patient. And while their views are solicited and are important to the law, the decision is not theirs to make.

The traditional model of the common law with a judge making the decision to treat or withhold treatment has been followed in a series of Massachusetts cases. The Supreme Judicial Court of Massachusetts is firm in its view that primary responsibility remains with the judiciary:

> We do not view the judicial resolution of this most difficult and awesome question—whether potentially life-prolonging treatment should be withheld from a person incapable of making his own decisions—as constituting a "gratuitous encroachment" on the domain of medical expertise. Rather, such questions of life and death seem to us to require the process of detached but passionate investigation and decision that forms the ideal on which the judicial branch of government was created. Achieving this ideal is our responsibility and that of the lower court, and is not to be entrusted to any other group purporting to represent the "morality and conscience of our society," no matter how highly motivated or impressively constituted. (*Saikewicz* 370 N.E.2d at 435)

The New Jersey supreme court has taken a much less active role in these matters:

We consider that a practice of applying to a court to confirm such decisions would generally be inappropriate, not only because there would be a gratuitous encroachment upon the medical profession's field of competence, but because it would be impossibly cumbersome. (*In re Quinlan* 355 A.2d at 669)

The Case of Joseph Saikewicz

In April 1976 Mr. Saikewicz, a sixty-seven-year-old man who had been for all but fourteen years of his life a resident in Massachusetts state institutions for the mentally retarded, was found to have terminal leukemia. Chemotherapy might have prolonged his life by a few months or a year. Physicians testified that even with these limited chances of prolonging life, most people who could choose would, in those circumstances, choose chemotherapy. The treatment would cause nausea, bladder inflammation, and other discomfort, and it required intravenous administration, which for Mr. Saikewicz meant that he had to be strapped to a hospital bed. Mr. Saikewicz was "profoundly mentally retarded" with an intelligence quotient of ten and a mental age of three years. That immobilization would terrify him, a doctor on the staff testified.

The alternative to providing treatment was possibly to hasten his death and to save Saikewicz from pain. The superintendent of the Belchertown State School, where Mr. Saikewicz was a resident, decided to administer the treatment, but some doctors on the staff argued against it. The probate court was requested to order treatment in May 1976. The trial judge appointed to represent Mr. Saikewicz a lawyer who initially argued that his client should receive the treatment. The entire proceeding was, not surprisingly, marked by uncertainty. Influenced by those physicians arguing against treatment, the court-appointed lawyer abandoned his position and maintained instead that Mr. Saikewicz should be allowed to die. The judge's uncertainty is reflected in the transcript (quoted in Burt 1979):

> The Court: There is evidence chemotherapy treatment is apparently the only treatment but by giving it to him he may have some discomfiture at the time of the treatment that may prolong his life. . . . I am inclined to give treatment.

Immediately following this tentative conclusion these exchanges occurred:

> Dr. Jones [a staff physician]: One thing that concerns me is the question about his ability to cooperate. I think it has been made

clear that he doesn't have the capability to understand the treatment and he may or may not be cooperative, therefore greatly complicating the treatment process. . . . That has to be weighed, whether [the treatment] could be administered.

The Court: Dr. Davis, do you agree?

Dr. Davis: I think it is going to be virtually impossible to carry out the treatment in the proper way without having problems. You have to see him. When you approach him in the hospital, he flails at you and there is no way of communicating with him and he is quite strong: so he will have to be restrained and that increases the chances of pneumonia, to restrain him if he can't be up and around.

Mr. Melnick [the court-appointed guardian who concurred in the physicians' determination to withhold treatment]: With no treatment he may live longer; with treatment, the treatment itself may terminate his life sooner. There is some risk because of the toxic nature of the treatment, so in effect, by ordering the treatment there is a possibility that you may shorten his life and there is a chance that you may be prolonging it.

The Court: Maybe I should change my judgment.

The trial court did not order chemotherapy, and that decision was affirmed by the Supreme Judicial Court of Massachusetts on July 19, 1976. Mr. Saikewicz died on September 9.

The values of autonomy and patient welfare that channel decision making for competent patients have been roughly translated in the case of incompetent patients into two standards: "substituted judgment" and "best interest." Both were taken from the law of trusts and estates, where they were originally used to make decisions involving the disposition of property belonging to incompetents. The substituted-judgment standard directs that a surrogate decision maker choose as the now incompetent patient would if able to choose. It is thought to preserve, as much as possible, the patient's own interest and self-determination. The other, the best-interest standard, is more objective. It does not rest on the value of autonomy but on the protection of the patient's welfare. When there is no evidence of a patient's wishes and consequently no guidance for a surrogate to make a decision based on substituted judgment, he or she must rely on the best interest of the patient.

The Massachusetts supreme court attempted to base its decision on what Mr. Saikewicz would have wanted if he could have decided for himself. But that was an impossible task. Unlike the Karen Quinlan case—involving a comatose young woman whose parents asked that her life support system be turned off after several years of no improvement—where there was some evidence of what the patient would have decided, Mr. Saikewicz had never been competent to make decisions for himself. The objective evidence was that most people would accept chemotherapy under those conditions.

If the court had chosen instead a best-interest standard, would that have solved the problem in a better way? I don't think so. It would merely have relocated it and forced the court or the family to engage in an impossible calculus, balancing the benefit of a life with pain from treatment versus a shortened life free from that pain.

How could anyone facing that choice decide? Were I called on to make a decision to accept chemotherapy for myself, I like to think that I would consider what my family and friends wanted. I like to think that they would be with me in my deciding and that they would not abandon me if I made a choice they would not have made. But any utilitarian calculus, no matter how refined, would be inadequate to weigh in precise terms such mysteries as suffering and death.

My colleague Thomas Shaffer (1979:658) has applauded the *Saikewicz* decision as "a remarkable and largely positive example of moral decision. . . . The advocates and judge attempted to understand Saikewicz . . . and tried to decide what Saikewicz would want." I am less certain. The transcript reflects that the trial judge changed his mind when given the powerful image of Mr. Saikewicz flailing his arms in his resistance to treatment. Perhaps there would have been no way to secure his acquiescence in the treatment. But it is possible to read the transcript as the court's distancing itself from pain and suffering. Did the court and the advocates speak for Joseph Saikewicz, or did they abandon him in his suffering under the guise of preserving his autonomy?

I do not think the decision to withhold treatment from Mr. Saikewicz was wrong. I think it is just as I would want it for myself, but I do not wish to pretend that the law was merely carrying out Joseph Saikewicz's wishes. To deny that "we" or the court thought that he should die is to deny the position of dominance that the Massachusetts court held. It is to deny the power of its own act. Any account that denies the silence of Joseph Saikewicz and attempts to deny the hierarchical nature of the decision seems an abdication of moral responsibility.

The Case of Claire Conroy

In contrast to the rather overpowering professional imprint on decision making in *Saikewicz,* the recent New Jersey decision *In re Conroy* holds out the possibility of a shared decision involving family, friends, and medical personnel.

Claire Conroy, who had lived a simple and private life, died in a most complicated way and with great notoriety. Ms. Conroy was a Roman Catholic. She never married. For nearly fifty years she worked for a cosmetics company and had lived in the same home from childhood until she was placed in a nursing home in her seventy-ninth year. She had very few friends. Although she had been very close to her three sisters, her only surviving blood relative was her nephew, Thomas Whittenmore.

In 1979 she was suffering from an organic brain syndrome that manifested itself in her showing periodic confusion. At his own request her nephew was designated her general guardian. At the same time she was placed in the Parkview Nursing Home. Although she was confused when she entered Parkview, she could converse and was in relatively good physical condition. Her condition rapidly deteriorated. In 1982 she was hospitalized for dehydration, and it was discovered that she had gangrenous ulcers as a complication of diabetes. By this time she was unable to maintain a conversation because of her extreme confusion. She could, however, respond to verbal commands. She could not swallow enough food and water to sustain herself; doctors inserted a nasogastric tube so that she could receive nutrients and medicine. Except for a two-week period during which she was fed by hand, this tube remained in place until her death.

In January 1983, Ms. Conroy's guardian petitioned the Superior Court of New Jersey to have the tube removed so that she could die. The trial court appointed a special guardian to represent her interests in the litigation; this guardian opposed the petition. At that time she was not brain dead, not comatose, and not in a chronic vegetative state. A physician testified that her mental state was "severely demented" and she could not respond to verbal stimuli. She could follow movement with her eyes and use her hands. When her hair was combed she would smile.

The physicians agreed that there was no chance of improvement in her condition. One physician, however, observed that because none of her medical conditions was fatal, it could not be predicted when, or from what cause, Ms. Conroy would die. According to all medical evidence, if the nasogastric tube were removed, she would die of dehydration and starvation in about a week. After a full trial the court declared that her nephew had the right to cause the removal of the nasogastric tube. An appeal was taken, and the judgment of the superior court was stayed pending appeal.

The appellate division reversed the decision and held that the right to terminate life-sustaining treatment based on the substituted judgment of a guardian should be limited to cases involving terminally ill patients who were brain dead, comatose, or vegetative and who would gain no medical benefit from continued treatment. Her nephew appealed. While the appeal was pending, Ms. Conroy died with the nasogastric tube in place.

The New Jersey supreme court reversed the appellate division and took the occasion to delineate the conditions under which nourishment could be withheld. The court outlined appropriate substantive guidelines for making these treatment decisions for incompetent patients and described what procedures should be followed in making them.

As to the substantive elements, the court held that life-sustaining treatment may be withheld or withdrawn from an incompetent patient when one of three tests is satisfied. The first is the so-called substituted-judgment, or subjective, test. This test is to be applied when clear and convincing evidence, such as a living will, shows that a particular patient would have refused the treatment under the existing circumstances. The second is a "limited-objective" test based on the best-interest standard. When there is no clear and convincing evidence of the patient's desires but there is some reliable evidence that the patient would have refused the treatment, and if the medical evidence establishes that the burdensome nature of the patient's continued life with the treatment outweighs the benefits of that life for the patient, the patient's best interest would permit withholding treatment. The third is a "pure-objective" test, also based on a best-interest standard. But this test is to be applied when there is no trustworthy evidence to establish whether the patient would have declined treatment. If the medical evidence establishes that the net burdens of the patient's life with the treatment clearly and markedly outweigh the benefits that the patient derives from life and, further, that the patient's pain with the treatment is so severe and unavoidable that administering life-sustaining treatment would be inhumane, treatment may be withheld. Almost as an incidental comment on the evidence in the case, the court found the record insufficient to satisfy any of the three tests it had outlined.

The court also outlined the necessary procedures for proxy decision making in cases like Ms. Conroy's. Previously the New Jersey court in *Quinlan* had established a procedure requiring the concurrence of the guardian, family, attending physician, and hospital prognosis committee. That procedure, said the *Conroy* court, was inadequate for patients such as Claire Conroy who are confined to nursing homes. The vulnerability of nursing home residents, their general isolation from family and friends, and the significant distinctions between hospitals and nursing homes were seen to mandate more formal procedures. The court outlined a series of steps to be followed in these cases.

Guidelines from the Conroy Case

First, a necessary prerequisite to surrogate decision making is the requirement of a judicial determination that the patient is incompetent to make decisions for himself or herself and designation of a guardian for the incompetent patient if one has not already been designated. It must be established by clear and convincing medical evidence that the patient will not regain the ability to make decisions. This requires a judicial determination even if the patient has already been adjudicated incompetent and a guardian has been appointed. When a patient already has a guardian, the court must determine the suitability of that guardian to represent the patient's best interests in regard to the medical decision in question.

Next, the patient's guardian, family, attending physician, or official of the nursing home is required to notify the state ombudsman if any of the above believes that withholding life-sustaining treatment would fulfill an incompetent patient's wishes or would be in his or her best interest. The ombudsman is required to investigate the case and report it within twenty-four hours to the head of the state's human services department and to any other government agency that regulates and operates the nursing care facility.

Third, at least two physicians other than the attending physician must confirm the patient's medical condition and prognosis. If all of the above conditions are satisfied, the guardian, with the concurrence of the attending physician, may withhold or withdraw life-sustaining medical treatment if he or she believes in good faith, based on the medical evidence and any evidence of the patient's wishes, that the subjective test or either of the two limited-objective tests is satisfied. The ombudsman must also concur in the decision to withhold or withdraw treatment. If either the limited-objective or pure-objective test is used, the patient's family members must also concur in the decision.

The New Jersey court refused to rest sole decision-making power either with itself or the medical profession. Instead it sought a wider community and a conversation outside the courtroom. That is an important innovation, for when people confront the mystery of death as equals with one another, the conversation is likely to be richer than when they address each other through the formal presence of a judge. The medical community is not cut out of the conversation, but it does not dominate it, for the decision maker is the patient's guardian. The court is not cut out, for it retains the role of overseer.

The Model Health-Care Consent Act

The Model Health-Care Consent Act is a proposed legislative solution to some of the procedural aspects of the termination of treatment problem.[2] It is purposefully narrow. It attempts to provide a means for an advance conversation and to provide an answer to the question of who speaks for the now silent patient. In addition, it establishes certain substantive standards to guide a surrogate decision maker.

The act is far from perfect. It reflects the uncertainty of society about one person speaking for another. The turf fights between patients' rights advocates and the professionals are not resolved by the act; they are sometimes openly acknowledged, but often covered over. The act was severely weakened, perhaps fatally so, by the effort of the drafting committee to protect physicians and surrogate decision makers from risk and to provide an order to the decision-making process when there is no underlying order in this particular corner of the world of health care decision making. Nonetheless, the act does, I think, make some important contributions to this ongoing debate in American law about who speaks for the now silent patient.

The act embraces four major concepts. First, it designates those who may consent to health care for themselves. These provisions are largely a restatement of the common law and are relatively uncontroversial.

Second, the act provides a triggering mechanism to determine when an individual is incapable of making health care decisions. The initial determination that one is incapable of consenting is made by a physician. The effect of that decision, however, is not to bypass consent but to shift the decision making to a third party. While this was to most a relatively uncontroversial provision, it troubled the more vocal advocates of the patients' rights movement, who saw it as an invasion of patient autonomy. Many health care providers, on the other hand, found fault with the requirement that they look to third parties in the event of incapacity of the patient. They saw this requirement as cumbersome and as an invasion of their professional domain. That this section of the act conformed to already existing laws made little impression on either group of opponents.

Third, the act provides a scheme for determining a proxy or surrogate decision maker to act for one who is incapable of consenting. At common law, parents were entrusted with making health care decisions for their children. The state's power to care for an incompetent adult was traditionally exercised through guardianship. That much is clear in existing law. However, unless the person in need of health care is an infant or has been afforded protection through a formal adjudication of incompetency, the common law provides no clearly established authorization for one family member to act for another. Courts and legal writers have long assumed that authorization from a spouse or close family member is permissible. While that accords with custom, actual judicial authority to that effect is sparse. The act seeks to legitimate that custom. It provides that guardians, parents, and other family members can act for one incapable of consenting and establishes a priority among those surrogate decision makers.

The fourth—and most unique—feature of the act is the mechanism by which an individual can appoint a health care representative for himself or herself—the "advance directive" provision. Most surrogate decision makers obtain their power by authorization of law or by virtue of relationship to the patient—spouse, parent, child, or other family member. Traditionally a surrogate designated by the law was charged with acting in the patient's "best interest." Incompetent or incapacitated persons are, like minor children, wards of the state, and the state's power supports the authority of its courts to allow decisions to be made that serve the incompetent's best interest. The health care representative appointed under the act takes his or her directions from the patient.

In more recent cases, beginning with the New Jersey decision *In re Quinlan*, surrogate decision makers have been authorized to render their best judgment of what the now incompetent patient would decide if able to choose. This so-called substituted-judgment standard is thought to preserve, as much as possible, the patient's own interests and self-determination. The provision for appointment of a health care representative in the act (Section 6) directs that the one making the appointment "may specify [the] terms and conditions considered appropriate" and that the health care representative is to "act in the best interest of the appointor consistent with the purposes expressed in the appointment."

One of the major criticisms of the act by the President's Commission for the Study of Ethical Problems in Medicine and Biomedical and Behavioral Research (1983:148) is that the act "failed to specify which standard should guide a health care representative (best interest or substituted judgment)." In fact, that particular criticism is unwarranted. The act does provide standards. They just do not fit the either/or choice the President's Commission thought appropriate.

The court decisions draw a distinction between the best-interest and substituted-judgment standards. The drafting committee, however, believed that the best way to ensure patient dignity was to shed the labels that had in some instances been reduced to dangerous fictions and deprived of significant meaning. One of the landmark cases purporting to apply the substitute judgment standard is the *Saikewicz* decision. But one would have difficulty ascertaining what Joseph Saikewicz would have decided for himself had he been competent when the evidentiary record showed that Mr. Saikewicz had been severely retarded since birth and had the mental capacity of a three-year-old. Yet on that record the Massachusetts supreme court in deciding to withhold treatment concluded that

> the decision in cases such as this should be that which would be made by the incompetent person, if that person were competent. . . . Having recognized the right of a competent person to make for himself the same decision as the court made in this case, the question is, do the facts on the record support the proposition that Saikewicz himself would have made the decision under the standards set forth. We believe they do. (*Saikewicz* 370 N.E.2d at 431)

It may have been proper to withhold treatment for Mr. Saikewicz. However, there is no evidence in the opinion to support the court's finding. Rather than use language so debased by existing precedent, the legislation directs that the health care representative is to act in the best interest of the patient "consistent with the purposes expressed in the appointment." The commentary makes it clear that specific directives in the appointment are to control. But if there are none, the drafters saw no recourse but to fall back on the general best-interest standard.

The valuable feature of the model act is that it encourages conversation between the health care representative and the one who appoints him and entrusts to him decisional authority. The advocates of living-will legislation have picked up this advance directive provision in the second generation of the natural death statutes and see it as a means of providing evidence of a patient's wishes. It can serve that function, of course. More important, however, is its potential to allow people to talk through issues of death and dying. There is no guarantee that such a conversation or series of conversations will take place, but the act offers an important incentive. One appointed as a health care representative is required to take on the important commitment to listen to and be with the one who entrusts this authority. It is not an obligation to be taken lightly.

A Critique

One of the virtues of the law is its ability to sharpen issues for debate. That is also one of its vices. For in that sharpening there is also a narrowing and distancing from life. The termination of treatment decisions reflects this problem, as the issue is most often narrowed simply to autonomy versus paternalism. On the one hand we conjure up images of a brave Promethean individual asserting the right to die. This patient's world is a world of rights—rights to protect him or her from the tyranny of doctors, hospitals, and the state, from everything that stands in the way of exercising one's choice to die, alone. On the other side we see the detached but passionate professional—either a doctor or a judge—deciding in the patient's best interest. Both images appeal to powerful values. But neither gives a complete account of the issues involved in deciding whether to forgo medical treatment. We need to search for a third way—a way that allows us to be present and to listen for the voice of that now silent patient.

The Inadequacy of the Law's Vision

Any critique of the law must start, I think, with the vision of the human condition on which the law is based. The right-to-die movement, the termination of treatment decisions, and even the Model Health-Care Consent Act begin with a view of human beings that makes choice the normative center of social relationships. It is not much of a leap to say that to be fully human is to be able to choose. But that raises a problem, for what about those who in the eyes of the law cannot make choices—the young, the mentally disabled, the comatose?

We are, as philosopher-novelist Iris Murdoch says, "the heirs of the Enlightenment, Romanticism, and the Liberal tradition" (1961:16). Our dilemma, she continues, "is that we have been left with far too shallow and flimsy an idea of human personality." In her view this dilemma is caused by the joining of a materialistic behaviorism with a dramatic view of the individual as a solitary will. Our received picture is of a human being who is "rational and totally free," who rules over all and is totally responsible: "Nothing transcends him. His moral language is a practical pointer, the instrument of his choices, the indication of his preferences. We picture man as a brave, naked will surrounded by an easily comprehended empirical world" (1961:44, 46). We have accepted the liberal theory as it stands because we have wished to encourage people to think of themselves as free, at the cost of surrendering a history and a community. We have a questionable faith in technology and a romantic conception of the human condition. The law's vision is of a Rambo alone on a desert island with his personal computer doing cost-benefit analyses.

But the world is not populated by Rambos nor are we merely universal background. We are, I think, inherently schizophrenic. On the one hand we are all Rambos—selfish and alone; at the same time we are self-sacrificing and altruistic, we are good neighbors. Professor Lon Fuller, one of the giants of American law, points out that being human involves living with another in a relationship marked by "an uneasy blend of collaboration and resistance" (quoted in Teachout 1986:1130). We are at once competitive and communal beings, at the same time pursuing self-interest and enhancement of the larger community. Fuller rejects any

radical either/or vision of humankind. He views the tensions and contradictions and complexities of life as being at the very core of human
existence.

To deny those contradictions is to seek to be other than who we
are. It is to quarrel with God for not making us better people. As George
Bernard Shaw said in criticizing the Shakespearean comedies because
they indicted individuals and failed to call an oppressive society to account, "an indictment of human nature is really a quarrel with God for
not making men better." We ought to regard these tensions, contradictions, and complexities not just as negative or destructive forces, but as
the sources of energy and growth and life.

To be fully human lies not just in the capacity to embrace those tensions and contradictions, but in the ability to do so in a way that leads to a
stable appreciation of the underlying relationships we have with others.
It is not easy. But we really have no other choice if we want to participate
fully in life. Those contraries can, with effort, lead us to a truer vision and
deeper insight.

Another Vision: The Judeo-Christian Narratives

Our inadequate anthropology has left us with two serious problems: the illusion of innocence and the refusal of moral obligations.

If we are searching for a more adequate statement about what it
means to be human, we can look to the stories of Moses and Jesus. We
could affirm as our own the story of the Exodus, and we could celebrate
the fact that Jesus rose. In our telling of those stories to each other as the
Church we could learn something very important about ourselves and
about God.

The most important thing we can learn about God is that we aren't
God. That is often too profoundly simple for those in my profession who
administer, practice, and teach the law. It is, I suspect, likewise too simple
for many in the health care professions. We once "played God" by extending life with the most extraordinary measures; now we may be
"playing God" in a different way—by withholding nutrition from one
who is not dying but who is merely silent.

If we tell those stories of the Exodus and the death and resurrection
of Jesus we can also claim a power greater than our own. We can say that
we were created in the image of God. That would give some definition to
the question of life which is sorely lacking in the right-to-die movement.
Some of the more strident advocates of the right to die make this such an
important right that it comes to define for them what life means. Perhaps
we are so vehement in asserting a right to die because our identity is not
anchored in life but in death. Will Barrett in Walker Percy's novel *The
Second Coming* (1981:146) captures this malaise while ruminating about

his father's suicide: "How can it be that only with death and dying does the sharp, quick sense of life return?" But those whose identity comes from the stories of Moses and Jesus know that our lives are to be lived in obedience to the God who led his people out of the wilderness and the God who revealed his love for us on the cross.

If we continue with the concept of the image of God we would need to affirm that we do have obligations to our sisters and brothers who are dying and that they in turn have obligations to us. My assertion that the dying have obligations to us strikes many of my colleagues in the law as foolish. However, the law's prohibition of suicide is based on the interweaving of the fabric of society which in turn must be based on the biblical assumption that our lives are not ours alone but God's.

Those who claim the Judeo-Christian tradition as their own will also admit that something went radically wrong at the time of the Fall which we are incapable of fixing. We are benevolent, we are caring, but there is always a dark side. We are at war with ourselves. On the one hand, we want to control our destiny. On the other, we are always seeking. We do care about strangers, while at the same time we want to obliterate them. That is particularly true when they are suffering and in pain.

To face this inner darkness, knowing that much of it is not controllable, requires a strong spiritual discipline. I wish I could affirm my intellectual commitment to nonviolence from my heart, but I know that there is, at some level, a killer in me. "My enemy is my mirror," says theologian Walter Wink (1987:30). "I project onto my enemy everything in myself I cannot stand, tolerate, acknowledge or accept."

Whatever caretaking arrangement we seek must account for our fallenness and must recognize our mutual vulnerability and interdependence. What we need be about in these termination of treatment cases is not so much developing procedures and standards to insure the right decision. There is often no right decision. What we must do is create conditions that encourage us to be vulnerable and to care for people even as they die.

The Curses of Order and Control

Operating in the law are important but unspoken values that distort what is at stake in termination of treatment cases. The law (perhaps all professions) places a high value on order and control; this is evidenced in the Model Health-Care Consent Act and in most of the court decisions involving the termination of treatment. We all want order. We all want clear lines of decision. But at what cost?

Although the stated ethical value in the substituted-judgment standard is individual autonomy, I think all too often the real value is efficiency or finality. Although the best-interest standard is concerned with assuring patient welfare, the balancing called for in that test may well encourage flight from the dying patient. Again the real value may be order, a false order—a flight from uncertainty and doubt.

Professionals always want order and clear lines of responsibility. The Massachusetts court in *Saikewicz* saw the decision-making process as a turf fight between professionals, between "the domain of medical expertise" and that of "judicial resolution." It opted for the latter: "[S]uch questions of life and death seem to us to require the process of detached but passionate investigation and decision that forms the ideal on which the judicial branch of government was created. Achieving this ideal is our responsibility. . ." (370 N.E.2d at 425).

But it is not an either/or decision. If we locate responsibility in a single party—the court, the physician, a particular family member—we tend to let others off the hook. Those others can avoid suffering and vulnerability all too easily. If we also then make the decision risk free for the one left with responsibility, we allow that person to avoid vulnerability. By contrast, to diffuse the responsibility and leave no one free of risk means that all are bound in a community of vulnerability.

One of the potentially liberating aspects of the procedure outlined by the *Conroy* court is the thrust to involve a wider community. While the guardian is charged with final decision making, family, physicians, and the state ombudsman must concur. That procedure has been described as "complex and restrictive" (Levant 1985:1351). It is, if it is viewed through the lens of professionalism. The same critic goes on to recommend review mechanisms "so that decisions to forgo life-sustaining treatment can be made properly and efficiently without overburdening the court system" (1985:1354). But if we were less concerned with efficiency and crowded court dockets and more concerned about providing an opportunity for being with one who is dying, we might view the matter differently. Of course the law cannot force us to care, but it can encourage us to be present.

If we worried less about our professional values of order, control, and lofty detachment and actually sought to inquire about the dignity of the silent patient, we would perhaps learn something about ourselves as well. This would require that we recognize, as did the New Jersey court, that when we don't know the patient's wishes it is "naive to pretend that the right of self-determination serves as a basis for substitute decision-making" (486 A.2d at 1231). We as lawyers would have to search for justice and would no longer equate justice with law. We would have to remember that justice is something we get not from the state, but from each other. Justice is not power, but what we discover as we walk together and give to each other, and as we listen for the voice of our now silent sister or brother.

A Plea for Particularity

How can we inject a more profound humanitarianism based on the values of our religious tradition into the law? I am inclined to think that first we will need to abandon the quest for universal principles or creedal statements. Our common heritage is not just the Enlightenment, nor is it merely a common religious tradition. The secular values of the Enlightenment and the principles of our religious traditions are ultimately nourished by two powerful stories: the story of the Exodus and the story of Jesus' passion and resurrection. It is our connectedness to those stories to which I think we need to return. As we generalize we float free of our experiential ground. We lose our rootedness. This is not a plea for a narcissistic vision but an affirmation that we live in a narrative-bound universe.

We cannot expect a secular and pluralistic world to adopt our stories, but we can nonetheless tell them to ourselves and in that telling have something to offer in the search for another way. We might recount a story about blindness and insight—of Jesus telling his people, after he had healed the blind beggar, "For judgment I came into this world, that those who do not see may see, and that those who see may become blind" (John 9:39). We would tell the law that "one *sine qua non* of human goodness is the ability to see things just as they are; and to see things as they are is a morally difficult task" (MacIntyre 1983:13).

To see things as they are requires that we free ourselves of self-deception and refrain from trying to impose an order where there is none. We would admit that we don't know how to decide whether to terminate treatment for Claire Conroy. But to do that we would have to give up our innocence and our claim that we can see. Only if we accept that we really do not know can we begin to see. And when we can really see, we can love and have compassion.

We might tell the story of Job, which is also a story of transformed perspectives. And in that story we may learn something about the mystery of suffering. We might also in that story learn something of the limitation of the law's power.

We know that we cannot know the answer to most of the questions of life and death. We do know that our lives are not our own but are to be lived in obedience to God. We know that we need not hang onto life or the quality of life as the only alternatives to nothingness. We also know that suffering is a reality and that we cannot dispense with that reality by eliminating the sufferer.

We may not, indeed do not, know what to do in most of these cases. But if we talk about who we are, if we tell our stories not merely for remembering but for repentance, for making amends as well as for giving thanks, we may just figure out what to do.

One thing we can do is resist the profession's quest for order as a substitute for justice. For another, we can look for a third way in this world which sees fight or flight as the only alternatives to death. We can seek a way to care, to develop the calluses to face death without becoming callous. We need to search for an order based on compassion.

NOTES

1. See *In re Quinlan.* 70 N.J. 10, 355 A.2d 647, *cert. denied,* 429 U.S. 922 (1976); *In re Conroy,* 188 N.J. Super. 523 (1983), 190 N.J. Super. 453, 464 A.2d 303 (App. Div. 1983), 98 N.J. 321, 486 A.2d 1209 (1985); and *Superintendent of Belchertown State School v. Saikewicz.* 370 N.E.2d 417 (Mass. 1977).

2. The act was drafted by a committee of the National Conference of Commissioners on Uniform State Law (hereafter the Uniform Law Conference). The Uniform Law Conference is a law reform organization composed of representatives from the legal profession and the legislative bodies of all fifty states. Its general charter is to draft and promulgate uniform legislation for the American legal system. The drafted Model Health-Care Consent Act was adopted by the Uniform Law Conference as a model act and recommended for enactment in all the states. Portions of the act have been adopted in several states.

REFERENCES

Burt, Robert A. 1979. *Taking Care of Strangers.* New York: Free Press.

Destro, R. A. 1986. "Quality of Life Ethics and Constitutional Jurisprudence: The Demise of Natural Rights and Equal Protection for the Disabled and Incompetent." *Journal of Contemporary Health Law and Policy* 2:71–130.

Goldberg, Michael. 1985. *Jews and Christians: Getting Our Stories Straight.* Nashville: Abingdon Press.

Hauerwas, Stanley. 1986. *Suffering Presence.* Notre Dame: University of Notre Dame Press.

Levant, S. 1985. "Comment, Natural Death: An Alternative in New Jersey." *Georgetown Law Review* 73:1331–54.

MacIntyre, Alasdair. 1983. "Moral Philosophy: What Next?" In *Revisions: Changing Perspectives in Moral Philosophy,* ed. Stanley Hauerwas and Alasdair MacIntyre, 1–15. Notre Dame: University of Notre Dame Press.

May, William F. 1983. *The Physician's Covenant.* Philadelphia: Westminster Press.

Meilaender, G. 1986. "The Confused, the Voiceless, the Perverse: Shall We Give Them Food and Drink?" *Issues in Law and Medicine* 2:133–48.

Murdoch, Iris. 1983. "Against Dryness: A Polemical Sketch." In *Revisions: Changing Perspectives in Moral Philosophy,* ed. Stanley Hauerwas and Alasdair MacIntyre, 43–50. Notre Dame: University of Notre Dame Press.

Percy, Walker. 1981. *The Second Coming.* New York: Washington Square Press.

President's Commission for the Study of Ethical Problems in Medicine and Biomedical and Behavioral Research. 1983. *Deciding to Forego Life-Sustaining Treatment.* Washington, D.C.: Government Printing Office.

Shaffer, Thomas. 1979. "Advocacy as Moral Discourse." *North Carolina Law Review* 57: 647–58.

Teachout, P. R. 1986. "The Soul of the Fugue: An Essay on Reading Fuller." *Minnesota Law Review* 70:1073–1148.

Wink, Walter. 1987. *Violence and Nonviolence in South Africa: Jesus' Third Way.* Philadelphia: New Society Publishers.

Yoder, John H. 1984. *The Priestly Kingdom.* Notre Dame: University of Notre Dame Press.

17 *Informed Demand for "Non-Beneficial" Medical Treatment*

Steven H. Miles, M.D.

Stephen Miles, M.D. is in practice at the Hennepin County Medical Center in Minneapolis, Minnesota.

An 85-year-old woman was taken from a nursing home to Hennepin County Medical Center on January 1, 1990, for emergency treatment of dyspnea from chronic bronchiectasis. The patient, Mrs. Helga Wanglie, required emergency intubation and was placed on a respirator. She occasionally acknowledged discomfort and recognized her family but could not communicate clearly. In May, after attempts to wean her from the respirator failed, she was discharged to a chronic care hospital. One week later, her heart stopped during a weaning attempt; she was resuscitated and taken to another hospital for intensive care. She remained unconscious, and a physician suggested that it would be appropriate to consider withdrawing life support. In response, the family transferred her back to the medical center on May 31. Two weeks later, physicians concluded that she was in a persistent vegetative state as a result of severe anoxic encephalopathy. She was maintained on a respirator, with repeated courses of antibiotics, frequent airway suctioning, tube feedings, an air flotation bed, and bio-chemical monitoring.

In June and July of 1990, physicians suggested that life-sustaining treatment be withdrawn since it was not benefiting the patient. Her husband, daughter, and son insisted on continued treatment. They stated their view that physicians should not play God, that the patient would not be better off dead, that removing life support showed moral decay in our civilization, and that a miracle could occur. Her husband told a physician that his wife had never stated her preference concerning life-

This article first appeared in The New England Journal of Medicine *325 (15 August 1991): 512–515.*

sustaining treatment. He believed that the cardiac arrest would not have occurred if she had not been transferred from Hennepin County Medical Center in May. The family reluctantly accepted a do-not-resuscitate order based on the improbability of Mrs. Wanglie's surviving a cardiac arrest. In June, an ethics committee consultant recommended continued counseling for the family. The family declined counseling, including the counsel of their own pastor, and in late July asked that the respirator not be discussed again. In August, nurses expressed their consensus that continued life support did not seem appropriate, and I, as the newly appointed ethics consultant, counseled them.

In October 1990, a new attending physician consulted with specialists and confirmed the permanence of the patient's cerebral and pulmonary conditions. He concluded that she was at the end of her life and that the respirator was "non-beneficial," in that it could not heal her lungs, palliate her suffering, or enable this unconscious and permanently respirator-dependent woman to experience the benefit of the life afforded by respirator support. Because the respirator could prolong life, it was not characterized as "futile."[1] In November, the physician, with my concurrence, told the family that he was not willing to continue to prescribe the respirator. The husband, an attorney, rejected proposals to transfer the patient to another facility or to seek a court order mandating this unusual treatment. The hospital told the family that it would ask a court to decide whether members of its staff were obliged to continue treatment. A second conference two weeks later, after the family had hired an attorney, confirmed these positions, and the husband asserted that the patient had consistently said she wanted respirator support for such a condition.

In December, the medical director and hospital administrator asked the Hennepin County Board of Commissioners (the medical center's board of directors) to allow the hospital to go to court to resolve the dispute. In January, the county board gave permission by a 4-to-3 vote. Neither the hospital nor the county had a financial interest in terminating treatment. Medicare largely financed the $200,000 for the first hospitalization at Hennepin County; a private insurer would pay the $500,000 bill for the second. From February through May of 1991, the family and its attorney unsuccessfully searched for another health care facility that would admit Mrs. Wanglie. Facilities with empty beds cited her poor potential for rehabilitation.

The hospital chose a two-step legal procedure, first asking for the appointment of an independent conservator to decide whether the respirator was beneficial to the patient and second, if the conservator found it was not, for a second hearing on whether it was obliged to provide the respirator. The husband cross-filed, requesting to be appointed conservator. After a hearing in late May, the trial court on July 1, 1991, appointed the husband, as best able to represent the patient's interests. It noted that no request to stop treatment had been made and declined to speculate on the legality of such an order.[2] The hospital said that it would continue to provide the respirator in the light of continuing uncertainty about its legal obligation to provide it. Three days later, despite aggressive care, the patient died of multisystem organ failure resulting from septicemia. The family declined an autopsy and stated that the patient had received excellent care.

Discussion

This sad story illustrates the problem of what to do when a family demands medical treatment that the attending physician concludes cannot benefit the patient. Only 600 elderly people are treated with respirators for more than six months in the United States each year.[3] Presumably, most of these people are actually or potentially conscious. It is common practice to discontinue the use of a respirator before death when it can no longer benefit a patient.[4,5]

We do not know Mrs. Wanglie's treatment preferences. A large majority of elderly people prefer not to receive prolonged respirator support for irreversible unconsciousness.[6] Studies show that an older person's designated family proxy overestimates that person's preference for life-sustaining treatment in a hypothetical coma.[7-9] The implications of this research for clinical decision making have not been cogently analyzed.

A patient's request for a treatment does not necessarily oblige a provider or the health care system. Patients may not demand that physicians injure them (for example, by mutilation), or provide plausible but inappropriate therapies (for example, amphetamines for weight reduction), or therapies that have no value (such as laetrile for cancer). Physicians are not obliged to violate their personal moral views on medical care so long as patients' rights are served. Minnesota's Living Will law says that physicians are "legally bound to act consistently within my wishes within limits of reasonable medical practice" in acting on requests and refusals of treatment.[10] Minnesota's Bill of Patients' Rights says that patients "have the right to appropriate medical . . . care based on individual needs . . . [which is] limited where the service is not reimbursable."[11] Mrs. Wanglie also had aortic insufficiency. Had this condition worsened, a surgeon's refusal to perform a life-prolonging valve replacement as medically inappropriate would hardly occasion public controversy. As the Minneapolis *Star Tribune* said in an editorial on the eve of the trial,

> The hospital's plea is born of realism, not hubris. . . . It advances the claim that physicians should not be slaves to technology— any more than patients should be its prisoners. They should be free to deliver, and act on, an honest and time-honored message: "Sorry, there's nothing more we can do."[12]

Disputes between physicians and patients about treatment plans are often handled by transferring patients to the care of other providers. In this case, every provider contacted by the hospital or the family refused to treat this patient with a respirator. These refusals occurred before and after this case became a matter of public controversy and despite the availability of third-party reimbursement. We believe they represent a medical consensus that respirator support is inappropriate in such a case.

The handling of this case is compatible with current practices regarding informed consent, respect for patients' autonomy, and the right to health care. Doctors should inform patients of all medically reasonable treatments, even those available from other providers. Patients can refuse any prescribed treatment or choose among any medical alternatives that physicians are willing to prescribe. Respect for autonomy does not empower patients to oblige physicians to prescribe treatments in ways that are fruitless or inappropriate. Previous "right to die" cases address the different situation of a patient's right to choose to be free of a prescribed therapy. This case is more about the nature of the patient's entitlement to treatment than about the patient's choice in using that entitlement.

The proposal that this family's preference for this unusual and costly treatment, which is commonly regarded as inappropriate, establishes a right to such treatment is ironic, given that preference does not create a right to other needed, efficacious, and widely desired treatments in the United States. We could not afford a universal health care system based on patients' demands. Such a system would irrationally allocate health care to socially powerful people with strong preferences for immediate treatment to the disadvantage of those with less power or less immediate needs.

After the conclusion was reached that the respirator was not benefiting the patient, the decision to seek a review of the duty to provide it was based on an ethic of "stewardship." Even though the insurer played no part in this case, physicians' discretion to prescribe requires responsible handling of requests for inappropriate treatment. Physicians exercise this stewardship by counseling against or denying such treatment or by submitting such requests to external review. This stewardship is not aimed at protecting the assets of insurance companies but rests on fairness to people who have pooled their resources to insure their collective access to appropriate health care. Several citizens complained to Hennepin County Medical Center that Mrs. Wanglie was receiving expensive treatment paid for by people who had not consented to underwrite a level of medical care whose appropriateness was defined by family demands.

Procedures for addressing this kind of dispute are at an early stage of development. Though the American Medical Association[13] and the Society of Critical Care Medicine[14] also support some decisions to withhold requested treatment, the medical center's reasoning most closely follows the guidelines of the American Thoracic Society.[15] The statements of these professional organizations do not clarify when or how a physician may legally withdraw or withhold demanded life-sustaining treatments. The request for a conservator to review the medical conclusion before considering the medical obligation was often misconstrued as implying that the husband was incompetent or ill motivated. The medical center intended to emphasize the desirability of an independent review of its medical conclusion before its obligation to provide the respirator was reviewed by the court. I believe that the grieving husband was simply mistaken about whether the respirator was benefiting his wife. A direct request to remove the respirator seems to center procedural oversight on the soundness of the medical decision making rather than on the nature of the patient's need. Clearly, the gravity of these decisions merits openness, due process, and meticulous accountability. The relative merits of various procedures need further study.

Ultimately, procedures for addressing requests for futile, marginally effective, or inappropriate therapies require a statutory framework, case law, professional standards, a social consensus, and the exercise of professional responsibility. Appropriate ends for medicine are defined by public and professional consensus. Laws can, and do, say that patients may choose only among medically appropriate options, but legislatures are ill suited to define medical appropriateness. Similarly, health-facility policies on this issue will be difficult to design and will focus on due process rather than on specific clinical situations. Public or private payers will ration according to cost and overall efficacy, a rationing that will become more onerous as therapies are misapplied in individual cases. I believe there is a social consensus that intensive care for a person as "overmastered" by disease as this woman was is inappropriate.

Each case must be evaluated individually. In this case, the husband's request seemed entirely inconsistent with what medical care could do for his wife, the standards of the community, and his fair share of resources that many people pooled for their collective medical care. This case is about limits to what can be achieved at the end of life.

REFERENCES

1. Tomlinson T, Brody H. Futility and the ethics of resuscitation. JAMA 1990; 264:1276–80.

2. In re Helga Wanglie, Fourth Judicial District (Dist. Ct., Probate Ct. Div.) PX-91-283. Minnesota, Hennepin County.

3. Office of Technology Assessment Task Force. Life-sustaining technologies and the elderly. Washington, D.C.: Government Printing Office, 1987.

4. Smedira NG, Evans BH, Grais LS, et al. Withholding and withdrawal of life support from the critically ill. N Engl J Med 1990; 322:309–15.

5. Lantos JD, Singer PA, Walker RM, et al. The illusion of futility in clinical practice. Am J Med 1989; 87:81–4.

6. Emanuel LL, Barry MJ, Stoeckle JD, Ettelson LM, Emanuel EJ. Advance directives for medical care—a case for greater use. N Engl J Med 1991; 324:889–95.

7. Zweibel NR, Cassel CK. Treatment choices at the end of life: a comparison of decisions by older patients and their physician-selected proxies. Gerontologist 1989; 29:615–21.

8. Tomlinson T, Howe K, Notman M, Rossmiller D. An empirical study of proxy consent for elderly persons. Gerontologist 1990; 30:54–64.

9. Danis M, Southerland LI, Garrett JM, et al. A prospective study of advance directives for life-sustaining care. N Engl J Med 1991; 324:882–8.

10. Minnesota Statutes. Adult Health Care Decisions Act. 145b.04.

11. Minnesota Statutes. Patients and residents of health care facilities; Bill of rights. 144.651:Subd. 6.

12. Helga Wanglie's life. Minneapolis Star Tribune. May 26, 1991:18A.

13. Council on Ethical and Judicial Affairs, American Medical Association. Guidelines for the appropriate use of do-not-resuscitate orders. JAMA 1991; 265:1868–71.

14. Task Force on Ethics of the Society of Critical Care Medicine. Consensus report on the ethics of foregoing life-sustaining treatments in the critically ill. Crit Care Med 1990; 18:1435–9.

15. American Thoracic Society. Withholding and withdrawing life-sustaining therapy. Am Rev Respir Dis (in press).

18 Balancing Moral Principles in Federal Regulations on Human Research

TERRENCE F. ACKERMAN

Terrence F. Ackerman is Professor and Chairman, Department of Human Values and Ethics, College of Medicine, University of Tennessee, Memphis, Tenn.

W hile considerable study is devoted to particular moral issues in clinical research, comparatively little attention is focused on the moral presuppositions that inform the analysis of specific problems. Although some consensus exists regarding the relevant moral principles, disputes arise about their precise formulation. Even less agreement is evident regarding the weight to be assigned different principles in situations of conflict.

This latter problem is crucially important in the development of research ethics. The resolution of specific issues often turns on the weight assigned to different moral factors. Consider, for example, research protocols whose design requires withholding information relevant to the consent of prospective subjects. If duties emanating from respect for autonomy require full satisfaction, these protocols ought not to be approved. On the other hand, if promoting the general welfare is assigned greater weight under certain circumstances, protocols that alter basic consent requirements may be permissible within specified limits. More generally, the adequacy of federal regulations on clinical research depends on whether a defensible strategy is utilized to weight diverse moral considerations. Because these regulations articulate basic conditions for approvable research, but also specify allowable exceptions, they suggest the use of an underlying weighting pattern. One commen-

This article first appeared in IRB: A Review of Human Subjects Research *14 (January/February 1992): 1–6.*

tator has suggested that the approach articulated in *The Belmont Report* and adopted in federal regulations fundamentally errs in its assumption that relevant moral principles should be "balanced" against one another in determining research guidelines.[1] Whatever the merits of this argument, proper evaluation of the conditions and exceptions formulated in federal regulations requires that we establish and critically assess the pattern for assigning weight to moral principles that informs them.

This undertaking involves four questions. First, what are the factors whose conflict creates the moral issues? Second, what pattern for weighting these factors is presupposed in federal regulations? Third, what are the merits of this approach compared to alternative weighting strategies? Lastly, how does clarifying this strategy facilitate assessment and interpretation of federal regulations?

Moral Issues in Clinical Research

The moral structure of clinical research reflects the diverse consequences of using medical procedures with human subjects to produce generalizable knowledge. On one hand, we may enhance the general welfare of society by expanding our body of generalizable knowledge. On the other hand, the design, procedures, or circumstances involved in research studies may necessitate compromising the interests of subjects in some measure. The key issues concern the extent to which the interests of subjects may be compromised, if at all, in pursuing the social good of expanded medical knowledge.

The relevant interests of subjects fall into three categories: in exercising the capacity for autonomous choice, in protecting and promoting personal welfare, and in fair treatment. The interest in exercising autonomous choice is reflected in the obligation to respect the capacity of persons to deliberate about and act on their life plans. In the research setting, this obligation issues in several specific requirements, such as duties to secure informed consent, to respect the privacy of persons, and to protect the confidentiality of data linked to identifiable subjects.

The interest of persons in protecting and promoting their welfare is reflected in several categories of obligations directed toward individuals. These might be called obligations of individual beneficence.[2] They include duties to avoid harming, prevent harm to, remove harm from, and promote the welfare of specific persons.[3] Each category is relevant in the context of clinical research. The duty to avoid harming others suggests that subjects who are unable to consent or are otherwise especially vulnerable should not be exposed to interventions involving more than minimal risk that are not intended for their benefit. The obligation to prevent harm to individuals generates the duty to minimize risk of harm to subjects consistent with sound research design. Obligations to prevent and remove harms suggest that a therapeutic procedure utilized in clinical research should have a harm/benefit ratio that is at least as advantageous as any alternative treatment acceptable to the subject.[4]

The interest in fair treatment is reflected in obligations of justice. Justice requires that the benefits and burdens of cooperative social endeavors be distributed in ways that provide persons with an equal opportunity to pursue their life plans. In the research setting, this obligation requires that the selection of subjects not impose special burdens on specific classes of persons rendering them less able to pursue their life plans. It also requires that subjects with special vulnerabilities be accorded stronger protections than less vulnerable subjects.

Finally, research activities are sustained by the interest in promoting the general welfare of society. The importance of this interest is reflected in categories of obligations similar to those of individual beneficence, although focused on the welfare of groups of persons. Thus they might be called duties of social beneficence. Again, each category of obligation is relevant in the context of human research. For example, the obligation to avoid causing harm to groups of persons generates a duty to assess the safety and efficacy of standard medical procedures whose value is uncertain. Similarly, obligations to prevent and remove harms generate duties to test new therapies for curing or ameliorating diseases that affect groups of persons.

This description of the relevant interests and obligations suggests several important points for framing the question of weighting. First, it is obvious that the key problem concerns how to balance pursuit of the general welfare against duties to subjects. Although conflicts between duties to subjects arise,[5] the basic issues in clinical research involve the conflict between these factors and considerations of social beneficence.

Second, this description of the moral structure of research assumes that there are duties to promote the general welfare through research activities. This view is accepted in *The Belmont Report*, but respected commentators, such as Hans Jonas, have argued that although clinical research is highly desirable, it is morally optional.[6] Jonas claims that while we have an obligation to avoid activities that cause harm to future generations, our descendants have no right to the development of new medical treatments. Although the logic of his claim cannot be fully explored, several points suggest its inadequacy. Jonas accepts the claim that we have a duty not to cause harm. But he fails to recognize that clinical research may be necessary to fulfill this duty. Physicians have often used treatments, such as high concentration oxygen therapy for premature infants, that unknowingly cause a net balance of harm to patients. Minimization of harm-causing practices requires formal evaluation of the safety and efficacy of controversial standard treatments in clinical trials.[7]

Moreover, it is difficult to sustain the claim that not causing harm to others is obligatory but that preventing or removing harms is not. Not causing harm and preventing or removing harm have precisely the same objective: minimizing the extent of harm that may occur to persons.[8] Also, the amount and type of effort required to prevent or remove harms may often be no different from that required to avoid causing harm. These points are illustrated in the setting of clinical research. Protocols that result in improved medical treatments provide means to prevent or alleviate the disabling sequelae of disease. Protocols designed to evaluate controversial standard therapies facilitate the identification of harm-causing medical practices. In both cases, the objective of clinical research is to minimize the extent of harm that might occur to patients. Furthermore, the process that must be undertaken to identify improved treatments or to expose current harm-causing therapies is precisely the same—formal evaluation of these interventions in well-designed clinical trials. Thus, if clinical research is necessary to satisfy the obligations to avoid causing harm, it seems reasonable to maintain that it is also required in fulfilling obligations to prevent and remove harms.

Finally, it is generally agreed that society is obligated to assure persons access to basic goods needed to pursue their life plans, such as food, housing, and gainful employment. Because seriously disabling or life-threatening diseases substantially compromise the ability of persons to pursue their life plans, availability of adequate medical treatment should also be considered a basic good. When safe and effective therapy is not available, the obligation to provide access to basic goods requires that clinical research be undertaken to develop the generalizable knowledge essential for improving treatment. Thus, various considerations support the claim that at least some research activities are required by general obligations of social beneficence.

Third, recognizing that there are obligations to conduct clinical research prevents us from viewing the weighting issue as a matter of balancing duties to subjects against merely desirable gains in medical knowledge. If the latter view were accepted, the weighting issue would be settled at the outset. Pursuit of optional research goals would be properly constrained by full satisfaction of duties to subjects. Once we admit that there are duties to conduct research, weighting strategies other than one assigning absolute priority to full satisfaction of duties to subjects merit consideration.

Fourth, some commentators incorrectly assume that the only conceptual alternatives are to require complete satisfaction of subject-related duties *or* to permit their total subjugation to obligations of social beneficence.[9] However, the nature of the interests and obligations at stake allows compromises of degree between conflicting moral duties. For example, a research study whose design requires withholding relevant information from prospective subjects violates the duty to secure informed consent. The information withheld may compromise in greater or lesser measure the ability of persons to deliberate about and act on their life plans. Similarly, an investigation that employs nontherapeutic procedures involving more than minimal risk with subjects unable to consent violates the obligation of individual beneficence to avoid causing harm. The risks involved may exceed the level of minimal risk to a greater or lesser extent. Thus, we might accept a weighting strategy that allows some compromise of degree in duties to subjects without embracing wholesale violations. The limits set on these compromises would necessitate correlative compromises of degree in the fulfillment of duties to promote the general welfare through research activities.

Finally, the structure of moral issues in research does not preclude adopting a weighting strategy that assigns different weight to the respective categories of duties to subjects *vis-à-vis* obligations to conduct clinical research. For example, a weighting strategy might permit limited compromises in fulfillment of duties to protect the welfare of subjects, but prohibit compromises in the fulfillment of obligations of fair treatment and respect for personal autonomy.

Thus, the key issue concerns the proper weighting of duties to subjects against duties to conduct human research. However, the nature of these duties admits a variety of options among potential weighting strategies.

THE WEIGHTING STRATEGY OF FEDERAL REGULATIONS

In exploring the weighting strategy embedded in the research regulations of the Department of Health and Human Services (45 CFR 46), it need not be assumed that their authors consciously articulated and applied a specific approach. Rather, the analysis can be viewed as formulating a plausible interpretation of the moral commitments implicit in the regulatory requirements. In constructing this interpretation, it is useful to review two points: first, the basic rules delineated for IRB approval of research protocols; and second, some specific exceptions allowing research that does not satisfy basic requirements.

Each category of subject-related duties is addressed in the basic conditions for IRB approval of research protocols, some of which are described in § 46.111. Duties to respect personal autonomy are reflected in the requirements that "Informed consent will be sought" and that adequate provisions be made "to protect the privacy of subjects and to maintain the confidentiality of data." Duties of fair treatment are represented in requirements that "the selection of subjects [be] equitable" and that "appropriate additional safeguards [be] included" to protect subjects especially vulnerable to coercion or undue influence. Several conditions are intended to implement duties of individual beneficence, such as the requirements that "risks to subjects [be] minimized," that "risks to subjects [be] reasonable in relation to anticipated benefits," and that adequate provisions be made "for monitoring the data collected to insure the safety of subjects." In addition, a beneficence duty generally acknowledged in sections on special subject populations is that nontherapeutic procedures involving more than minimal risk may not be used with subjects who are unable to consent or are otherwise especially vulnerable.

Moreover, § 46.111 specifies that to approve research "the IRB shall determine that all" of the requirements therein listed "are satisfied." This statement suggests that duties to subjects set prior constraints on research activities which must be fully satisfied before IRB approval can be granted. Thus, this section appears to adopt a weighting strategy that assigns absolute priority to the fulfillment of duties to subjects.

However, other sections introduce exceptions that undermine the plausibility of this initial interpretation. For example, § 46.116 specifies that consent requirements may be altered or waived provided that

(1) The research involves no more than minimal risk to the subjects; (2) the waiver or alteration will not adversely affect the rights and welfare of the subjects; (3) the research could not practicably be carried out without the waiver or alteration; and (4) whenever appropriate, the subjects will be provided with additional pertinent information after participation.

When these conditions are met, research may be undertaken even though informed consent requirements are not fully satisfied. Similarly, § 46.406 formulates conditions under which nontherapeutic procedures involving more than minimal risk may be used with children. Research employing such procedures may be approved only if (1) the risk represents a minor increase over minimal risk, (2) the intervention presents experiences commensurate with those inherent in the life-situation of the subjects, and (3) the intervention is likely to yield vitally important knowledge about the subjects' disorder or its treatment. When these conditions are satisfied, the use of nontherapeutic procedures may be

292   TERRENCE F. ACKERMAN

approved even though the rule that prohibits exposure of vulnerable subjects to more than minimal risk of harm unrelated to their own welfare is not satisfied.

These basic conditions and exceptions for IRB approval of research suggest a weighting strategy that involves two main components. On one hand, presumptive priority is assigned to duties to subjects, requiring their full satisfaction in most circumstances. On the other hand, this presumptive priority may be overridden provided that certain necessary conditions are satisfied. Several candidates are suggested by the regulatory formulation of exceptions. One is that it must not be practicably possible to conduct the research unless the exception to full satisfaction of duties to subjects is allowed. For example, the regulations specify that waiver or alteration of consent requirements can be permitted only if "the research could not be practicably carried out" without it. Similarly, the regulations on research with children allow the use of nontherapeutic procedures involving more than minimal risk only when the research is likely to produce knowledge of "vital importance" that cannot otherwise be secured. A second condition for permitting exceptions is that compromise in the fulfillment of duties to subjects must be narrowly circumscribed. For example, alteration or waiver of consent requirements is permitted only if it does not "adversely affect the rights and welfare" of subjects and the research imposes only "minimal risk." Likewise, use with children of nontherapeutic procedures involving more than minimal risk is permitted only if the risk "represents a minor increase" over minimal risk. A third necessary condition for permitting exceptions might be the requirement that the knowledge generated through the research be important in preventing substantial harms to groups of persons. For example, the use with children of nontherapeutic research procedures involving more than minimal risk is permitted only if the knowledge to be developed will be vitally important for understanding or ameliorating the subjects' disorder or condition. (However, the conditions for waiver or alteration of consent do not include a similar requirement.) Whatever the precise set of conditions necessary for approval of exceptions, protocols that meet these requirements may be conducted even though duties to subjects are not fully satisfied.

Further refinements would be necessary to give a fully satisfactory account of the operative weighting strategy. For example, the regulations on research with fetuses and children permit research that is not approvable under the basic rules and exceptions, provided the moral principles relevant to research are satisfied.[10] A substantial digression would be required to explore how this provision might be integrated into the presumptive weighting strategy as outlined. However, these refinements will be bypassed in order to compare the presumptive weighting strategy with other conceptual alternatives.

ALTERNATIVE WEIGHTING STRATEGIES

There are four basic approaches for weighting duties to conduct research *vis-à-vis* duties to subjects: duties to conduct research assume absolute priority; the respective sets of duties possess equal weight; duties to subjects assume absolute priority; or each of the competing duties is assigned some weight in the resolution of issues, but not in equal amounts.

The first alternative can be quickly dismissed. It would allow the extent of compromise in the fulfillment of duties to subjects to be determined entirely by the impact in fostering or impeding clinical research. Carried to its logical conclusion, it would clearly permit unacceptable violation of the rights and welfare of subjects.

A second alternative is to assign equal weight to subject-related duties and duties to conduct human research. Resolution of particular issues would involve striking a balance between the requirements of the competing moral duties.[11] This weighting strategy encounters a fatal dilemma. On one hand, its most obvious interpretation would result in research guidelines that offer inadequate protection for the rights and welfare of human subjects. If we begin with competing duties possessing equal weight, then striking a balance should involve compromising the requirements of each to an equal degree. However, it is generally agreed that the rights and welfare of human subjects should be broadly protected in the conduct of research, while pursuit of the general welfare must be narrowly constrained by regard for these interests. Thus, the idea of an evenly balanced compromise between the competing duties is not tenable. On the other hand, we might interpret this weighting strategy as assigning equal moral force to the competing duties only in the abstract, with the resolution of conflicts proceeding by compromises of unequal degree in their respective requirements. Although this revision avoids the prior unacceptable result, it engenders a loss of clarity. The metaphor of striking a balance between duties of equal weight loses its directive power, providing no guidance regarding the extent to which competing duties should be compromised in resolving conflicts between them.[12] Thus, this second weighting strategy either leads to clearly unacceptable results for protection of the rights and welfare of subjects or must be assigned an interpretation that lacks prescriptive clarity.

The third weighting strategy overcomes both difficulties. It assigns absolute priority to the fulfillment of duties to subjects. The clearest interpretation of "absolute priority" is Rawls' lexical ordering strategy:

the requirements of duties assigned higher priority must be fully satisfied before meeting the requirements of duties possessing lower priority.[13] Applied to human research, this means that pursuit of the general welfare through research activities must be constrained by full satisfaction of duties to subjects.

The basic rationale for this approach involves two points. On one hand, it offers a weighting strategy that secures a firmly grounded protection for the rights and welfare of subjects. On the other hand, it assures that "No amount of good consequences can overwhelm the inherent moral requirements" of duties to subjects.[14] The result is achieved by closing the door on any consideration of the beneficial consequences of research activities until the requirements of duties to subjects are fully satisfied.

Despite the initial attractiveness of this weighting strategy, it suffers from fatal difficulties in an important range of situations. It is widely agreed that individuals have duties of beneficence to prevent substantial harms to other specific persons when doing so will involve no more than modest costs to their own interests.[15] By extension, it is reasonable to maintain that individuals have similar "duties of rescue" when they can prevent serious harms to groups of persons at modest costs to their own interests. Similarly, when persons organized collectively can prevent serious harms to groups of persons at modest costs to their own interests, collective duties of rescue can be posited.[16] In the context of human research, situations occur in which compromises in fulfilling duties to subjects may be necessary in order to undertake research activities that may prevent substantial harms to other groups of persons. If these compromises represent only a modest cost to the interests of individual subjects, the analogy with duties of rescue suggests that they are morally justified. Since this conclusion is inconsistent with the weighting strategy that gives absolute priority to duties to subjects, the latter approach should be rejected.

The last weighting strategy involves some degree of recognition for each set of competing duties, but not in equal proportion. One version of this approach is a presumptive weighting strategy like that represented in the federal regulations. Presumptive priority is assigned to duties to subjects, requiring their full satisfaction in most circumstances. However, this presumption may be overridden if it is necessary to undertake research activities that may prevent substantial harm to others and there will be no more than minor compromises in protections for the rights and welfare of subjects.

This position possesses several advantages while avoiding the liabilities of alternative approaches. First, it recognizes the preeminent importance of protecting the rights and welfare of human subjects. Full satisfaction of duties to subjects is required in most situations. Moreover, compromises in the fulfillment of these duties may involve only minor infringements on the interests of subjects. Thus, this approach avoids the laxness or lack of clarity regarding subject-related protections that undermines the position assigning equal weight to the competing sets of duties.

Second, the presumptive weighting strategy acknowledges the pertinence of duties of rescue within the context of human research. That is, it recognizes that circumstances occur in which substantial harms to groups of persons can only be prevented through research activities that involve modest costs to the interests of human subjects. Insofar as subjects acting collectively can prevent these harms, duties are engendered to accept minor compromises in their interests. The presumptive weighting strategy supports the legitimacy of research rules that reflect these duties. In this regard, it takes more complete account of our obligations than the strategy that assigns absolute priority to duties to subjects.

More generally, the presumptive weighting strategy takes better account of the moral import of "pursuit of the general welfare." Too often this phrase conveys the image of a mechanically summed quantity of benefit not belonging to specific individuals. In the context of clinical research, however, pursuit of the general welfare includes the prevention of substantial harms resulting from injury or illness that will be visited upon specific, if not now identifiable persons. The harms to which these individuals may succumb demand moral recognition if we have regard for their equal status as persons with the capacity for suffering. Such respect requires our collective assistance when it can be rendered at modest costs to our own interests as research subjects.

Third, while the presumptive weighting strategy allows pursuit of the general welfare to partly constrain fulfillment of duties to subjects, it does not permit substantial undermining of subject-related protections. Compromises in these protections are permitted only when they are practicably necessary to the conduct of research. Moreover, they must involve no more than minor infringements on the requirements of duties to subjects. Finally, these compromises are permitted only if the research may generate knowledge that prevents substantial harms to others. Thus, concern for the welfare of others is assigned limited weight in resolving moral issues in clinical research, without functioning as the predominant factor.

This weighting strategy involves the exercise of judgment in determining legitimate exceptions to the presumption favoring full satisfaction of duties to subjects. Key phrases, such as "minor compromise in the requirements of duties to subjects," "prevention of substantial harms to others," and "necessary for the conduct of research activities" require interpretation. Concern may arise that too much latitude is thereby permitted in determining the extent to which protections for the rights and welfare of subjects may be attenuated. However, assuming a more rigid approach to protection of human subjects precludes proper recognition of duties of social beneficence requiring us to prevent substantial harm to others when it can be accomplished at modest costs to our own interests. Thus, this latitude is inescapable if our weighting strategy is to acknowledge fully all dimensions of the moral landscape bearing on the resolution of research issues.

CRITIQUE AND INTERPRETATION

Clarification of the appropriate weighting strategy for balancing moral duties provides a basis for both assessing the adequacy of federal regulations and interpreting components of the guidelines that lack clarity.

The critical function can be illustrated by recurring to provisions on the alteration or waiver of consent requirements. The four conditions specified define circumstances under which deception or withholding of information may be permitted as an element in research protocols.[17] The weighting strategy suggests two important problems. On one hand, the allowable circumstances in which consent requirements may be waived or altered are too broad. The regulatory threshold for considering this exception is crossed when "the research could not practicably be carried out" without alteration or waiver. However, our weighting strategy also suggests that compromises in duties to subjects should only be considered when necessary to prevent substantial harm to other persons. Research whose goal is to expand generalizable knowledge without contributing to the prevention or removal of substantial harms should not qualify for the waiver or alteration of consent requirements.[18] By contrast, rules permitting the use with children of non-therapeutic research procedures involving more than minimal risk are properly restricted to studies that may develop "vitally important" knowledge for understanding or ameliorating the disorder afflicting the subjects.

On the other hand, the conditions for waiving or altering consent requirements are also too narrow. They specify that the waiver or alteration must "not adversely affect the rights" of subjects. However, it is patently unclear how key elements of information needed by a reasonable person in deciding about participation in research can be withheld without compromising the subject's right to give informed consent. Literally interpreted, this condition forecloses use of the waiver or alteration exception.[19] It is more reasonable to acknowledge that withholding consent information compromises the rights of subjects, but to require that the waiver or alteration not seriously undermine the opportunity of persons to deliberate about and act on their life plans. The presumptive weighting strategy would loosen the relevant condition to permit the waiver or alteration if it involves no more than a minor impairment in subjects' opportunity to make autonomous choices.

As formulated, the weighting strategy also allows interpretation of regulatory requirements that are not fully specified. Basic conditions for IRB approval of research include the requirement that "risks to subjects [be] reasonable in relation to anticipated benefits, if any, to subjects . . . "[20] However, the regulations do not clarify what further conditions are necessary to establish "reasonableness." With regard to treatment for a serious illness provided in a clinical trial, individual beneficence requires that the therapy offered be thought likely to have as favorable a harm/benefit ratio as any alternative treatment acceptable to the patient. The presumptive weighting strategy requires that this rule normally be satisfied. However, minor compromises of the rule are permitted when it is necessary to undertake research studies whose results may prevent substantial harm to others. This application of the weighting strategy provides interpretive content for determining whether the risks of therapeutic procedures are "reasonable" in relation to anticipated benefits for subjects.

One application of this gloss on "reasonableness" concerns the use of placebo controls in randomized trials. For example, there are currently many placebo-controlled trials of drugs for the treatment of uncomplicated mild-to-moderate hypertension that include discontinuation of treatment in control subjects for eight to twelve weeks. Because 50 percent of the control subjects return to their baseline hypertension within this period, a question arises as to whether they are subjected to increased risk of morbid sequelae.[21] Annualized rates of increased risk of morbid events in untreated hypertensives suggest a major increment in risk for control subjects.[22] However, the absence of statistically significant differences in the occurrence of morbid events between treatment and placebo groups in these short-term studies, as well as the fact that the physiological changes leading to morbid events in untreated hypertension usually develop over an extended period of time, suggest that the increment of risk for these events in control subjects is rather modest. Thus, if the use of placebo controls is shown to be necessary in conducting these studies, the presumption in favor of using only treatments with the same net therapeutic advantage could be overridden.

Formulation of an appropriate weighting strategy for resolving conflicts does not assure easy resolution of moral issues in clinical research. As indicated above, application of the presumptive weighting approach requires interpretation of key terms such as "modest cost" and "necessary for the conduct of research studies." Moreover, important disagreements may occur about the precise formulation of the duties to subjects and duties to conduct research that constitute the framework for conceptualizing the moral issues. Nevertheless, formulation of a defensible approach to weighting moral principles is essential to assess and interpret satisfactorily federal guidelines on clinical research. This need is satisfied by the presumptive weighting strategy.

REFERENCES

1. Marshall, E: Does the moral philosophy of the Belmont Report rest on a mistake? *IRB: A Review of Human Subjects Research* 1986; 8(6): 5–6.

2. Obligations of beneficence include various classes determined by their focus and source. Obligations of *individual* beneficence focus on the welfare of specific persons, while obligations of *social* beneficence focus on the welfare of groups of persons. Obligations of *role-specific* beneficence derive from specific roles or institutional arrangements, while obligations of *general* beneficience devolve upon persons independently of roles or institutions. Moreover, the classification of beneficence obligations determined by focus cuts across the classification determined by source. For example, a public official may have a role-specific, but social obligation of beneficience that derives from the assumption of elected office and focuses on the welfare of his or her constituency as a group.

3. Frankena, WK: *Ethics* (Englewood Cliffs, N.J.: Prentice Hall, 1973, 2nd ed.), p. 47.

4. Cf. World Medical Association Declaration of Helsinki: In Levine, RJ: *Ethics and Regulation of Clinical Research* (Baltimore: Urban and Schwarzenberg, 1986, 2nd ed.), p. 429.

5. For example, see The National Commission for the Protection of Human Subjects of Biomedical and Behavioral Research: *Report and Recommendations: Research Involving Prisoners.* DHEW Publication No. (OD) 76-131, Washington, D.C.: U.S. Government Printing Office, 1976, pp. 5–7.

6. See The National Commission for the Protection of Human Subjects of Biomedical and Behavioral Research: *The Belmont Report: Ethical Guidelines for the Protection of Human Subjects of Research.* DHEW Publication No. (OS) 78-0012, Washington, D.C.: U.S. Government Printing Office, 1978; and Jonas, H: Philosophical reflections on human experimentation. In *Experimentation With Human Subjects,* ed. P. Freund (New York: George Braziller, 1969), pp. 13–14.

7. Cf. The National Commission for the Protection of Human Subjects: *The Belmont Report,* p. 8.

8. Cf. Feinberg, J: *The Moral Limits of the Criminal Law: Harm to Others* (New York: Oxford University Press, 1984), pp. 126–86.

9. See, for example, Veatch, RM: *A Theory of Medical Ethics* (New York: Basic Books, 1981), pp. 299–300.

10. *Code of Federal Regulations,* Title 45, Part 46, §§ 46.211 and 46.407.

11. Cf. Beauchamp, TL, and Childress, JF: *Principles of Biomedical Ethics* (New York: Oxford University Press, 1989, 3rd ed.), pp. 51–54; and Levine: *Ethics and Regulation of Clinical Research,* p. 12.

12. Cf. Marshall, E: Does the moral philosophy of the Belmont Report rest on a mistake?, p. 6.

13. Rawls, J: *A Theory of Justice* (Cambridge, Mass.: Harvard University Press, 1971), pp. 42–44.

14. Veatch: *A Theory of Medical Ethics,* p. 300.

15. Cf. Beauchamp and Childress: *Principles of Biomedical Ethics,* pp. 200–203; and Feinberg: *Harm to Others,* pp. 126–86.

16. See Goodin, RE: *Protecting the Vulnerable* (Chicago: University of Chicago Press, 1985), pp. 134–44.

17. *Code of Federal Regulations,* Title 45, Part 46, § 46.116 (d).

18. It could be argued that this further condition for allowing compromises in the fulfillment of consent-related duties is overly restrictive. For example, some epidemiological studies cannot be conducted without waiving the requirement for explicit consent of subjects to the use of their medical records. Moreover, these studies are sometimes concerned to develop knowledge that is useful, but may not be needed to prevent substantial harms. If we accept the judgment that such studies ought to be permitted, problems arise for the weighting strategy outlined above. Several approaches are available for resolving the issue, but their consideration must be deferred to another occasion. This point was called to my attention by Robert Levine.

19. Cf. Veatch, RM: *The Patient as Partner: A Theory of Human-Experimentation Ethics* (Bloomington, Ind.: Indiana University Press, 1987), pp. 103–106.

20. *Code of Federal Regulations,* Title 45, Part 46, § 46.111(a)(2).

21. William Applegate, MD (personal communication).

22. See Levine, RJ: The use of placebos in randomized clinical trials. *IRB: A Review of Human Subjects Research* 1985; 7(2): 1–4.

19 Building a New Consensus: Ethical Principles and Policies for Clinical Research on HIV/AIDS

CAROL LEVINE, M.A., NANCY NEVELOFF DUBLER, LL.B., AND ROBERT J. LEVINE, M.D.

Carol Levine, M.A., is Executive Director of the Citizens Commission on AIDS for New York City and Northern New Jersey. Nancy Neveloff Dubler, LL.B., is Director of the Division of Law and Ethics, Department of Epidemiology and Social Medicine, Montefiore Medical Center/The Albert Einstein College of Medicine, Bronx, N.Y. Robert J. Levine, M.D., is Professor of Medicine, Yale University School of Medicine, and Chair of the Yale Human Investigation Committee.

Safe and effective drugs to treat AIDS and HIV infection are urgently needed. Without them, an increasing number of men, women, adolescents, and young children will face suffering, disability, and death. The process of developing and approving new drugs in the United States over the past thirty years has typically been long, laborious, and often frustrating. Some of the delays are inherent in the scientific method. Others reflect the particular structure of the drug regulation process in the United States, and the history that shaped its implementation. The primary statutory and regulatory emphasis has been on assuring that drugs are safe and effective before they are widely marketed. Patients' access to possibly beneficial but still unproven drugs has been seen as an interest to be accommodated where possible, but not as a right or a major goal.

This article first appeared in IRB: A Review of Human Subjects Research 13 *(January/April 1991): 1–17.*

As the demand for new and better HIV/AIDS drugs mounts, the process by which these drugs move from the laboratory to the pharmacy has come under intense and extraordinary scrutiny. Academic research institutions and government agencies—the traditional centers of scientific and regulatory power—have been targets of political protest, including slogans, picketing, marches, and sit-ins. Individuals have demanded access to experimental drugs. In some trials subjects analyzed their medications to see whether they were active agents or placebos, shared the active agents with other individuals, and took additional, unapproved medications, thereby violating the terms of the protocol and possibly compromising the validity of the data. Furthermore, the underrepresentation of some groups affected by HIV in trials has been increasingly seen as discrimination against them rather than protection from risk or exploitation.

At the very least, the spirit of mutual respect and cooperation that should be at the heart of the investigator-trial participant relationship has been challenged; public and professional confidence about the adequacy of the drug approval process has been shaken. Regulators' attempts to respond through new or revamped mechanisms are attacked both by those who view them as too timid and those who see them as too drastic.

Controversy has never been absent from the drug development process; nor is the ethics of human subjects research a closed topic. Nonetheless, whatever carefully crafted (albeit tenuous) consensus once existed has broken down. The new context of increased advocacy and empowerment of potential subjects requires a reappraisal of the ethical balance between protecting the rights and welfare of subjects and expanding their options for access to possibly beneficial but still unproven drugs.

This report represents the beginnings of a new consensus, a broad framework of agreement on basic principles and policies that ought to guide HIV/AIDS clinical research. It also identifies some areas where consensus is fragile or where emphases differ. These recommendations, which were developed by a multidisciplinary group representing diverse professional, public, and social interests, are intended to clarify the ethical issues, further the creation of scientifically valid and ethically justifiable protocols, and encourage the kind of meaningful community consultation that will result in more rapid accumulation and dissemination of the high-quality data that is so urgently needed to enhance patient care. Although these recommendations concern HIV/AIDS, we hope that they will stimulate researchers, clinicians, and potential subjects concerned with other diseases to re-examine their own practices and priorities.

The recommendations are directed at several audiences: researchers, governmental officials, drug company sponsors, members of Institutional Review Boards (IRBs), trial participants, and AIDS advocacy organizations. The recommendations cover five main areas: research design, community consultation, rights and obligations of participants and investigators, informed consent and inducements to participate in research, and additional considerations for research involving four special populations (children and adolescents, women, prisoners, and people with mental disabilities).

We intend the recommendations to be seen as a coherent whole, with each section building on the previous ones and leading logically to the next. Failing to look at the clinical trial process in its entirety leads to confusion and misunderstanding; for example, in seeking to understand why some subjects fail to comply with the terms of a protocol, one must determine whether the problem lies in unrealistic or unacceptable conditions in the research designs, in social and economic deprivations that make compliance difficult, or in individuals' suspicions or apprehensions about the research. Many problems can be avoided or ameliorated by careful planning and sensitivity to concerns about the studies as expressed by potential subjects and community advocates.

In focusing on protocol development, review, and implementation, we recognize that several important areas of ethical concern are not covered. These include the setting of the research agenda itself (that is, which drugs are chosen for development and how and to whom research funds are allocated); the entrepreneurial aspects of drug development (the high costs of drugs, the links between researchers and industry, and third-party coverage of experimental drugs); and, particularly, the absence of a national health program to ensure adequacy of basic medical care for all Americans. All these issues, and others, require sustained analysis but would be a diversion from the main focus of these recommendations.

HIV/AIDS research is conducted in a context of standards already set by law and ongoing regulatory and professional practice. In some cases the recommendations of this group suggest changes in these standards. In most cases, however, the proposed modifications can be implemented by greater sensitivity and mutual understanding among all the participants in the research process.

DEFINITIONS AND KEY CONCEPTS

Language is important in all discussions of HIV/AIDS. In this section, we define the most important terms used in the report.

Ethical Principles

The generally accepted source of the definitions of the ethical principles that should guide research involving human subjects is the Belmont Report, published by the National Commission for the Protection of Human Subjects of Biomedical and Behavioral Research in 1978. These principles form the basis for our ethical analysis:

Respect for persons. Respect for persons incorporates at least two ethical convictions: first, that individuals should be treated as autonomous agents, and second, that persons with diminished autonomy are entitled to protection.

Beneficence. Persons are treated in an ethical manner not only by respecting their decisions and protecting them from harm, but also by making efforts to secure their well-being. . . . Two general rules have been formulated as complementary expressions of beneficent actions . . . (1) do no harm and (2) maximize possible benefits and minimize possible harms.

Justice. Who ought to receive the benefits of research and bear its burdens? This is a question of justice, in the sense of "fairness in distribution" or "what is deserved." Justice is relevant to the selection of subjects of research at two levels: the social and the individual.

Individual justice in the selection of subjects requires researchers to be fair; that is, they should not offer potential benefit only to some favored patients or choose "undesirable" persons for risky research. Social justice extends the principle of fairness to groups; that is, groups should not be included in research merely because it is expedient to do so, nor should groups be excluded from a fair share of the benefits of research.

Research and Treatment

Research is a category of activity designed to develop or contribute to generalizable knowledge—the theories, principles, or relationships that can be corroborated by scientific observation or inference.

Medical practice (also called "care" or "treatment") is a class of activities solely intended to improve the health and well-being of an individual patient.

"Nonvalidated practices" or "innovative therapies" are activities that are intended to improve the health and well-being of an individual patient but that have not been proved to be safe or efficacious. Some practices may be too new for sufficient data to have been collected or they may be applications of a validated therapy in a different population or for a different indication.

Differences between research and treatment. Research protocols for drug trials present evidence from laboratory or animal studies or other human trials that justifies the study, the study design, exclusion and inclusion criteria, and procedures for carrying out the study and analyzing the results. Protocols outline a formal regimen that cannot be revised to meet individual needs, unless the design specifically provides for variation. Some, but not all, research studies may involve elements of medical care, but providing care is not their primary purpose. (See "Informed Consent and Access to Research," below.)

Medical care does not have many of the constraints of research. In the course of treatment, a physician may alter drug dosages to meet individual needs, prescribe drugs for indications other than those that are FDA-approved, and in many other ways adjust patient care. Patient benefit is the foremost concern.

Nonvalidated drug therapies may be studied through research protocols, particularly when the goal is to develop knowledge that will allow the drug sponsor to submit data to the FDA for marketing approval. Some nonvalidated therapies, however, do not require formal research protocols. For example, pediatricians prescribe many drugs for their patients without the benefit of data from formal clinical trails, because trials have been conducted only on adults.

Human subjects. The traditional science and ethics literature and federal regulations refer to individuals involved in research as "subjects." Many advocates prefer the term "trial participants" because it avoids the negative connotations of being "subjected" to something or someone and emphasizes the co-equal status of the individual and the investigator. In this document we will use both terms synonymously, recognizing both the prevailing usage in the research community and the importance of treating "subjects" as moral equals.

Justifications for Starting Clinical Trials

The **null hypothesis** is a formal statement of equivalence (no difference) regarding the primary endpoints (outcome measurements) of a clinical trial. Ethically the term is used in a different sense, to justify the beginning of a randomized clinical trial (RCT). An ethical null hypothesis (also termed "theoretical equipoise" by Benjamin Freedman) is a statement that there are no differences among all relevant outcomes, including the *balance* of risks and benefits and quality of life. It is impossible to *prove* a null hypothesis, since to do so, one would have to prove that treatment A and treatment B are equal in all patients with a specific condition. It is, however, possible to *reject* a null hypothesis, i.e., to observe a difference between A and B that is unlikely to have occurred by chance. Thus, if the P (probability) value is less than .05, there is less than a 5 percent likelihood that the observed difference is due to chance. The goal of clinical trials is to reject the null hypothesis.

Clinical equipoise, also Freedman's term, refers to the situation in which there is a current or likely dispute among expert members of the clinical community as to which of two or more therapies is superior in all relevant respects. An ethically justified RCT, then, is one that can reasonably be expected to resolve the dispute. Trial participants are entitled to the information that has created a state of clinical equipoise; this may require investigators to state their belief that A is better than B and also the opposing view and rationale.

The Federal Regulations Governing Research with Human Subjects

Review of the ethical aspects of research involving human subjects is governed by two parallel (but slightly different) sets of rules. One set applies to research conducted or funded by the Department of Health and Human Services (DHHS); the other applies to drug studies that will result in submissions for marketing approval to the Food and Drug Administration (FDA). Although technically the DHHS regulations apply only to federally funded projects, in practice almost all institutions that conduct research, whatever the funding source, have adopted these rules for all projects. In addition, some states have laws, mostly modeled on the federal regulations, that set standards for the ethical conduct of research.

The federal regulations require prior ethical review of protocols by institutional review boards (IRBs). Most of these committees are created by, and are responsible to, the institutions where research is conducted; there are also some independent or company-based IRBs. IRBs have diverse memberships, including laypersons from the community in addition to scientists associated with the institutions. Despite the mandatory inclusion of nonscientists on IRBs, the membership of IRBs typically does not reflect the cultural and ethnic mix of the study populations, particularly the HIV/AIDS populations.

The primary mission of IRBs is to protect the rights and welfare of subjects. They review, among other things, the ratio of benefits to risks, the confidentiality protections in the protocol, the informed consent process (with particular attention to the informed consent document), and the selection of subjects to ensure that it is equitable. Their ultimate power (rarely exercised) is to withhold approval, without which a protocol cannot go forward. They can suggest changes but cannot force an investigator or sponsor to make them.

The Sources of the Protectionist Stance in Research Regulation

The current regulations were adopted in 1981 with some subsequent modifications; the regulations on fetal research, which affect research involving pregnant women, date from 1975. However, the present debate about the appropriate balance between protecting individuals and furthering the social good of research originated in the period immediately following World War II. Revelations at the Nuremberg trial of the Nazi doctors described atrocities committed on unconsenting prisoners—Jews, gypsies, homosexuals, and other people deemed "unworthy to live"—in the name of science and the military medical needs of the Third Reich.

Subsequent scandals in the United States included the Jewish Chronic Disease Hospital case, in which elderly patients were injected with live cancer cells without their knowledge or consent; and the Willowbrook Hospital vaccine studies, in which retarded, institutionalized children were deliberately infected with hepatitis B virus. In 1966 in a now-classic article in the *New England Journal of Medicine*, Henry Knowles Beecher, a well-known Harvard anesthesiologist, described a series of unethical research studies conducted at major medical institutions. This article made it clear how widespread the problems really were. In the 1970s the public was particularly outraged by news reports about the Tuskegee syphilis studies, which had been going on since the 1930s and had been extensively reported in the professional literature. Poor black men enrolled in a U.S. Public Health Service study of the natural history of the untreated disease were not told the true purpose of the study, were subjected to research procedures that were described as "treatment," and were not treated for their disease, even when penicillin became available.

The experience that has most shaped the protectionist stance concerned the sedative thalidomide, and is typically referred to as the "thalidomide disaster." Thalidomide was synthesized by a West German company and approved for marketing in that country in 1958. Among the twenty countries that approved the over-the-counter sale of thalidomide were Canada, Great Britain, Australia, and Sweden.

While thalidomide was being widely distributed in these countries, physicians noted an alarming increase in the number of children being born with an unusual and extremely rare set of deformities. The most prominent feature was phocomelia, a condition in which the hands are attached to the shoulders and the feet attached to the hips, superficially resembling the flippers of a seal. By 1962, when the link between these birth defects and thalidomide was established, about 8,000 children had been affected.

The harm done to women and their infants by thalidomide was not the result of participation in research; it was the result of inadequate research (even by contemporary standards), corporate greed, and physicians' uncritical acceptance of promotional claims. Animal tests that would have proved thalidomide was teratogenic were not in general practice at the time. However, those that were available would have clearly established the strong possibility of teratogenicity, and it was well known that some drugs could cross the placental barrier and affect the fetus.

In the United States, a cautious FDA official, Dr. Frances Kelsey, delayed marketing approval for thalidomide as an antidote to nausea in early pregnancy. Nevertheless, over 1,200 doctors did give their patients thalidomide as an "investigational" drug. Several thalidomide babies were born in this country as a result, and many more women whose fetuses were affected miscarried.

As a result of publicity about thalidomide, the 1962 Kefauver-Harris amendments to U.S. drug approval laws institutionalized a rigorous pre-approval process. Before these amendments new drugs could be marketed after the drug company submitted safety data, unless the FDA prohibited it. After 1962 no new drug could be marketed until the FDA had judged, after review of the submitted data, that the drug was both safe and efficacious. Equally important, the powerful emotional impact of the thalidomide experience created a political and cultural aversion to risk-taking in drug research.

By the 1970s critics of the slow and cumbersome pre-marketing approval process resulting from the 1962 amendments claimed that a "drug lag" prevented American patients from receiving drugs in as timely a fashion as patients in Europe, where more emphasis was placed on post-marketing surveillance. The FDA's procedures were modified in 1983 in an attempt to speed up the process. At the same time the perception that being a research subject was highly risky was changing, as studies showed that very few subjects had been injured in the course of their participation.

Thus, the AIDS epidemic arrived at a point of transition in the process. The direction was already established—away from protectionism and toward more rapid approval of safe and effective drugs—but the pace was slow. As a new, fatal, stigmatizing, infectious disease primarily affecting young adults, the majority of them gay men, AIDS was the catalyst for change. Those who took the lead in a sustained critique of the government's slow response came from a generation accustomed to "miracle drugs" and rapid explanations of epidemiological puzzles. Their arguments were imbued with the language and ideology of the civil rights movement, especially the gay rights movement. They became skilled in the use of political protest to change governmental policy. Their arguments carried particular force because they coincided with the pharmaceutical industry's desire for change. As it became increasingly apparent that no cure was in sight and that the traditional clinical trial process, designed to develop scientific knowledge, was failing to meet the needs of desperately ill and dying patients, the advocacy movement turned in full force toward changing the rules, the pace, and the direction of research.

Mechanisms of Access to Experimental Drugs

At present individuals can obtain access to experimental HIV/AIDS drugs in several ways. The following processes have different goals, standards, and levels of accessibility:

Clinical trials. The drug development process has three phases: Phase I typically involves ten to fifty patients, and studies the way in which the drug is tolerated, metabolized, and excreted. Phase II generally involves fifty to 200 patients and is directed primarily at determining whether there is evidence of efficacy. Phase III expands the patient population to 1,000 or more patients and is designed to expand on the safety and efficacy data obtained in the earlier stages. Phases I and II are sometimes combined. Only Phase II and III are formal research studies designed to study the efficacy of various drugs or combinations of drugs.

a. **AIDS Clinical Trials Group (ACTG).** This system, sponsored by the National Institutes of Allergy and Infectious Diseases (NIAID), includes forty-one research institutions or AIDS Clinical Trial Units (ACTUs) around the country. Some of the institutions conduct research at several sites. As of January 12, 1990, there had been a total of ninety-nine ACTG trials involving 9,206 subjects. The majority (85.8%) of all subjects were involved in trials of antiretroviral drugs, mainly zidovudine (AZT), alone or in combination with other drugs. The next highest category—opportunistic infections—involved 17 percent of the subjects, and the majority of these were trials for prophylaxis of *Pneumocystis carinii* pneumonia.

The ACTG system is government-controlled, conducted through well-established academic research institutions, and relies heavily on traditional research designs and procedures. Typically the inclusion criteria are strictly defined to make the population as homogeneous as possible; as a result, many people are ineligible, particularly those who are very sick or who do not exactly fit the medical profile. Patients are generally referred through private physicians; however, some recruitment may take place in other ways. Although the ACTG is a national system, many areas with large potential subject populations are not included.

b. Community-based research. The community-based research movement grew out of dissatisfaction with the fragmentation, pace, and focus on antiretroviral therapies in the ACTG clinical trials. The prototypes are the San Francisco Community Consortium (a group of community-based physicians closely collaborating with researchers based at San Francisco General Hospital and the University of California-San Francisco) and the New York City Community Research Initiative (a patient/community-physician directed group). Some community-based research efforts have been funded by the American Foundation for AIDS Research (AmFAR) and by NIAID through the Community Programs for Clinical Research on AIDS (CPCRA); many are still in the formative stages.

These groups already conduct or intend to organize studies that do not require hospitalization or sophisticated laboratory backup. They are more receptive than the ACTG system to testing novel therapeutic approaches and to focusing on therapies for opportunistic infections (the most urgent need of current patients) rather than on antiretroviral therapies. Because of their community connections and acceptance, they may be able to recruit and retain participants more easily and may be better able to reach previously excluded groups. They have begun to establish a national database of clinical patient information. They perform an important educational function, by informing potential participants about trials and drugs and enhancing their access to whatever is available in the community. For the most part, community physicians have not been involved in clinical trials as investigators; the special tensions that arise from the dual roles of caregiver-investigator are discussed in "Compliance and Obligations of Participants and Physicians," below.

"Compassionate Use" or "Single-Patient" IND. There are no regulations governing the "compassionate use" or "single-patient" IND. By the late 1960s an informal FDA policy permitting individual physicians to have access to experimental drugs for a particular patient came to be known as a "Compassionate Use IND." The term "open-label or open-enrollment IND" came to be used synonymously in the 1970s. Under this mechanism, the sponsor decides on a case-by-case basis whether a physician can have access to an experimental drug.

Treatment IND. All companies, organizations, or individuals seeking approval from the FDA to market and sell new drugs in the United

States must file a New Drug Application (NDA). An Investigational New Drug Application (IND) allows the sponsor to test the drug in humans to develop the data needed to file an NDA. In June 1983 the FDA issued proposed regulations for a "treatment IND," which included a very broad interpretation of the use of investigational drugs for therapeutic purposes. On May 22, 1987, after protracted negotiations between AIDS activists and the FDA, the agency announced final regulations for a Treatment IND, that is, a mechanism under which drugs could become available prior to marketing approval to persons who might benefit (52 Federal Register, p. 19466). The Treatment IND regulations provide that a sponsor may seek the FDA's approval to distribute the drug provided that the disease is serious or life-threatening, there are no satisfactory alternatives, the drug is under investigation in a controlled clinical trial under an IND or trials have been completed, and the sponsor is actively pursuing marketing approval. A Treatment IND requires a protocol, inclusion and exclusion criteria, and reporting of adverse effects. The primary purpose of the Treatment IND is to facilitate the availability of promising new drugs after NDA application but before marketing approval; a secondary purpose is to obtain additional data on the drug's safety and effectiveness.

As of March 1990, eighteen Treatment INDs had been approved. Six are AIDS/HIV drugs, although three are already marketed for other indications. The Treatment IND, originally conceived of as a way to provide access to experimental drugs early in the approval process, has evolved into a mechanism that typically serves as a bridge between the late phases of clinical trials and FDA approval.

Parallel track or expanded access. The primary purpose of the "parallel track," a concept that originated among AIDS advocacy groups and a term coined by Dr. Anthony Fauci, director of NIAID, is to expand the availability of selected investigational therapeutic agents at a very early stage in the clinical trials process. The goal of "parallel track" is to make certain promising drugs available simultaneously both through clinical trials and through expanded access for those who are not eligible for the protocol because of medical or other exclusionary criteria or who live outside the catchment area of a trial site.

The proposed policy statement on parallel track was developed by the National AIDS Program Office, in collaboration with AIDS advocacy groups, industry representatives, and researchers (Federal Register, 21 May 1990). It would not require regulatory change (except to allow the FDA to stop distribution of a drug if it deems such an action necessary). The policy would require promising evidence of efficacy based on an assessment of laboratory and clinical data; evidence of reasonable safety, taking into consideration the use and the patient population for which the drug is intended; and sufficient information to recommend an appropriate starting dose. There should also be preliminary pharmacokinetic and dose-response data and, ideally, data about interactions with other drugs commonly used in the intended patient population.

Other factors are evidence of a lack of satisfactory alternative therapies, a description of the patient population, assurance that the manufacturer is willing and able to produce sufficient drug product for both the controlled clinical trials and the expanded access process, a statement of the status of the controlled clinical trial process, an assessment of the impact of the parallel track study on recruitment for the clinical trial, and finally, information on the educational efforts to be taken by the manufacturer to ensure that participating physicians and potential recipients have sufficient knowledge of the potential risks and benefits to assure that they can make an adequate decision. The proposed policy statement also calls for the creation of a national human subjects protections review panel; local IRBs would have the option of also reviewing parallel track protocols.

Thus far only two drugs—dideoxyinosine (ddI) and dideoxycytidine (ddC)—have been distributed under "parallel track" conditions, even though the ground rules for that process are still not finally approved. The drug ddI is obtained under a Treatment IND, issued at the request of the sponsor, Bristol Myers Squibb. At present over 7,300 patients have been enrolled; about 700 have enrolled in the clinical trials, which have a total target of 2,400 subjects. The rate of recruitment for the trials is generally believed to be about average. In June 1990 ddC became available, under similar but very limited conditions, from its sponsor, Hoffmann-La Roche. Only a small number of patients who cannot tolerate the side effects of AZT or ddI are eligible.

Importing unapproved drugs. The FDA will allow individual patients to import for their personal use small quantities of unapproved drugs from foreign countries on what it calls a "pilot" basis, unless there is evidence of unreasonable risk or fraud. The patient must supply the name of a physician who will be responsible for his or her treatment, and no commercial distribution or promotion is permitted.

Underground studies. Beyond these more or less formal processes, groups of patients, physicians, or advocates may organize to provide unapproved drugs or substances solely as "treatment," or primarily as treatment with a secondary goal of gathering data on adverse effects or efficacy. Many patients who use unapproved medications do so on an individual basis and are not participants in underground studies.

CONSENSUS STATEMENTS

Research Design

1. The randomized clinical trial (RCT) is properly regarded as the most reliable scientific design for the evaluation of new therapies or new medical interventions. This point notwithstanding, there are circumstances in which other designs are more appropriate.

The RCT is the most reliable method for developing information about the effects of therapies, preventions (e.g., vaccines), and diagnostic tests. It is more reliable primarily because random allocation mitigates the effects of bias in the assignment of subjects to one or another of its "arms," or regimens. (Some RCTs have three or more arms. For convenience, in the remainder of this report, we refer to the simplest case, the two-armed RCT.) For example, when assignment is not randomized, investigators may consciously or unwittingly assign patients with the best prognoses to what they believe to be the superior therapy. Furthermore, the RCT is reliable because unknown variables (attributes of patients) that might influence the outcome of therapy tend to be distributed evenly among the two or more "arms." This further reduces bias in the results.

To be scientifically acceptable, a clinical trial must be controlled. In addition to a group of subjects who receive the therapy or other intervention being evaluated, another group of subjects do not. Randomization helps assure that there is a high degree of homogeneity in the relevant characteristics of the subjects at the outset of the clinical trial. Sufficient numbers of subjects should be enrolled in each arm to ensure statistical validity of the results. There should also be a very high degree of similarity in the way the subjects are treated during the clinical trial; ideally, all treatments, diagnostic tests, monitoring, and so on should be identical except that one group will not receive the therapy or other modality being evaluated. The need for a high degree of similarity in treatment during the clinical trial creates a presumption in favor of concurrent rather than historical controls, either published ("literature") or unpublished (anecdotal case reports).

Control groups, then, differ primarily (and ideally, only) in that they do not receive the therapy being evaluated. Instead they may receive another active therapy ("active control"), a lower or higher dose of the same drug ("dose-response design"), no therapy, or placebo, to name some examples. Placebos (inert substances) are used in two main categories of trials: those testing whether the active agent retards the disease process and those testing whether the active agent relieves symptoms without altering the disease process.

Randomization is justified only when the treatments (or nontreat-ment) in each of the arms can be said to be in a state of clinical equipoise (a legitimate dispute as to which treatment or nontreatment is superior). It is ethically unjustifiable to assign sick persons to receive a therapy known to be inferior. Moreover, if there is no legitimate dispute and no question to be answered, there is no scientific justification for random-ization.

Ethical justification of an RCT requires in addition that there be no other therapy known to be more effective than that being studied in the RCT. This requirement obtains unless the population of research sub-jects will consist of either those in whom the superior alternative has been tried and failed or individuals who are aware of the superior alter-native and, for various reasons, have refused it.

To the extent that the conditions of clinical equipoise are not satis-fied, it is appropriate to consider nonrandomized clinical trial designs. If the new therapy is being considered for a disease for which there is no known effective therapy, one should, in this case, consider the use of his-torical or literature controls—i.e., comparison of the effects of the new therapy with past experiences in the treatment of patients before the introduction of the new therapy. To the extent that the new therapy is designed to prevent death or serious disability, the ethical justification for historical or literature controls is increased. For example, critics of the Phase II AZT trials felt that the drug had already shown sufficient evidence of efficacy, compared to nontreatment, to preclude use of a placebo arm. Another example of a recently proposed RCT criticized on grounds that it did not meet the conditions of clinical equipoise was the case of ganciclovir versus no treatment in patients with Cytomegalovirus (CMV) retinitis. Critics of the trial argued that preliminary evidence for efficacy based upon uncontrolled clinical experience was so strong that there was no reasonable doubt of this drug's superiority to no treatment. Since the purpose of ganciclovir is to prevent loss of vision, the argu-ment continued, all eligible patients should receive the drug and the results should be compared with outcomes in patients who had devel-oped CMV retinitis before the advent of ganciclovir (historical controls).

In some cases, other nonrandomized designs may be considered. For example, when the nonvalidated therapy is widely used and widely recognized as "the treatment of choice," an observational case-con-trolled design may be considered. Such designs are beyond the scope of this discussion. Suffice it to say that there are alternatives to randomiza-tion that should be considered in the absence of clinical equipoise.

Although the use of a nonrandomized design is often associated with some loss of confidence in the reliability of the results of a clinical trial, when used appropriately, nonrandomized designs can provide sufficient confidence for the purposes at hand. There is, for example, sufficient confidence that penicillin is effective for treating pneumococcal pneumonia, that appendectomy is effective for appendicitis, and that digitalis is effective for congestive heart failure to conclude that randomized clinical trials are not justified.

Part of the scientific tradition requires independent confirmation of the results of any important experiment. Insistence upon independent confirmation of the results of an RCT, however, can present serious ethical problems. When the null hypothesis has been rejected in an adequate RCT, the conditions of clinical equipoise required to justify a second RCT usually do not exist. Thus, when such independent confirmation is necessary, one should conduct the two (or, if necessary, more) RCTs concurrently.

2. In addition to scientific validity, the ethical values of respect for persons, individual beneficence, and justice must be considered in research design.

A high level of confidence in the validity of the results of an RCT is often the dominant consideration in its design. Validity is a value arising from considerations of social, not individual, beneficence. In the design of clinical trials other values must be taken into account. Two other values grounded in social beneficence are often in competition with traditional concepts of validity and with each other: generalizability (the results are widely applicable) and efficiency (the trial is affordable and resources are left over for patient care and other health research).

In the interests of efficiency, clinical trialists often select as subjects patients who are at high risk of developing the outcome measures or endpoints promptly (see below for further discussion of endpoints). Such practices often compromise generalizability. For example, the Lipid Research Clinic (LRC) RCT studied the effects of lowering cholesterol levels on the rate of heart attacks in men who had already had a heart attack. Consequently, this trial cost less money and took less time than it would have if it had included subjects at lesser risk. By the nature of its design, therefore, it left open the question of whether women or men who had not had previous heart attacks could profit from lowering cholesterol levels. Also in the interests of efficiency, clinical trialists may reduce the number of subjects to be studied in an RCT. This has obvious implications for validity in that it increases the likelihood of both "type 1 errors" (falsely concluding that a drug is effective) and "type 2 errors" (failing to find that a drug is effective).

Implicit in the prevailing practice of trading off RCT design features in the interests of validity, generalizability, and efficiency is a concept we call "sufficient validity for our purposes." This concept permits such statements as "While we would have more confidence in the result if the p value were less than .01, we shall settle for a p value of less than .05 because it is not worth the additional \$500,000 the additional confidence would cost." Similarly, we may refer to "sufficient generalizability for our purposes." Hence, although men who had not had heart attacks and women were excluded from the LRC trial, doctors recommend that they lower their cholesterol levels, reasoning that these patients are sufficiently like the study subjects to justify the recommendation.

Just as it is essential to balance the demands of validity, generalizability, and efficiency against each other in the design of clinical trials, it is equally essential to balance each of these against considerations grounded in individual beneficence, patient's desires (respect for persons) and equitable distribution of both burdens and benefits.

One element of the consensus that prevailed before the advent of AIDS remains intact: *A research proposal must be justified on grounds other than social beneficence in order to be ethically acceptable.* Just as it is unethical to place subjects at any risk in a study whose design is so flawed it cannot yield valid data, it is unethical to ignore subjects' welfare and rights to conduct a flawlessly designed study. Although it would enhance the efficiency of RCTs to dispense with the informed consent requirement, it is generally agreed that such an action would be an unacceptable violation of patients' rights to self-determination (respect for persons). Similarly, a proposal to withhold known effective therapy to do a placebo-controlled RCT of a drug designed to inhibit HIV replication should be rejected as an unacceptable disregard for patients' well-being (individual beneficence) even though such an RCT would be more efficient than one having an active drug control. Exclusion of representatives of groups of prospective subjects who are believed to be noncompliant (e.g., intravenous drug users) may arguably enhance validity and efficiency; however, such exclusions are unacceptable on grounds of both generalizability and the requirement for equitable distribution of both burdens and benefits (distributive justice).

Scientists and clinicians are accustomed to accepting data obtained by many types of research designs to establish efficacy of various types of therapies. These differences are not simply matters of taste or preference. Rather, they reflect a balancing of the requirements of the various relevant values. For example, studies of cancer chemotherapy generally use active controls—comparing one active agent against another—instead of placebos. Studies of the efficacy of antibiotic therapy for systemic infection generally use historical or literature controls. Since patients would not knowingly accept sham surgery, studies of surgical techniques may use historical controls, "no treatment" controls, or comparisons with patients who either elect or who are randomly assigned to medical management rather than surgery. Evaluations of psychotherapy may use "waiting list" controls.

Wherever possible, participant choice should be incorporated into the design of an RCT. For example, in the Studies in the Ocular Complications of AIDS (SOCA) trial, patients with peripheral retinitis are randomized to one of two drugs but elect whether to have immediate or delayed treatment. In this design, the investigators are trying to answer two questions: the relative efficacy of the two drugs and the impact of immediate or delayed treatment. The first question, considered the most important, involves randomization; the second permits patient choice.

Although the established mechanisms of IRB and peer review have heightened awareness of the values of justice, respect for persons, and beneficence, and have undoubtedly improved the ethical conduct of clinical trials, these processes generally involve review and revision of already designed RCTs. The recommendations in this report are designed to enhance the likelihood that each of the relevant values will be given due consideration during the initial stages of research design with the expectation that such early consideration will improve both the design and the implementation of clinical trials.

3. In order to assure that adequate consideration is given to the relevant values (Recommendation 2) and to alternative research designs (Recommendation 1), community consultation should be routinely considered in the early stages of the design of clinical trials and during their implementation.

Community consultation is defined, described, and discussed in detail below ("Community Consultation"). The routine use of community consultation will reduce efficiency in the planning stages of clinical trials. We expect, however, that in the long run the net result will be an improvement in efficiency as a consequence of increased community support, more rapid recruitment, and enhanced cooperation on the part of subjects as well as primary care doctors. It will also enhance generalizability.

4. Placebo controls are especially difficult to justify ethically when the endpoints of an RCT are death or serious disability.

As noted earlier, justification of an RCT requires a condition termed "clinical equipoise." When the outcome is death or serious disability, by the time an RCT reaches the organizational stage, preliminary evidence almost always suggests strongly that the new therapy is more effective than placebo. In such cases, considerations of individual well-being and respect for self-determination generally require use of an active control when such is available or, when there is no known effective therapy, a historical or literature control. Although active and historical controls are generally associated with reduced efficiency and validity, these are often appropriate trade-offs.

Dose-response designs can be justified only when there is legitimate uncertainty or controversy regarding the relative efficacy of the two or more doses. Dose-response designs in which an active dose is compared with a dose so low that it is not expected to have a therapeutic effect—a "camouflaged placebo"—are equally difficult to justify in RCTs having death or disability as their endpoints.

5. Placebo-controlled RCTs can be justified under certain well-defined conditions.

In some highly limited circumstances, placebo controls may be justified in RCTs having as their endpoints death or serious disability. A necessary but not sufficient condition for all such RCTs is that there is either no known effective therapy or subjects will be only those patients who cannot profit from the known effective therapy—e.g., those who have become refractory to its therapeutic effects. (Known effective therapy for purposes of this discussion is not the same as FDA-approved-for-this-specific-indication.) Then placebo controls may be justified if the new therapy is so scarce that only a limited number of patients can receive it. (We assume legitimate, not artificial, scarcity.) It is generally agreed that a lottery is a fair way to allocate scarce benefits among equally qualified petitioners. In an RCT, the random allocation system has the same relevant features as a lottery. The major difference is that prospective subjects agree that if they do not receive the active drug, they will accept the placebo.

Placebo-controlled RCTs having as endpoints death or serious disability may also be justified (some of the time) in diseases for which there is great variability in or uncertainty about prognosis. In such cases historical control data may be nearly impossible to interpret.

In addition, placebo controls can be justified in RCTs having endpoints other than death or disability, particularly when the trials are of short duration and when there are grounds for reasonable confidence that participation will not impair the subject's long-range prognosis by delaying access to effective therapy. In such cases, if the new drug proves effective, all participants should have continuing access to the new drug at the conclusion of the RCT.

318   CAROL LEVINE, NANCY NEVELOFF DUBLER, ROBERT J. LEVINE

6. Whenever possible, meaningful endpoints other than death, disability, and disease progression should be incorporated in the design.

We recommend that the development of such endpoints, often called "surrogate endpoints," be given a very high priority on the national research agenda. The Institute of Medicine recently reached a similar conclusion. The goal should be the development of a prognostic indicator (e.g., T-4 lymphocyte levels) that will serve as carcinoembryonic antigen (CEA) does in cancer of the colon.

7. Criteria for inclusion in phase II and III clinical trials should be based on a presumption that all groups affected by the research are eligible, regardless of gender, social or economic status, use of illicit drugs, or stage of illness unless the study is specifically designed to look at a particular stage of illness.

Phase I studies involve small numbers of subjects and are not designed to determine efficacy; therefore, questions of equity or generalizability do not arise. In phase II and III studies, however, the burden of proof should rest with those who would set narrow and strict exclusion criteria. Inclusion criteria should reflect the realities of the demographics of patient populations and of clinical needs. Some protocols are designed to study certain stages of illness or specific populations, for example, the action of prophylactic agents in HIV-infected, asymptomatic individuals or the effects of a drug on patients with a specific opportunistic infection. In such cases exclusion criteria related to the stage of illness can be justified.

This recommendation is designed to foster the equitable distribution of the benefits of research. It is essential that data be developed to serve the well-being of all groups affected by the research. In the case of HIV infection this includes men, women (including those having the biological capacity to become pregnant), children, intravenous drug users, prisoners, racial and ethnic minorities, persons with mental incapacities, and others. Thus, the overall plans for development of a new therapy should include plans for studies in each of these populations.

In addition, it is necessary to assure equitable access to clinical trials for all affected groups within particular communities. This does not necessarily mean that each and every protocol must be open to all affected groups. It would be unreasonable, for example, to require that a protocol conducted in a children's hospital be open to adult intravenous drug users. It does mean, however, that there should be a general presumption in favor of including persons from all affected groups within particular communities and that any exceptions be rigorously justified.

In the design of clinical trials, it must be recognized that some (indeed, many) members of affected groups routinely use a variety of drugs (licit as well as illicit) and will continue to do so during the conduct of the clinical trial; some take medications that they believe will help combat HIV infection. Such behaviors should not constitute grounds for exclusion unless there is evidence to support specific exclusions—e.g., a known drug interaction that would threaten the subject's safety. Clinical trials should attempt to adapt to these drug-taking behaviors. They should encourage patients to be candid about their drug use and refrain from penalizing their candor. They should also monitor the effects of concomitant medications and, when appropriate and feasible, introduce "stratifications" into the randomization assuring that equal numbers of users of a particular drug are stratified into each arm of the RCT.

Also to be avoided are such "boiler-plate" exclusions as abnormal liver function tests or low hemoglobin levels. Such exclusions may result in unwarranted exclusion of some prospective subjects such as drug users or hemophiliacs. Like other exclusion criteria, these must be justified rigorously in the protocol design and must be reviewed by IRBs to ensure their acceptability.

8. Each RCT should be monitored by an independent data safety and monitoring board (DSMB), which has the authority to make recommendations regarding early cessation of the RCT.

The DSMB is a committee charged with the responsibility of periodically examining the results of an RCT with the aim of deciding whether those results indicate a need for action before the expected date of termination of the RCT. Actions it may recommend include (but are not limited to) termination of a trial (e.g., because it has accomplished its purpose of demonstrating efficacy of a therapy at the desired level of confidence or because of an unacceptable level of adverse reactions), changing the design of a trial, or changing the consent process or forms. Although the authority of the DSMB is generally limited to making recommendations to the executive or steering committee of the sponsoring organization, usually its recommendations are accepted.

Members of the DSMB are pledged to secrecy. They agree to withhold information about emerging trends in the data from all others including investigators, sponsors, and subjects as well as the general public. Such secrecy is essential. General knowledge about emerging trends in data suggesting efficacy could destroy the validity of randomization and blinding and result in failure of the clinical trial owing to diminished willingness of investigators or subjects or both to continue.

In general, the DSMB makes its decisions within the framework of "stopping rules" developed with regard to the specific RCT. An example of a typical stopping rule is: The trial will be stopped if the null hypothesis with regard to the primary endpoints is rejected at the level of p less than .01 the first time the group examines the data.

It is now customary to have a DSMB for large, multicentered RCTs. We recommend that they also be established routinely for small RCTs conducted in only one location.

9. Information about significant developments in clinical trials should be communicated in a timely and effective fashion to concerned clinicians, trial participants, patients, investigators, and community groups.

Significant developments in clinical trials are data about safety or efficacy that is likely to influence decisions made by doctors and patients. Based on such information, patients may decide, for example, to seek access to a therapy or to withdraw from a clinical trial.

The methods and timing of communication should be appropriate to the nature of the information. Care must be taken to avoid premature release of unsubstantiated data that may create false expectations about new therapies. It is equally important to avoid unwarranted delays in the release of negative information; for example, critics point to a delay in releasing data that dextran sulfate is ineffective. Whether positive or negative, accurate information is needed urgently by sick patients and their doctors.

At times the public's need to know urgently may conflict with the scientific tradition of publishing in peer-reviewed journals, generally a prolonged process. Such conflicts should be resolved in a spirit of cooperation by all concerned parties. In cases of irreconcilable conflicts, which we hope will be rare, the public's need to know should generally have first priority.

10. Clinical trial protocols should include procedures for monitoring investigators' and participants' experiences and reporting both adverse events and practical difficulties to appropriate agencies, whether that be the IRB, the sponsor, the FDA, or some combination of these.

Adverse effects are routinely reported to the IRB, the FDA and the sponsor. Such routine reporting commonly results in prompt and effective responses—e.g., modifications in consent procedures and forms. We suggest that monitoring for and reporting of practical difficulties be made similarly routine. An example of such a practical difficulty would be failure of patients to keep appointments because of transportation or child care difficulties. Prompt remedial action in response to such problems could be vitally important in preventing the failure of an RCT.

11. Procedures should be developed to collect and coordinate data in relation to all uses of investigational new drugs.

Increasingly, investigational new drugs are being made available to patients through such mechanisms as expanded access, treatment and compassionate INDs, and the parallel track. The primary purpose of making drugs available in such fashions is therapeutic. However, collection of data regarding safety and efficacy in conjunction with such uses would contribute to the drug development process. Some community-based trial centers are offering technical assistance in data gathering and reporting to physicians who use these mechanisms; such efforts should be expanded.

There is concern, however, that such collection of data might interfere with making investigational new drugs available to sick persons. In particular, doctors might be unwilling to assume the burdens of paperwork that would be associated with securing investigational new drugs for their patients. We recommend, then, that data collection activities be conducted in a fashion that does not undermine the primary therapeutic goal of these programs.

12. Physicians and investigators should collect data in a systematic way on patients who self-medicate.

The purposes and implications of this statement are similar to those provided for in Recommendation 11.

13. Underground protocols that fail to meet contemporary ethical and scientific standards must be discouraged.

Without independent scientific and ethical review it is difficult to have confidence in a protocol's capacity to obtain scientifically valid data. Participants may be subjected to risks without commensurate benefits and there is a danger of fraud and exploitation. Our reference to contemporary ethical and scientific standards is not intended to be construed as a requirement for filing an IND, which is a regulatory standard.

Underground protocols are a response to a perception that the system has failed either to test a specific drug adequately or speedily or to develop therapies for particular conditions. If the recommendations concerning research design (Nos. 1–12) and community consultation (below, Nos. 14–19) are followed, there should be less perceived need to initiate underground protocols.

COMMUNITY CONSULTATION

14. Prior and ongoing community consultation should be an integral part of the planning and design of clinical trials of nonvalidated therapies.

Community consultation consists of a formal meeting between investigators and prospective subjects or their representatives. Ideally, the prospective subjects should be persons who have the attributes that would make them eligible for participation in the clinical trial (inclusion criteria). In addition, they should also include a broad representation of the intended beneficiaries of the clinical trial—those for whom the therapy would be recommended if it proves effective. During the course of the community consultation it may be decided to extend the inclusion criteria to incorporate additional groups of intended beneficiaries.

In addition, it will usually be appropriate to include sponsors, advocates for the prospective subject and intended beneficiary populations, physicians who provide their primary care, community leaders, and IRB members.

The purpose of community consultation is to negotiate the design of the clinical trial and to assure a suitable balancing of the relevant values (Recommendation 2) in the design and conduct of the clinical trial. In the context of community consultation, there should be reasonable assurance that discussions reflect the priorities of prospective subjects and intended beneficiaries as well as those of the investigators and sponsors. Community consultation is designed to share decision-making power among all interested parties at a time when decisions can influence research design, plans for informed consent, inclusion and exclusion criteria, and related matters.

The objective of community consultation is to learn whether the proposed research can be conducted in such a way that it will not only measure up to scientific standards ("sufficient validity for our purposes," as defined in the commentary following Recommendation 2) but also be found acceptable by most members of the population of prospective subjects and intended beneficiaries. If a substantial number of prospective subjects disapprove the plan for the study, it is reasonable to predict that it cannot be conducted successfully.

The ongoing community consultations should address problems that arise during the conduct of the clinical trial (see e.g., Recommendation 10).

15. Community consultation should not be seen as a way to obtain acceptance of an already agreed-upon protocol; to be successful, it must be a partnership.

16. The primary responsibility for initiating and conducting community consultation rests with the investigator.

Ultimately, investigators are legally and ethically responsible for the way in which trials are designed and conducted; therefore, they should also bear the primary responsibility for integrating community consultation into their procedures. The main purpose of consultation—the initiation of an ongoing dialogue—requires, however, that those who are being consulted also have the opportunity to begin the discussions.

Prior community consultation should have already been conducted before the investigators prepare a protocol for review by the IRB. A summary of the discussions conducted and agreements reached at the prior community consultation should be incorporated in the protocol. IRBs should take this information into account as they make their judgments about risks and benefits and their balance, the adequacy of the plans for informed consent, the equity of the plans for selection of subjects, and so on.

In some cases the investigators may request the IRB either to waive the requirement for community consultation or to substitute a less formal consultation that might consider a reduced number of issues. In some circumstances the IRB may approve such requests, if it determines that the issues raised by the proposed research are not sufficiently weighty or controversial to merit full community consultation. The new research proposal may, for example, be very similar in most relevant respects to a clinical trial previously conducted in the same community without problems. Approval of such requests for waiver or alteration should be granted only with the concurrence of the standing advisory committee, discussed below (Recommendation 17).

17. Institutions that regularly conduct clinical trials of therapies for HIV infection should have standing community advisory committees.

Standing advisory committees should include among their membership representatives of the various communities of intended beneficiaries of clinical trials for therapies for HIV infection, community leaders, investigators, and sponsors. The purpose of the standing advisory committee is to provide continuing advice to the institution through researchers or the IRB on matters germane to the conduct of clinical trials of therapies for HIV infection. It should be so constituted as to be an effective voice for the concerns of the various communities of prospective subjects and intended beneficiaries of such clinical trials.

Among the topics that are appropriate for the agenda of the standing advisory committee are:

a. Priorities in the research agenda—e.g., which problems are seen as most pressing for patients, nonvalidated therapies that are being used by the community, or substances that the community desires to test.
b. Conflicts between the needs of current patients and benefits for future patients, when both groups may come from the same community or when they do not.
c. Suspicion on the part of potential trial participants of researchers or of the research establishment based upon history of past abuses—e.g., the Tuskegee study—or bad experiences with health care institutions.
d. The need for primary care facilities in the community and how the institution might work most effectively to accomplish the objectives set forth in Recommendation 29.

Standing advisory committees should also participate in the planning and conduct of prior and ongoing community consultation. They should also have the authority to ratify or veto the IRB's recommendations to approve requests for waiver or alteration of the requirement for community consultation (Recommendation 16).

In some circumstances, standing advisory committees should recommend the holding of open forums on community concerns relevant to the clinical trial program.

18. When there is no clearly defined community of prospective subjects and intended beneficiaries, or when different groups claim to represent the community, community consultation may be problematic. This does not absolve the investigator of the responsibility to accomplish the purposes of community consultation.

Even in situations where no formal community-based organizations exist that might plausibly serve to represent potential subjects' interests, individuals who have long experience in the community can be consulted to identify particular concerns and other knowledgeable people.

Through such contacts it should be possible to assemble a credible standing advisory committee. This standing advisory committee can provide advice on how the investigators may accomplish the purposes of community consultation in regard to particular proposed clinical trials.

19. IRBs that regularly review HIV/AIDS research should seriously consider including among their members representatives of or advocates for populations of prospective subjects and intended beneficiaries.

There was considerable disagreement in the working group on this issue. A majority felt that imposing a specific membership requirement on IRBs would be unwieldy, unlikely to accomplish the purpose of greater sensitivity to the concerns of particular groups of subjects, and inequitable unless other groups of vulnerable subjects were similarly represented. However, a minority of the participants dissented. They argued that true empowerment of affected communities can only occur when IRBs have members with full voting powers to represent the communities' views.

In the section on IRB membership, the federal regulations (CFR 46.107a) state: "The IRB shall be sufficiently qualified through the experience and expertise of its members, and the diversity of the members' backgrounds including the racial and cultural backgrounds of members and sensitivity to such issues as community attitudes, to promote respect for its advice and counsel. . . ." The requirement for a nonscientist member and a member not affiliated with the institution is not linked to the requirement for sensitivity to community attitudes, and in practice lay members are not usually "community" representatives but lawyers, clergy, or other professionals. Furthermore, the regulations continue, "If an IRB regularly reviews research that involves a vulnerable category of subjects, including but not limited to subjects covered by other subparts of this part, the IRB shall include one or more individuals who are primarily concerned with the welfare of these subjects."

These statements can be read to support the view that IRBs that regularly review HIV/AIDS research must include a community representative. However, in practice most IRBs do not follow this regulation in regard to other vulnerable groups and the Office of Protection from Research Risks does not enforce it.

This issue will be most significant for IRBs at large institutions that review many categories of research. IRBs that rarely review HIV/AIDS research will not need a regular member and may rely on community consultation; IRBs that solely review HIV/AIDS research are likely to include one or more community representatives as a matter of principle.

COMPLIANCE AND OBLIGATIONS OF PARTICIPANTS AND PHYSICIANS

20. Implementation of the recommendations set forth in this report should decrease the incidence of misrepresentation to gain entry to clinical trials.

It is commonly said that some patients, often with the aid of their primary care doctors, misrepresent themselves as meeting the inclusion criteria for various clinical trials for one or both of the following reasons: It is the only way available to them to gain access to investigational new drugs or to adequate health care. Since these and other factors to which misrepresentation is attributed are addressed in recommendations calling for community consultation, broadened inclusion criteria, acceptance of the use of non-protocol drugs, and provision of adequate primary health care facilities both inside and outside the clinical trials, we expect implementation of these recommendations to result in fewer instances of this type of undesirable behavior.

21. If the recommendations in this report are implemented, participants who enroll in clinical trials, after having given a valid informed consent, are more likely to honor their ethical obligations to comply with the protocol.

Subject compliance was the most difficult issue in this group's process of reaching consensus, and the consensus statement is a predictive rather than a normative statement. One position—articulated by the majority of the group—bases its support of compliance on the strong ethical proscriptions against lying and breaking promises. Persons who lie or break promises take advantage of the trust placed in them by other persons, thus violating the autonomy of others. In this view, trial participants violate the trust of researchers and wrong them by engaging in noncompliant behavior. Trial participants can also harm the interests of current and future patients because the trial may result in scientifically invalid data and have a negative effect on their care. Moreover, subjects who engage in noncompliant behavior may harm other, compliant trial participants' interests because if the trial results in invalid data, all participants have been placed at risk for no benefit. Invalid trials also incur considerable economic and social costs.

On the other hand, several members of the working group focused on political and social realities, emphasizing that the legacy of injustice in the research and health care system against gay people and communities of color is a deep sense of alienation and suspicion. People who feel that their lives are not highly valued have no incentive to comply with protocol requirements, especially if research is their only access to potentially life-saving drugs. Many aspects of the traditional research process, as has already been pointed out, are disincentives to compliance. In this context it becomes even more important for investigators and all those concerned with drug development to develop a relationship of trust and honesty with potential trial participants.

If participants experience difficulties in compliance based on the protocol requirements, they should describe them to the investigator. The investigator has an obligation to take the problem to the appropriate agency, which may be the executive committee of the ACTG, the clinical monitor, or the IRB. If the problem appears to be inherent in the protocol and not related to a particular subject's experience, and a protocol revision is deemed necessary, the IRB's approval is required. Participants who cannot comply with a protocol should withdraw; investigators should assist them in gaining alternative access to the drug if possible or to an alternative therapy. (The obligations of investigators toward participants who withdraw are discussed below, "Informed Consent and Access to Research.")

22. In their role as caregivers, physicians have an ethical obligation to act in their patients' best interests. Physicians also have professional and social responsibilities to provide accurate information about patients' eligibility for clinical trials.

Under the current system many physicians also experience disincentives to fulfill their ethical obligations to: (a) present honestly inclusion criteria to enroll patients in clinical trials; (b) advise subjects not to enter clinical trials for the sole purpose of obtaining a particular drug and to withdraw from the trial if randomized to a different arm. If the recommendations in this report about research design and inclusion criteria are followed, these disincentives will be decreased.

23. Physicians who act as investigators are obligated to fulfill the terms of the protocol.

In the practice of medicine, physicians typically alter drug schedules, dosages, and other aspects of therapy to provide the best possible care for individual patients. However, physicians who agree to act as investigators, either in a hospital or in a community-based trial, undertake a different obligation—that is, to abide by the protocol requirements or to inform the appropriate agency or individual that the protocol requirements do not conform to acceptable standards of patient care. If mutually agreeable adjustments are not possible, the physician should withdraw from the role of investigator.

328   CAROL LEVINE, NANCY NEVELOFF DUBLER, ROBERT J. LEVINE

24. Community-based physicians who act as investigators should receive assistance and training, where necessary, to help them fulfill the special obligations for record keeping, reporting, and so on.

It is the obligation of the sponsor, whether industrial or governmental, to provide or to arrange for the provision of such assistance. They may in some cases enlist the aid of experienced investigators in research institutions to conduct educational programs. The pharmaceutical industry can be a source of expertise and technical assistance.

INFORMED CONSENT AND ACCESS TO RESEARCH

25. Accepted standards of informed consent must be maintained rigorously.

The life-threatening and infectious character of HIV/AIDS does not justify any suspension of rights of subjects to full information, voluntary participation and withdrawal from the study, protection of confidentiality, and all other elements of informed consent as set forth in federal regulations.

A valid informed consent must be voluntary, informed, and given by a competent person. However, we caution against setting excessively high standards for determinations of the validity of consent or of the capacity of persons to give a valid consent. For example, to interpret the requirement for voluntariness to mean that the person must be as unconstrained as the typical, independent, free-living adult would result in a rejection as invalid of all consents given by prisoners, students, employees of drug companies, hospitalized patients, and some other institutionalized or dependent persons. Similarly, excessively high standards for comprehension would tend to exclude too many persons with minor impairments of cognitive function.

The following statements of the President's Commission support this view:

> How deficient must a decision-making process be to justify the assessment that a patient lacks the capacity to make a particular decision? Since the assessment must balance possibly competing considerations of well-being and self-determination, the prudent course is to take into account the potential consequences of the patient's decision. When the consequences for well-being are substantial, there is a greater need to be certain that the patient possesses the necessary level of capacity. When little turns on the decision, the level of decision making capac-

ity required may be appropriately reduced (even though the constituent elements remain the same) and less scrutiny may be required about whether the patient possesses even the reduced level of capacity. Thus a particular patient may be capable of deciding about a relatively inconsequential medication, but not about the amputation of a gangrenous limb.

26. Informed consent is an ongoing process that requires investigators and participants to communicate with each other about information that may affect the health and well-being of the participant or the validity of the findings of the study.

27. The inadequacy of primary health care and psychosocial supports in many poor communities seriously affected by HIV/AIDS may compromise the voluntariness of participation and the adequacy of consent.

In the introduction to this report (section entitled "The Source of the Protectionist Stance in Research Regulation"), there is a brief explanation of why the consensus in research ethics expressed in the Belmont Report and in the ensuing federal regulations placed a great emphasis on voluntariness. Because of cases of fraudulent, forced, or uninformed enrollment in research, the emphasis on voluntariness was considered essential so that individuals could exercise their right to self-determination and refuse to be research subjects.

One's capacity for self-determination may be weakened or overcome by conditions other than force, fraud, or ignorance. Of particular concern in the context of this report is "inducement." An inducement consists of an offer to a person of something of value in exchange for his or her agreement to do something that he or she might not do without the inducement. A simple example of an inducement is a cash payment. A cash payment so large that it overwhelms other relevant considerations—e.g., risk/benefit assessment—in the decision to be or to continue to be a research subject is called an "undue inducement."

In addition to direct inducements such as cash payments, there are implicit inducements, i.e., things of value that a person receives as an integral part of enrollment in a research program. Unlike direct inducements, they are not offered as a quid pro quo. Rather, enrollment entails receipt of the thing of value, a thing that has value to the subject apart from the purpose of the research; one such thing is primary medical care.

Primary medical care is often and quite appropriately provided free of charge to persons who enroll in a clinical trial. Persons who are sick and thus require primary medical care and who lack the resources to secure it by any other means, may be induced to enroll in a clinical trial simply as a means to secure primary medical care. Their need for primary medical care may overwhelm other considerations such as risk or inconvenience that might otherwise lead them to refuse to participate or to withdraw from a clinical trial. In this sense, the provision of primary medical care may be considered at least potentially an implicit undue inducement.

The following two statements are designed to be responsive to this concern.

28. The relationships between patient and physician and between subject and investigator are different and may be ambiguous when a physician acts as both primary care doctor and investigator.

The central ethical responsibility of a primary care physician is to act for the benefit of the patient in accord with the patient's wishes. The physician who acts solely as an investigator in a clinical trial has an obligation to contribute to the development of generalizable knowledge through conformity to the specifications of the protocol. Informed consent to participation in a trial should make it clear whether a physician is assuming the limited role of investigator or the more complex role of physician-investigator. In the former case, the prospective subject must be advised that he or she should seek primary medical care outside the clinical trial.

Physicians who act as physician-investigators assume all the legal and ethical responsibilities of primary care physicians. Among these responsibilities is the proscription against abandonment. When patient-subjects withdraw from clinical trials either because it is in their best medical interests to do so or because they are exercising their rights to withdraw without loss of benefits to which they are otherwise entitled, the physician-investigator should follow these individuals to the end of the trial, both to provide medical care and to obtain data. If this is not feasible, they should ensure that these individuals have been referred appropriately. They should continue to provide medical care until the participants are accepted as patients by other health professionals.

Many participants in clinical trials have continuing relationships with multiple health professionals—not only investigators or physician-investigators within the clinical trial program but also primary care professionals and consultant specialists outside the program. These professionals must make every effort to maintain timely and effective communications with one another. Such communications serve the interests of both the patient-subjects and the research program.

29. Institutions in which members of the medical staff serve as physician-investigators in clinical trials should assure that primary medical care is provided for patient-subjects who withdraw from clinical trials.

In some cases physician-investigators may leave the institution to accept positions elsewhere. In recognition of this possibility, institutions should adopt policies and procedures that provide for a continuation of primary medical care and, as appropriate, an orderly and effective system of referral as set forth in Recommendation 28.

Health care institutions that conduct research, as centers of medical, economic and political power, bear an ethical responsibility either to provide or to advocate for adequate primary care for their communities.

SPECIAL POPULATIONS

30. No group should be categorically excluded, on the basis of age, gender, mental status, place of residence or incarceration, or other social or economic characteristics from access to clinical trials or other mechanisms of access to experimental therapies. Special efforts should be made to reach out to previously excluded populations. However, people who are vulnerable for any of these reasons require special consideration in the design and implementation of trials.

We recognize that many people fall into more than one of these groups, and that each group has different needs and interests. These factors must receive special consideration if all of those infected are to have equitable access to clinical trials. The special needs of each group should receive the kind of sustained analysis offered in this report on research design, community consultation, compliance and obligations of participants and physicians, and informed consent. Such an in-depth consideration was beyond the scope of this project. Therefore, the following sections should be seen as an outline of some key issues rather than definitive conclusions about them.

In the following discussion, we assume that the federal regulations governing research with human subjects represent the baseline standards. The consensus statements presented below reflect some of the most important issues that are not covered in the regulations.

Children and Adolescents

Children have historically been underrepresented in clinical trials; as a result, treatment options must frequently be determined by extrapolating from data on adults. The federal regulations governing research on children, promulgated in 1983, are entitled, "Additional Protections for Children Involved as Subjects in Research." The regulations reflect the prevailing consensus that government's primary roles were first, to protect human subjects from the risks of research; and second, to restrict the conditions under which research may be conducted, especially on children who are not capable of providing legally or ethically valid informed consent. In a time of escalating numbers of HIV-infected children, government's ethical responsibility now includes facilitating protocols that may benefit them.

The goal of public policy should be to strike an appropriate moral balance between protectionism and the research imperative. This balance must accommodate the moral interests of children:

- protection of the welfare of child subjects;
- provision of adequate, knowledgeable, aggressive and continuous advocacy;
- equitable selection and participation of HIV-infected child-subjects.

Children Under 13

31. Until there are reliable tests generally available to detect true HIV infection in seropositive but asymptomatic babies under 15 months, in general these children are not appropriate candidates for studies of drugs to treat HIV infection or AIDS.

Trials designed to study the efficacy of drugs or procedures to treat confirmed or symptomatic HIV infection or AIDS may involve serious risks and burdens. Since the majority (at least two-thirds) of HIV-positive, asymptomatic children under fifteen months are not infected and do not have the condition for which the trial is indicated, they should not be subject to these risks and burdens. However, seropositive, asymptomatic children under fifteen months may be candidates for trials that do not involve serious risks or burdens; parents or guardians should be offered such options when appropriate. Furthermore, these children may be appropriate candidates for some vaccine trials or trials designed to study the prevention of opportunistic infections or developmental delays.

32. Since the time and precise mechanism of vertical HIV transmission is as yet unknown, perinatal trials of agents designed to prevent transmission may be ethically justified.

Because there is so much uncertainty in this area and scientific knowledge is advancing so swiftly, this option should be presented when appropriate.

33. Drugs or procedures intended to be used in all age groups should be tested in children only after Phase I/II studies have demonstrated safety and drug activity in adults. Phase II/III trials involving children should be conducted in parallel with Phase II/III trials on adults.

HIV disease in children has different manifestations from those in adults, and children often experience fewer toxicities than adults given the same agent. Therefore, studies involving children should not be delayed until all results from adult trials have been reported. However, Phase I clinical investigations are not designed to provide any benefit; therefore, there is no social obligation, on the grounds of beneficence, to enroll children unless that trial is studying a condition that occurs only in children or a drug that is intended for use only in children. Even in that case, parents and guardians should be clearly informed of the lack of expected benefit in Phase I studies.

34. Children should be entered in clinical trial protocols only after consultation with their primary care physician.

The primary care physician is able to evaluate the totality of the child's health care needs and to make an appropriate recommendation about the risks and benefits of entering a research protocol. Children who do not have a regular primary care physician should be evaluated by someone other than the investigator.

35. Trials should be conducted only in settings that provide an adequate level of medical and psychosocial support for the child and the child's caregivers.

Research involving children should take account of the context and contours of their lives—their needs for nurturing, emotional, social, and cognitive development. Most typically the necessary range of support systems will be available in comprehensive care centers; other settings, such as community health centers and community hospitals, may also be able to provide or coordinate the necessary services. Protocols should be designed to recognize the family as a unit.

Advocacy for Children Not in the Custody of Their Parents
36. To enhance access to trials and to ensure the ethical acceptability of the consent process, children not in the custody of their parents and therefore especially vulnerable should be provided advocates for this purpose.

The federal regulations do not require a formal advocate for children without parents, because the National Commission feared that such a requirement would act as a bureaucratic barrier to clinical trials. Nonetheless we suggest such a role precisely to pierce already developed barriers and to help ensure the ethical acceptability of the consent process for such especially vulnerable children. This advocate can help agency personnel, informal caregivers, and formally appointed guardians to negotiate the barriers to clinical trials; this person cannot and should not be a substituted consenter.

In practice, the advocate will probably be a health professional, such as a nurse, pediatric nurse practitioner, or social worker. However, lay persons with special backgrounds could also be effective advocates in special circumstances if previously provided with appropriate training. Different protocols may require different qualifications for the advocate.

37. The advocate should have the following characteristics:

a. **The ability to assess the medical needs of the child and judge the likely risks and benefits of a particular protocol considering the child's stage of disease and range of symptoms.**

Whereas an IRB makes generic judgments on risk/benefit ratio, the advocate must consider the "best interest" of an individual child in his or her social context and at a particular point in the disease process;

b. **The ability to be involved with the child and primary caregiver over time and to reassess the child's reaction to and progress in the clinical trial;**
c. **The ability to communicate effectively with health care personnel and the confidence to ask questions, seek additional advice, and make independent judgments in order to advise continuing in the trial, or suggest termination of a child's participation when appropriate.**

38. Each advocate should be responsible for a limited panel of children and must make an effort to be present each time the child is seen by the clinician or researcher.

39. Children should not be excluded from research because of the lack of an identified advocate.

A primary moral obligation of state child-welfare agencies is to devise reasonable, realistic, effective, and responsive systems that permit timely response to possible involvement in protocols.

Adolescents

Teenagers who engage in heterosexual or homosexual sex or drug use are at risk for HIV infection. Many HIV-infected adolescents are alienated from family, school, and society and are difficult to engage in any prevention, treatment, or research program. Many adolescents at highest risk for HIV infection are economically disadvantaged youngsters of color. This social context presents formidable challenges to investigators, but should not be a categorical bar to including adolescents in research.

40. States must establish clear rules to enable mature and emancipated minors to provide legally adequate consent for counselling, testing, treatment, and research.

Most states permit some youth before the legal age of consent (generally eighteen) to consent to medical care and other matters if they are emancipated (usually having borne a child or entered the armed services), or mature (demonstrated an independent life pattern). These categories tend to be vague and the criteria governing them uncertain. Clarification would remove many barriers to participation in research.

41. Even though adolescents may legally give consent, they should be encouraged to accept a knowledgeable, sympathetic adult as an advisor in the process.

Because adolescents, particularly those of younger ages, have developmental characteristics that distinguish them both from children and adults, they have special needs for sensitive guidance in making health care decisions, including the decision to enter a research protocol.

42. Research and treatment facilities must have counselor-advocates available in case no other responsible adult is acceptable to the adolescent.

43. Research should only be pursued in settings with adequate psychosocial support services.

Women

Women are at increasing risk for HIV infection. Whereas they constitute only 10 percent of reported AIDS cases, they represent the fastest growing segment of the infected population. In addition to the risks of sharing needles, any act of unprotected sexual intercourse with an HIV-infected partner is a risk-laden behavior for a woman. While most sexually active women are potentially at risk, the demography of the epidemic puts poor women, especially those of color, at greatest risk.

44. It is inequitable and discriminatory to exclude women, including women of reproductive age, from clinical trials.

Women have been systematically underrepresented in research since the thalidomide experience of the late 1950s, because of the fear of liability on the part of drug sponsors if the drug turns out to have teratogenic effects. (See Introduction.) Nevertheless, there are both scientific and ethical reasons to include women in clinical trials. Developing effective treatments for the range of disease manifestations in women requires that they be included in clinical trials. Furthermore, shielding women from the burdens of research and denying them its potential benefits fails to respect them as autonomous agents and fails to meet the standards of justice in the equitable distribution of burdens and benefits.

45. The concepts of community consultation should be applied to research on women; women should be asked to identify the barriers to participation and to help plan protocols that will reflect their needs.

Programs must be designed to permit and encourage women to enroll. Such programs should include: child care capacity at the research site; funds for care of a sick child who cannot be transported; plans for assistance to dependents (and men who are primary caregivers) should the side effects of treatment be debilitating to the women.

Pregnant Women
Most HIV-infected women are of childbearing age; many of those who are or become pregnant will choose to continue the pregnancy. While the inclusion of nonpregnant HIV-infected women in clinical trials is controversial, there is even less agreement about whether pregnant women should be enrolled in (a) all protocols despite known or unknown risks to future children; (b) in some protocols where there is no evidence of risk; or (c) in no protocols because of the possibility of an adverse birth outcome and the fear of subsequent institutional or investigator liability. In moral terms, the question is whether the interests of the future child override or are even relevant in decisions about including pregnant women. The moral dimensions of the problem are often lost as investigators, IRBs, and institutions are increasingly faced with two competing claims: the demand that HIV-infected pregnant women be eligible for all clinical trials; and the insistence on avoiding potentially risky situations that may lead to litigation.

To promote the values of beneficence, the prevention of harm, and justice, we recommend that:

46. Pregnant women should not be categorically excluded from Phase II/III protocols or from access to drugs under treatment INDs.

Pregnant women need not be included in Phase I studies, however, since there is no benefit likely to accrue to them and there are alternative subject recruitment plans that do not raise comparable possibilities of risks.

47. If a drug is potentially life saving, and no other treatment exists, a pregnant woman must be permitted access either to a Phase II/III trial or to a treatment IND.

48. The generalized presumption that pregnant women are eligible for trials can be rebutted only by a showing of serious risk to the future child; and either (a) the availability of a potentially equally effective alternative treatment for the woman; or (b) little expected benefit to her from the particular protocol.

We use the term "future child" to identify the subjects of our concern as fetuses who will be born rather than fetuses in general or at any particular stage of development. These statements represent the extremes of risks and benefits; while we recognize that most protocols would fall in the middle, we offer these recommendations to facilitate an exploration of the values at stake.

The informed consent process should raise issues of the possible danger to the future child with potential subjects. Once issues of possible harm to the future child have been raised with the woman, some argue that it should be left solely to her judgment to balance her need for access to the investigational drug against possible harm to her unborn child. Proponents of this position argue that society has no basis for intruding into the maternal-fetal relationship because the fetus has no moral or legal standing.

Others, including this group, argue that the lack of fetal standing does not preclude weighing the interests of the future child in public policy determinations and research regulation. Society may not have a relationship to the fetus but certainly will have a connection to the future child. Thus, in a trial where the benefit to the woman would be negligible and the harm to the future child devastating, common sense and prudent public policy dictate excluding the woman from the trial. In the real world it is virtually inconceivable that a woman would either seek access to or agree to participate in such a trial, but were such to be the case it would be appropriate to exclude her.

In the converse case—when the potential benefit to the woman is life-saving or life-enhancing and no other treatment exists—it seems entirely wrong to limit access even if the effect on the future child will be catastrophic, i.e., substantial irreversible injury which could lead to a life of suffering. In this instance the claim of a life-in-existence predominates.

There are, therefore, two ways of approaching the problem. One ascribes moral weight only to the claims of the mother and supports her autonomy as the primary value. The other, a more consequentialist analysis, recognizes the complexity of assigning moral value and permits a balancing of interests between the pregnant woman and her future child.

The working group recommends further study and clarification of the many issues raised but not resolved in this section.

Prisoners

Prisons and jails are settings of systematic deprivation; inmates live in circumstances characterized increasingly by overcrowding, and in general by lack of privacy and random violence. Examples of abuse of inmates in research received wide publicity in the 1960s and 70s. Because of the unsettled state of federal regulations governing prisoner research, researchers and research institutions have avoided prisons as research sites and prisoners as possible subjects.

Despite the inadequacies of prison health care services, the high prevalence of HIV infection among incarcerated populations argues for permitting Phase II and III drug trials in prisons. Inmates want to participate in clinical trials; the line between validated and nonvalidated therapies shifts quickly and inmates want access to potentially effective treatments. Moreover, permitting research will engage academic researchers and clinicians in the largely substandard health services and thus may assist in upgrading those services.

IRB Review

49. Because of the vulnerability of prison populations all clinical trials in correctional institutions should be reviewed by an IRB, constructed in accordance with federal regulations on research involving prisoners, in order to: protect confidentiality; ensure fairness; limit the possibility of further discrimination or stigmatization; and preclude any further deprivation of an already circumscribed ability to choose.

Informed Consent

50. Prisoners are able to provide informed consent to participation in Phase II/III clinical trials.

Prisons are settings of such systematic deprivation and intimidation that some argue that incarcerated persons can never provide truly voluntary informed consent. In addition, many prison health systems are inadequate and confidentiality is generally impossible to protect.

Nonetheless, we support the involvement of prisoners in Phase II/III clinical trials. To deny access to clinical trials because of the imperfect nature of the consent would be to punish inmates beyond the sentence imposed and to further deprive them of equitable treatment. The voluntary nature of the informed consent in prison may not reach an abstract standard of perfection; nonetheless this is a "good enough" consent to support subject participation.

51. Investigators should take special care to protect confidentiality.

52. Investigators should assist, if possible, in upgrading the prison health service so that adequate primary care is provided.

Mentally Ill or Disabled Persons

This section is intended to guide decisions about research involving those persons born with developmental disabilities, those who have developed a mental infirmity (mental illness) during life that affects decision-making ability, and those whose cognitive abilities are impaired because of AIDS-related dementia. These persons will have somewhat different needs and life situations. Many developmentally disabled individuals will have legally appointed guardians who regularly participate in their health care decisions; almost none of the mentally infirm or patients with AIDS dementia will have such a legal guardian.

Regulations governing research on mentally ill, developmentally disabled, and cognitively impaired persons were recommended by the National Commission for the Protection of Human Subjects of Biomedical and Behavioral Research but were never incorporated into the federal regulations. Therefore there are no special regulations to guide the consent process. Because the regulations fail to provide relevant and specific guidelines, investigators must struggle to create protective and fair mechanisms; they must try to do good with inadequate guidance.

Protocols with these populations regularly accept variations of surrogate consent. Some IRBs, notably the one at the National Institutes of Health, have made specific provisions for a consent auditor. None of these solutions meets the requirement for a "legally authorized representative" as provided for by the regulations.

53. Persons with mental or developmental disabilities should not be categorically excluded from HIV/AIDS research.

Increasingly, mentally ill persons have been granted the right to refuse medications, especially psychotropic medications. This right can only be overridden by specific institutional procedures or, in some jurisdictions, by the courts. If mentally ill persons have the right to refuse psychotropic medications, which professionals argue puts their physical and mental health in jeopardy, they should, with the help and support of research advocates and consent auditors, be able to choose to participate in research that may present equal or far less risk.

54. Developmentally disabled and mentally infirm persons, and those with AIDS-related dementia, should have advocates to evaluate on their behalf protocols for which they are eligible and to remain involved during the course of the trial.

Advocacy for mentally ill persons has become increasingly complex as federal and Supreme Court opinions have delineated the rights, duties, and obligations of caregivers, family, the patient, and state supervisory agencies. Given the complexity of research design and the sophistication of probabilistic reasoning, advocates should work with mentally ill persons who have not been declared incompetent to assist them in evaluating and choosing among various options.

These advocates should have characteristics similar to, and function like, advocates for children. They should always seek to inform the potential subjects, to the degree possible, and gain assent when appropriate.

55. No research should proceed over the objection of the subject.

56. Court-appointed guardians should be permitted to enroll their wards in clinical trials or obtain access to investigational drugs if the ward does not object.

If the ward objects the objection should be honored. If the guardian nonetheless wishes to proceed, only a judicial order could override the ward's objection. In general, judges should not order subject participation in clinical trials, but may consider ordering treatment under a treatment IND.

57. **The best routes for facilitating the participation of demented and cognitively failing persons, given the prevalence of these conditions associated with HIV disease, are (a) the design of long-term/long-range protocols that permit an HIV-infected person to consent, in advance of dementia, to later participation if and when appropriate; and (b) the use of Durable Powers of Attorney for health care decision-making, which permit the attorney-in-fact to consent to research for the patient.**

CONCLUSION

Consensus building, by its very nature, is a slow and searching process. It requires an exploration of basic assumptions and principles and a willingness to appreciate other points of view while holding firm to one's most deeply held values. As it has in so many other areas, HIV/AIDS has provided a lens through which to examine social processes, in this case, the development of new drugs and the involvement of human subjects in research. This document, and the process by which it was produced, support the values of equity, cooperation, scientific progress, and respect for the lives of all persons affected by HIV/AIDS.

20 *Is Consent Useful When Resuscitation Isn't?*

G‌ILES R. S‌COFIELD

Giles R. Scofield is a fellow in the Department of Psychology, Craig Hospital, Englewood, Colorado.

> At midnight
> I pondered on the beating of
>   my heart;
> One single pulse of anguish
> Raged in my heart
> At midnight.
>
> —*Gustav Mahler*

O‌ur increasing awareness that limitations of human knowledge, resources, and ingenuity impose finite horizons on medicine's ability to ward off disease, disability, and death has forced us to acknowledge that we must either limit medical interventions on a societal and individual basis or bankrupt ourselves.[1] Attaining a consensus about limiting treatment requires educating patients and society to understand that expectations once held about medicine no longer apply, or do so less categorically. Given our faith in medicine and its impact on personal well-being, adjusting ourselves to the realities of limited medical options will generate anxiety and a crisis in confidence, which will make shifting expectations even harder. How well we make this adjustment depends on how we make these decisions. If they occur or are perceived to occur in ways that generate suspicion and distrust, the ultimate decisions, no matter how fair or necessary they are, will prove unacceptable, and the process become paralyzed, protracted, fragmented, and counterproductive. We cannot avoid the effort reorientation involves or the disappointment unmet expectations create, but we can manage these difficulties and

This article first appeared in Hastings Center Report 21 *(November/December 1991): 28–36.*

enhance the prospects for responsible deliberation by carefully framing the decisionmaking dialogue.

How we structure that dialogue depends on how we define consent, since that will determine both the character of the deliberation and the kind and quality of consensus we ultimately obtain. We need the model of consent most likely to insure that meaningful communication occurs, yet it must also be closely connected to our most fundamental social values as decisions to withhold treatment become more commonplace.[2]

In truth, decisions to withhold treatment are and always have been ubiquitous and frequent. They occur whenever a physician weighs and ultimately decides against offering or recommending that a patient be admitted, tested, treated, or referred. Such decisions are not necessarily invidious and often represent prudent restraint. Doctors are expected to use the professional expertise derived from their education, training, and experience to make judgments about what they believe should or should not be done in a given situation.

What is troublesome about a decision to withhold treatment is how it occurs. Because it is low-profile in nature, it does not have the inherent visibility that triggers consent when intervening or withdrawing are at issue. Thus, the fact that it has occurred may be known only to the doctor and those colleagues involved in the patient's care. Although affected by it, the patient may not know how, why, or even that the decision was made. Whether the proper criteria were correctly applied to a particular decision is unlikely to be examined beyond professional circles, which makes withholding especially problematic in terms of the values consent is supposed to serve.

Given the special nature of decisions to withhold treatment, we should not assume that the model of consent developed to provide accountability in an era of therapeutic relentlessness will do the job as medicine begins to rein itself in. Because greater justification is required to withhold than to withdraw treatment,[3] finding the right way to make these decisions becomes especially critical as we adjust individual and social expectations to the new realities setting limits creates. Theoretically, the order not to resuscitate a patient (DNR order) defies withholding's usual pattern. This decision requires express authorization and documentation reflecting the consent of the patient or the patient's surrogate, or, as in the case of emergency medical services, a physician's permission to withhold resuscitation. Because resuscitation, commonly known as CPR, is the expected response to sudden death, if it is not provided someone has to account for why.

Articles discussing consent to DNR orders have exposed thought processes usually confined to professional enclaves. This provides an opportunity to consider how such decisions ought to be made in light of the values consent serves. Due to CPR's ubiquitous, symbolic, and momentous nature—each of us may well face a decision about being resuscitated or allowed to die—how we decide to limit resuscitation is critical to developing a model of consent suited to making other decisions about limiting treatment.

CPR: In Like a Lion, Out Like a Lamb?

It is difficult now to imagine the enormous impact of the introduction of CPR. Catastrophic trauma, life-threatening surgery, and failed hearts no longer meant certain death. Medicine could reverse death's surest sign—the heart that had stopped beating. With its promise of life after death, CPR transformed medicine, society, and our expectations about mortality.

Society affirmed CPR's significance by declaring it an emergency procedure, which exempted it from consent prior to use. Public perceptions about CPR came largely from the media, which usually portrayed it and medicine in glowing, heroic terms. CPR rapidly proliferated into ICUs, general wards, and even the public domain, as emergency medical teams, police officers, firefighters, lifeguards, and concerned citizens learned to provide basic life support in the event of a cardiac arrest.

The emergency exception eventually evolved into presumed consent to CPR, making it society's standing order against death. This shielded CPR from patient and public scrutiny, hid its realities from all but those involved in administering or receiving it, fostered its indiscriminate use, and excused physicians from seeking anything other than grateful ratification when it worked or heartfelt solace when it did not.

Presumed consent freed physicians from disclosing that CPR's success, however defined, depends on a number of factors. The patient's condition and the presence of pathology are important determinants. Other noteworthy factors include: where the arrest occurs (in an ICU or elsewhere, for example); the nature of the arrest; whether the arrest is witnessed or not; the time elapsed between arrest and the commencement of resuscitative measures; the availability of the equipment and drugs needed to provide advanced life-support; whether the equipment works; how long resuscitative measures are employed; and the training, skill, experience, and collaborative ability of the code team.[4] Although some patients would have found such information germane to a decision about submitting to CPR and its sequelae, presumed consent obviated the need to secure real consent. Even where an arrest was "not unexpected," physicians who were unwilling or unable to talk to patients about resuscitation needed only to wait for an "emergency" to materialize in order to act. Presumed consent to CPR was medicine's license to intervene at will.

As time and experience brought balanced insight into CPR's benefits and limitations, perceptions about its life-saving powers yielded to the awareness that its effectiveness could no longer be categorically presumed nor its burdensomeness denied. Discussions about limiting CPR through DNR orders found their way into the literature and the courts.

Yet fast upon recognizing the need to make decisions about forgoing this not always beneficial treatment came attempts to exempt physicians from obtaining consent to a DNR order. Some contended that because consent prevents uninvited contact, there was no duty to secure consent not to commit a battery, a view that has been rejected.[5] Recent discussions concede that DNR orders require consent, but argue that there is no duty to secure a patient's consent when CPR is medically futile; when it would be futile to attempt resuscitation, consent to a DNR order may be presumed.

One need only translate presumed consent into its oxymoronic synonym—unilateral consent—to appreciate how radically it departs from the goal of collaborative decisionmaking. Although a DNR order is about *doing* nothing, it's not about nothing; nor is it about not doing something that no sensible physician would ever do. It reflects a physician's considered judgment that a patient is going to die and reverses society's standing order to preserve life against death. It has profound social, personal, and professional ramifications. To determine whether consent is useless when resuscitation is futile, we need to examine consent and futility more closely.

An Exercise in Futility

The argument that when CPR is futile consent is pointless rests on two prongs.[6] The first starts with the premise that what distinguishes physicians is the professional expertise that gives them the exclusive ability to make medical judgments. A physician's professional integrity lies in the ability to recognize and integrate what is known about a patient's medical condition with what medicine has to offer, and to exercise his or her best judgment about how or whether to proceed with treatment. That integrity and the value we place on such judgment are meaningless if patients may freely ignore or override it out of fear, irrationality, or ignorance. Because only physicians can evaluate whether an intervention is medically futile, they must have unilateral authority to make and act on judgments about matters that fall exclusively within the domain of their expertise.

The second prong analyzes futility according to the patient's autonomy interest. Without discounting autonomy's value, it argues that this interest is not unlimited. Patients may not demand treatment, especially treatment that would accomplish nothing. Similarly, physicians have no duty to provide and a patient may not successfully sue for the failure to provide futile treatment. Patient autonomy and consent are irrelevant to a decision about CPR when it offers no potential benefit.

Moreover, involving patients in deliberations about useless treatment confuses and upsets them. Some, believing that a discussion about CPR implies that it must be of some benefit (otherwise, why mention it?), will ask or insist that it be administered. Others will find such discussions disturbing because their hopeless condition has left them emotionally drained and vulnerable; they will think that seeking consent is cruel or demand CPR out of desperate fear. Instead of elevating form over substance, we should acknowledge that a patient's right to choose ends where futility begins.

These arguments seem so sensible, internally consistent, and authoritatively supported that their conclusion appears ineluctable. They seem to strike a reasonable balance between patient and physician autonomy and accommodate society's legitimate interest in not wasting resources. To suggest that decisions about futile treatment require consent sounds ludicrous; doctors have better things to do than discuss pointless therapy. Patient autonomy needs sensible limits, and authorizing doctors to enter DNR orders unilaterally when CPR is futile seems legally and ethically sound.

The apparent soundness of this conclusion evaporates upon close examination. In reality the futility exception is a dishonest solution to the tragic choice that decisions to limit treatment represent. It purports to respect, but in fact departs from the fundamental values consent is intended to serve. It will not generate the conversation we need if we are to attain a consensus about limiting treatment; nor will it make physicians sensitive in their dealings with patients, especially dying patients. It promotes a model of consent that is antithetical to setting limits in a democratic, caring manner.

The argument that physician expertise at judging futility justifies unilaterally entered DNR orders rests on several assumptions: agreement on what resuscitation means; a definition of what constitutes "futile" (and successful) treatment; concurrence that physicians can make such judgments accurately, reliably, and consistently; and agreement on what a DNR order means. Before empowering physicians to decide these matters unilaterally, we should analyze each of these assumptions.

The global pronouncement that resuscitation won't work obscures its subtle realities. Many people who stereotypically imagine resuscitation as a chest-thumping, bone-crushing, electrifying experience would be shocked to learn that depending on the clinical situation it defines a range of interventions.[7] Less invasive measures include drug support and fluid resuscitation. Thus, when a physician says that resuscitation is futile we cannot know what is meant, and will remain ignorant if nothing more is said. Even were we to agree that compression and defibrillation would be futile, pharmacological support with proper monitoring might be useful.

Implicit in the judgment that CPR is medically futile is a definition of medical success. Even assuming that physicians can predict whose CPR will succeed and whose won't, how they define success and whether their definition comports with the patient's, the family's, or the larger society's are legitimate questions. Presumed consent presupposes that only the physician's perspective matters.

Even if a physician's judgment that CPR won't work is sound and comports with the patient's perspective (difficult to accomplish if the patient is not involved in the decision), *why* it won't is significant, especially because CPR's success can depend on factors other than the patient's physiology or pathology. It's one thing to conclude that nothing more can be done, and something else to believe that we can do nothing more for you here. If patients might be better off elsewhere, presumed consent hides knowledge about that option from them.

The belief that physicians know futility when they see it is an illusion.[8] There is no set definition of medical futility, only suggested parameters that vary widely. Even if medicine could define medical futility, trusting physicians to make unilateral judgments assumes that they know what the definition is and can apply it accurately, consistently, and reliably. Medical judgment involves recognizing and integrating relevant data correctly, an uncertain process that inevitably involves false positives and negatives, erroneous judgments, and differing interpretations. The same doctor may view data about prognostically indistinguishable patients differently, and different doctors, depending on their specialty and experience, may assess the same patient's chances differently.[9] Presumed consent assumes a world of medical certainty that does not exist.

Moreover, futility is not some objective, value-free fact that jumps up and announces "Here I am." It is a concept, that is, a way of judging facts. We are concerned about futility precisely because we value not wasting resources. Whether it is futile "in fact" to attempt to keep someone alive may depend on whether that person is a potential organ donor, a potentially viable fetus, or worth salvaging for some socially or otherwise informed reason. Presumed consent assumes that in making medical decisions we can separate observer from observed, facts from values, and individuals from context, an assumption that is doubtful at best.[10] Among themselves physicians do not uniformly understand what a DNR order connotes,[11] putting aside whether their understanding agrees with the patient's. Some physicians equate a DNR order with a decision to withhold or withdraw other and sometimes all means of life support. A DNR order does not and was never meant to concern itself with anything other than resuscitative measures, but the fact that not all physicians know this, or that some who do nonetheless regard or treat a DNR order as authority to forgo other treatment argues against one-sided consent.

Finally, even if physicians *could* exercise judgment with the certainty they claim, that would not mean that they *should* make such decisions unilaterally. After all, if physicians cannot avoid the consent process where a treatment is "clearly" beneficial, why should they do so when it is "clearly" futile? And although a physician may not be held liable for failing to provide futile care, whether he or she actually exercised proper judgment in a given case is a question a court may decide.[12] A physician whose futility defense might ultimately prevail against the claim that CPR was wrongfully withheld must nonetheless defend against it, which should make even the most confident physician uneasy about presumed consent.

The second prong of the argument fares no better than the first. Its essential assumption—that because autonomy triggers the duty to secure consent, the absence of an autonomy interest excuses it—puts the ethical cart before the horse. Autonomy is important, but it is neither the sole nor the primary principle of medical ethics. It is derivative of and subordinate to the overarching obligation that we show respect for persons.[13] Respecting autonomy is simply one way of respecting persons. The futility exception ends its analysis where it ought to begin. By not asking whether excluding patients from deliberations about their fate demonstrates respect for them, presumed consent mistakenly equates ignoring persons with respecting them.

Presumed consent gives autonomy undue prominence because it erroneously assumes that autonomy is all there is to consent. Yet consent concerns itself with matters beyond autonomy. Among them: respecting human dignity; promoting rational decisionmaking; encouraging professional self-scrutiny; avoiding deceit and coercion; and educating the public.[14] Under this view of consent, futility looks different.

Given the variability, uncertainty, and biases that influence the physician, talking with patients forces a doctor to get clear on what lies beneath the judgment that resuscitation would be futile before giving this news to the person to whom it means the most. This fosters professional self-scrutiny and helps assure that the determination that CPR is medically futile does not become a sterilized way of unilaterally classifying patients as "pointless to treat," that is, not *worth* treating.

Presumed consent thwarts the legitimate goal of avoiding deceit and coercion. Unless physicians explain futility to patients we cannot determine if they do so accurately, deceptively, or manipulatively.[15] Imposing on patients consequences they have not assumed is a form of coercion. When what the patient believes and what the chart denotes do not reflect one another and the staff must act out the charade of hiding from the patient how close death is, deceit occurs.

Rational decisionmaking is a process of shared understanding and collaborative planning. It is not irrational to give patients the opportunity to agree with the assessment that CPR is futile; if anything, it is irrational *not* to afford them that chance. Decisions about CPR can open the door to other matters, assure the patient that "no code" does not mean "no treatment," and clarify to all concerned what DNR means, including that it can be reassessed. Rational decisionmaking cannot occur absent patient involvement, unless, of course, all decisions are to be made unilaterally.

Educating the public is an integral function of consent; as we educate patients we can educate and reorient society. Most patients and their families are unaware of medicine's recent change of heart about CPR. The best way to debunk the myths, fears, and misperceptions they may harbor from whatever source is by being candid with them in the course of making treatment decisions. Word will get around, and discussing beforehand why CPR won't work minimizes the chances for hurt feelings and possible recriminations if relatives later wonder why a loved one died without heroic efforts.

Respect for human dignity requires truth-telling. Most patients know something is wrong with them. They do not know how bad that something is and what, if anything, can be done about it. They are entitled to know that; presumably that is one reason they went to the doctor. Not acquainting patients with what is known and believed about their prospects and disenfranchising them from deliberations about their fate denigrates them.

Presumed consent's disrespect for personhood is reflected in its meager concept of autonomy, which it defines as a "negative right"—to be let alone. This simply repackages the already rejected view that consent to a DNR order is never required. It also suggests that patients need information only when medical choices need to be made. Nothing could be further from the truth.

Patients need medical information to make choices that have nothing to do with medicine, especially when no medical options exist. However commonplace DNR orders are to physicians, most patients cross this Rubicon only once, and need to know—in order to plan a funeral, say farewell to friends, try to hold on for the arrival of a new grandchild, or simply look out the window with the knowledge—that time is drawing to a close. Patients are value systems, not organ systems, and consent serves a personal purpose even when it is medically useless.[16]

The futility exception's final arguments—that because patients will demand resuscitation or be so confused and upset by discussions about it they are best served by being excluded from such decisions—do not bear weight. Patients do not behave irrationally as frequently as some people fear, and the patient's first reaction may not last or be the last. Also, the idiosyncratic demands *some* patients may make do not justify a rule that excuses not talking with *all* patients. Finally, a doctor is always free to refrain from continuing to care for a patient whose demands for resuscitation violate his or her professional conscience, though separating from a patient at so critical a juncture should prod any physician to deep reflection. Similarly, the commonly invoked adage that candor hurts patients lacks the evidence to support the therapeutic privilege it creates. The truth is, many patients welcome and are relieved by the opportunity to be involved in such deliberations (which also gives those who want the chance to opt out).[17] The recommendation that physicians forgo consent when CPR is futile is usually based on studies in which patients were not adequately informed, or is made despite evidence that properly informed patients overwhelmingly agree with their doctor's recommendation. What these studies do establish is that physicians have trouble talking with patients. More silence is not the solution to that problem.

If a conversation intended to bring patients to a realistic understanding of their situation and of medicine's limited ability to postpone death confuses or hurts them (more so than silence bewilders or angers them), we should determine the cause and address it. Some patients will be upset because no one has ever been candid with them about their condition and prognosis; others because discussing death tongue-ties their doctor. The cure is not less, but more talk. Physicians need to converse more often, thoroughly, and carefully with their patients.

For such conversations to occur, physicians must regard them as integral to practicing good medicine. If they view consent as a form that patients must sign, instead of the ongoing process the form is supposed to substantiate, resuscitation decisions will elevate form over substance in a way that is insensitive and hurtful to patients. Physicians cannot pass patients along or avoid the responsibility for defusing situations their or their colleagues' silence creates. They need education, training, and support to ensure that these conversations occur appropriately and sensitively; which means learning how to converse candidly, comfortably, and sympathetically with patients about death and dying.[18]

Not conversing with patients about such matters should be the exception, not the rule. Indeed, if the expertise physicians gain from their knowledge and experience reveals anything, it is that there is rarely a good reason to wait until a crisis erupts or resuscitation is futile to determine what ought to be done. How often have physicians found their hands tied because they or one of their colleagues were too tongue-tied to plan ahead? If taking a patient's values history were as integral to clinical practice as the medical history is, physicians could establish early on in the relationship the foundation of knowledge and trust needed to discuss decisions concerning the sort of care and treatment patients want at the end of life.

HEADS I WIN, TAILS YOU LOSE

When viewed concretely, the futility exception loses much of the luster it generates in the abstract. It neither encourages advance planning nor discourages not talking with patients. It is unlikely to promote honest, shared decisionmaking or to demonstrate respect for persons and is antithetical to the values consent is supposed to serve. To appreciate the futility exception fully, however, we need to dig further.

The futility exception's latent significance appears when we compare it to its counterpart, the emergency exception. Whereas the futility exception arises partly out of solicitude for a patient's physical integrity, the emergency exception circumvents that integrity in theory and practice. What reconciles these contradictory exceptions is the doctrine of presumed consent, which each promotes. Presumed consent enables physicians "legally and ethically" to exclude patients from participating in decisions affecting them and to decide unilaterally whether to use or withhold resuscitation. What it protects is not a patient's physical integrity, but medicine's professional integrity. Lurking within the futility exception is the medical profession's desire to protect its autonomy against the threats posed by death and health care rationing.

Medicine's professional autonomy—its right to be let alone—rests on a belief in professional expertise that causes individuals and society to surrender to medical authority judgments about private and public health matters.[19] Among the most powerful sources of our faith in medicine is the belief that it can "do something" about death. Resuscitation, which transformed our view of medicine and death, symbolizes medicine's power and lies at the crux of its authority.[20]

For that authority to remain secure, medicine must maximize its control over how resuscitation is perceived and over decisions about when, where, how, and whether it will be used. Disclosing resuscitation's realities and permitting patients to participate in decisions about it diminishes that control and the professional power that comes with it. Because resuscitation decisions are about death, they are personally and professionally challenging. It is more attractive to gloss over or avoid conversations about death than to invite situations where physician or medical impotence is revealed through the overt confession, "There is nothing I (or we) can do."

The futility exception and presumed consent try to solve this problem in a way that does not seem to offend the values consent serves, thereby enabling medicine to retreat intact, as unaccountably as the emergency exception enabled it to advance. By completing the circle the emergency exception starts, the futility exception surrounds resuscitation with a model of consent that maximizes medicine's control over decisions about its use. With consent in favor of resuscitation already presumed, a physician who is unwilling or unable to talk to a patient about such matters need only delay determining a patient's DNR status until resuscitation is futile for the presumption to flip the other way. The decision gets made without the patient's ever knowing when, how, why, or even that it did. Between the emergency and futility exceptions, presumed consent gets patients coming and going.

The futility exception also enables medicine to control how resuscitation is perceived, and especially why it does not always work. Emphasizing the perception that some patients are simply "too far gone" for resuscitation to do any good helps hide the other truths about why and how often resuscitation fails. This preserves the heroic aura the emergency exception promotes. It also keeps the public from asking what all this suggests about whether pre-hospital use of CPR ought to remain unlimited; and whether cases such as Nancy Cruzan's raise as profound questions about CPR as they do about feeding tubes. For now, a conversation about an intervention that affects the public excludes it.

Additionally, the futility exception promotes the perception that physicians can (and therefore ought to) be trusted to limit medical resources unilaterally, especially to keep the health care system from being run into the ground by the demands of rapacious, irrational, idiosyncratic patients. Not only do doctors save lives, they save resources too. Setting limits, therefore, involves letting medicine set them for us.

The futility exception's suggestion of presumed consent will likely swallow the rule of actual consent in decisions to limit resuscitation, thereby enabling the medical profession to rein itself in unilaterally and unaccountably. It is medicine's license to withhold at will. It vests the profession whose accountability is at issue with the authority to determine when and whether that authority is properly exercised. It establishes a model of decisionmaking that purports to respect patients, when it actually rationalizes physician avoidance of death and legitimates medical authority.

If physicians are given the authority to enter DNR orders unilaterally when they believe resuscitation would be futile, nothing prevents their using the same reasoning to enter DNT (do-not-treat), DNH (do-not-hospitalize), or any other order denying treatment unilaterally when they believe it would be futile—whether "futile" means not medically effective, not cost effective, or not worth it for this patient. The futility exception sets limits to everything and everyone except the medical profession's autonomy.

The decisionmaking model it promotes is undemocratic and uncaring. By vesting the medical profession with the authority to make decisions that should be the product of open discussion and shared deliberation, it forecloses the conversation we must have if we are to arrive at a genuine consensus about setting limits.[21] The legal fiction of presumed consent is no substitute for the solid work we all must do if we are to adjust ourselves to the new realities these limits impose. There is no such thing as presumed consensus.

The futility exception is uncaring because it legitimates and perpetuates the practice of isolating dying patients from their physicians. By placing a wall of silence between them, presumed consent severs the dying from the human community before death actually takes them from the world. It offers social death and exclusion at the one moment when we most need the consolation of our fellow men and women.[22] It limits respecting persons to the tissue-thin perspective conveyed by the right to be let alone (a pretty pathetic way of respecting patients we have no intention of touching) and ignores the deeper human values that make us who we are. The morally barren and impoverished ethics of indifference promoted by isolating, disenfranchising, and abandoning patients is no way to treat them as persons.[23]

Is Consent Futile?

Given the unacceptable consequences that result if we adopt the futility exception and presumed consent, we must ask what kind of consent will enable us to make decisions we need to make in a way that preserves our fundamental social values. To do that we must acknowledge what the decision not to resuscitate represents in the debate about how we set limits at the clinical and societal levels. It asks us, individually and collectively, to arrive at a consensus on how to integrate death and decisions about it into the legitimating values of our moral universe. Deciding what kind of life we want involves deciding what kind of death we can face.

To a society whose faith in medicine and whose commitment to the fundamental values of life and liberty has led it to declare that death, once a matter of fate, is now a matter of choice, how we want to allocate death represents the quintessential tragic choice.[24] It strikes at the heart of our strongest values—the Rule of Rescue, the presumption in favor of life—and at our deepest fears. Just when we most need to rely on our basic values to resolve this tragic choice, we find that death and decisions about it overwhelm medicine, life, and liberty. It is a choice we need, but do not want to make; it concerns values we want to hold onto absolutely, but cannot; and it forces us either to admit a truth that seems unbearable or hide it beneath illusions that preserve the moral foundations of social collaboration.

The futility exception is one such illusion. It preserves our faith in medicine, harmoniously reconciles a fundamentally irreconcilable clash of values, and cloaks a decision about allocating death behind a decision about resuscitation. As we have seen, it is a dishonest solution and unless those basic values change it is only a matter of time before it is exposed for illusion. When that happens, the tragic choice resurfaces, as it did in the *Wanglie* case, and we grope for other subterfuges we hope will do the trick, of which denying the personhood of the unconscious is one and leaving these decisions entirely to "patient self-determination" is another.

Because we cannot make death go away, we cannot keep the tragic choice from resurfacing. This means that we must either adopt subterfuge after dishonest subterfuge—and accept the moral erosion each illusion's failure causes—or decide to make these decisions openly and honestly. If we wish to remain true to the values served by consent and respect for persons, we must opt in favor of candor. Once we opt in favor of candor the answer to our question becomes ironically clear: consent is useful *because* resuscitation is futile.

Difficult though saying no to patients is, the dangers that flow from saying nothing at all are far worse. Obscuring the basis of decisionmaking will generate fear and misunderstanding and lead to abuse, especially of those groups within society traditionally subjected to neglect and mistreatment. Deciding to withhold or limit resuscitation asks us to accept the self-limiting condition of our mortality; deciding to forgo consent asks us to deny the basic values that define us as a society.

Forging a consensus about matters of clinical and social importance requires trust and honesty, and the current posture of the debate suggests that no one trusts anyone to make these decisions. The truth is, however, that we must trust ourselves to make them together, setting aside our fear and mistrust, and conversing openly and respectfully with each other.

For that conversation to occur, we will have to talk in ways we are unaccustomed to. Patients can no more marginalize the legitimate concerns physicians have about their integrity and the need to set reasonable limits than physicians can dismiss patients through the futility exception. Each must give up some autonomy to overcome the barriers that currently serve only to separate us from each other and prevent us from making decisions we need to make together. We must integrate a relational perspective into how we see ourselves and each other.[25] Thus, we must talk about rights in a different way. Instead of trumping them out as conversation-stoppers, we must use them—and the values they express—as the starting point for a conversation about how we can best reconcile our individual wants with our collective needs.

We might well turn a conversation about futility to a useful purpose, by deciding to place less emphasis on death-defying interventions and to put more effort into life-enhancing ones, such as preventive and public health measures, chronic and rehabilitative care, and improved access to care. Not only would this be attentive to patient well-being and autonomy, it might also generate renewed and more heartfelt respect for medicine and physicians.

The question is not whether we can, should, or must make caring and conversation integral to how we decide matters of clinical and social importance, but whether we will. If we do, the hour of our death need no longer be anguished, angry, or lonely.[26]

ACKNOWLEDGMENTS

This article is dedicated to the memory of Shirley Katzenbach.

REFERENCES

1. Robert H. Block, *Rationing Medicine* (New York: Columbia University Press, 1988); Daniel Callahan, *Setting Limits* (New York: Simon & Schuster, 1987); Larry R. Churchill, *Rationing Health Care in America* (Notre Dame, Ind.: University of Notre Dame, 1987).

2. Howard Brody, "Transparency: Informed Consent in Primary Care," *Hastings Center Report* 19, no. 5 (1989): 5-9; Marion Danis and Larry R. Churchill, "Autonomy and the Common Weal," *Hastings Center Report* 21, no. 1 (1991): 25-29.

3. Bernard Lo and Albert R. Jonsen, "Clinical Decisions to Limit Treatment," *Annals of Internal Medicine* 93, no. 5 (1980): 764-68; President's Commission for the Study of Ethical Problems in Medicine and Biomedical and Behavioral Research, *Deciding to Forego Life-Sustaining Treatment* (Washington, D.C.: U.S. Government Printing Office, 1983), pp. 73-77.

4. George E. Taffet, Thomas A. Teasdale, and Robert J. Luchi, "In-Hospital Cardiopulmonary Resuscitation," *JAMA* 260, no. 14 (1988): 2069-72; Peter Safar, "Resuscitation from Clinical Death: Pathophysiologic Limits and Therapeutic Potentials," *Critical Care Medicine* 16, no. 10 (1988): 923-41; Richard O. Cummins, Kaye Chesemore, Roger D. White et al., "Defibrillator Failures," *JAMA* 264, no. 8 (1990): 1019-25.

5. President's Commission, *Deciding to Forego Life-Sustaining Treatment*, pp. 231-58.

6. Donald J. Murphy, "Do-Not-Resuscitate Orders: Time for Reappraisal in Long-Term-Care Institutions," *JAMA* 260, no. 14 (1988): 2098–2101; Leslie J. Blackhall, "Must We Always Use CPR?" *NEJM* 317, no. 20 (1987): 1281–84; Tom Tomlinson and Howard Brody, "Ethics and Communication in Do-Not-Resuscitate Orders," *NEJM* 318, no. 1 (1988): 43–46; Tom Tomlinson and Howard Brody, "Futility and the Ethics of Communication," *JAMA* 264, no. 10 (1990): 1276–80; J. Chris Hackler and Charles Hiller, "Family Consent to Orders Not to Resuscitate," *JAMA* 264, no. 10 (1990): 1281–83; Lawrence J. Schneiderman, Nancy S. Jecker, and Albert R. Jonsen, "Medical Futility: Its Meaning and Implications," *Annals of Internal Medicine* 112, no. 12 (1990): 949–54.

7. Peter Safar and Nicholas G. Bircher, *Cardiopulmonary Cerebral Resuscitation* (Philadelphia: Saunders, 1988); Jeffrey Hammond and C. Gillon Ward, "Decision Not to Treat: 'Do Not Resuscitate' Order for the Burn Patient in the Acute Setting," *Critical Care Medicine* 17, no. 2 (1989): 136–38.

8. John D. Lantos, Peter A. Singer, Robert M. Walker et al., "The Illusion of Futility in Clinical Practice," *American Journal of Medicine* 87, no. 1 (1989): 81–84; Lawrence J. Nelson, "*Primum Utilis Esse*: The Primacy of Usefulness in Medicine," *Yale Journal of Biology and Medicine* 51, no. 6 (1978): 655–67; Donald J. Murphy and David B. Matchar, "Life-Sustaining Therapy: A Model for Appropriate Use," *JAMA* 264, no. 16 (1990): 2103–8; AMA Council on Ethical and Judicial Affairs, "Guidelines for the Appropriate Use of Do-Not-Resuscitate Orders," *JAMA* 265, no. 14 (1991): 1869–71.

9. Robert M. Wachter, John M. Luce, Norman Hearst et al., "Decisions about Resuscitations: Inequities among Patients with Different Diseases but Similar Prognoses," *Annals of Internal Medicine* 111, no. 6 (1989): 525–32.

10. Daniel Callahan, "Values, Facts and Decisionmaking," *Hastings Center Report* 1, no. 1 (June 1971): 1.

11. Joan La Puma, Marc D. Silverstein, Carol B. Stocking et al., "Life-Sustaining Treatment: A Prospective Study of Patients with DNR Orders in a Teaching Hospital," *Archives of Internal Medicine* 148, no. 10 (1988): 2193–98.

12. *Payne v. Marion General Hospital,* 549 N.E.2d 1043 (Ind. Ct. App. 1990).

13. The National Commission for the Protection of Human Subjects of Biomedical and Behavioral Research, *The Belmont Report* (Washington D.C.: U.S. Government Printing Office, 1978), pp. 4–6.

14. Jay Katz and Alexander M. Capron, *Catastrophic Diseases: Who Decides What?* (New Brunswick, N.J.: Transaction Books, 1982), pp. 82–90.

15. Theodore J. Schneyer, "Informed Consent and the Danger of Bias in the Formation of Medical Disclosure Practices," *Wisconsin Law Review* (1976): 124–70; Dennis H. Novack, Barbara J. Detering, Robert Arnold et al., "Physicians' Attitudes Toward Using Deception to Resolve Difficult Ethical Problems" *JAMA* 261, no. 20 (1989): 2980–85.

16. Stuart J. Younger, "Who Defines Futility," *JAMA* 260, no. 14 (1988): 2094–95; Stuart J. Younger, "Futility in Context," *JAMA* 264, no. 10 (1990): 1295–96; Susan M. Wolf, "Conflict between Doctor and Patient," *Law, Medicine & Health Care* 16, nos. 3–4 (1988): 197–203.

17. Ronald S. Schonwetter, Thomas A. Teasdale, George Taffet et al., "Educating the Elderly: Cardiopulmonary Resuscitation Discussions before and after Intervention," *Journal of the American Geriatrics Society* 39, no. 4 (1991): 372–77.

18. Bernard Lo, "Unanswered Questions about DNR Orders," *JAMA* 265, no. 14 (1991): 1874–75; Raanan Gillon, "Deciding Not to Resuscitate," *Journal of Medical Ethics* 15, no. 4 (1989): 171–72; Giles R. Scofield, "Terminal Care and the Continuing Need for Professional Education," *Journal of Palliative Care* 5, no. 3 (1989): 32–36.

19. Paul Starr, *The Social Transformation of American Medicine* (New York: Basic Books, 1982), pp. 3–29; Eliot Freidson, *Professional Dominance: The Social Structure of Medical Care* (New York: Atherton, 1970).

20. Kathleen Nolan, "In Death's Shadow: The Meanings of Withholding Resuscitation," *Hastings Center Report* 17, no. 6 (1987): 9–14; Jay Katz, *The Silent World of Doctor and Patient* (New York: Free Press, 1984), pp. 213–25.

21. Eliot Freidson, *Profession of Medicine* (New York: Harper & Row, 1970), pp. 335–52; Michael Walzer, *Spheres of Justice* (New York: Basic Books, 1983), pp. 155–60, 284–90.

22. Michael Ignatieff, *The Needs of Strangers* (New York: Penguin Books, 1986), pp. 76–79.

23. Elizabeth V. Spelman, "On Treating Persons as Persons," *Ethics* 88, no. 2 (1978): 150–61.

24. Guido Calabresi and Philip Bobbit, *Tragic Choices* (New York: W.W. Norton & Co., 1978), pp. 17–28; Guido Calabresi, *Ideals, Beliefs, Attitudes and the Law* (Syracuse, N.Y.: Syracuse University Press, 1985), pp. 87–117; Peter L. Berger and Thomas Luckman, *The Social Construction of Reality* (New York: Doubleday, 1966), 101–2.

25. Daniel Callahan, "Autonomy: A Moral Good, Not an Obsession," *Hastings Center Report* 14, no. 5 (1984): 40–42; Martha Minow, *Making All the Difference* (Ithaca: Cornell University Press, 1990); Robert N. Bellah, Richard Madsen, William Sullivan et al., *Habits of the Heart* (Berkeley and Los Angeles: University of California Press, 1985).

26. William F. May, "On Not Facing Death Alone," *Hastings Center Report* 18, no. 1 (1971): 2–3; Philip Aries, *The Hour of Our Death* (New York: Alfred A. Knopf, 1981), pp. 611–14.

21 *Privacy and Disclosure in Medical Genetics Examined in an Ethics of Care*

DOROTHY C. WERTZ, PH.D. AND JOHN C. FLETCHER, PH.D

Dorothy Wertz, Ph.D. is at the Shriver Center for the Mentally Retarded in Waltham, Massachusetts. John Fletcher, Ph.D. is the Director of the Center for Biomedical Ethics at the University of Virginia Medical School.

INTRODUCTION

The progress of genetic knowledge magnifies existing ethical problems in medical genetics. Among the most troubling types of problems—for medicine, patients, and the larger society—are those of privacy and disclosure. Examples of the range of problems involving privacy and disclosure are: 1) disclosure of false paternity to an unsuspecting husband; 2) disclosure of a patient's genetic make-up to his or her unknowing spouse; 3) disclosure of information, against a patient's wishes, to relatives at genetic risk; 4) disclosure of ambiguous test results; 5) disclosure of adventitious nonmedical information, e.g., fetal sex; and 6) disclosure to institutional third parties, such as employers and insurers.

The Human Genome Project will fuel rapid progress to identify genes and understand their functions. Such progress will mean that problems like the ones above arise more often. Most medical information pertains only to the patient. However, genetic information is more often important to the entire genetic family. Patient/family genetic information will also be of great interest to third-party payers and possibly to employers. In nations where employers contribute heavily to health insurance, interest will doubtless be high. These problems are a subject for public policy[1] as well as for ethical reflection.

This article first appeared in Bioethics 5 *(July 1991): 212–232.*

In the literature, ethical problems like privacy and disclosure are frequently addressed as problems of "conflicting rights". Resolutions are sought by an examination to determine whose individual rights have priority. However, the very nature of genetic information, as something that is shared among family members, cuts against the grain of a rights-based approach. An approach that values the relationships of persons, rather than individual rights, may provide a richer understanding and source of guidance for such complex problems. Our experience in conducting an international study of medical geneticists that included cases on privacy and disclosure has brought us to this view.

An Ethics of Care in Clinical Practice

"Principlism" has been the source of many discussions of rules for confidentiality and disclosure in clinical practice. Guidance for classes of ethical problems is derived, often with skill and flexibility, from basic ethical principles, such as autonomy, non-maleficence, beneficence, and justice.[2] Such discussions can be very helpful on a broad canvas. However, when it comes to tangled cases in clinical practice and the needs of persons in them, ethical principles seem to remain hovering over the hardest knots and human needs. Approaches to resolution of problems are usually described in the language of individual rights and obligations also used in jurisprudence. Some writers, including some feminists, have criticized rights-based approaches as inadequate to the human dimensions of many medical dilemmas and have proposed an alternative.[3]

An ethical view construed as "care", or as we prefer, an ethics of responsibility to care for persons in their relationships, can provide for a richer treatment of these problems. This view emphasizes the role of emotions and character traits in ethics and the inseparability of emotions and reasoning. Essentially, to "care" means to identify with other persons, each of whom is unique, with a view toward nurturing the web of relationships they share or can share. Instead of seeing atomistic individuals in conflict and competing for space, a care-based ethics views patients and clinicians in terms of interactive relationships. The "patient" is a family, or rather several social and biological families. From this perspective, an ethics of care may be closer to the ethical beliefs of some African societies than to a dominant ethical tradition drawing heavily on individualism in Western society.[4]

We cannot develop a full argument here for an ethics of care. Our main task, using survey results on the moral reasoning of geneticists in many nations, is to discuss recommendations based upon an ethics of care in clinical practice for cases of privacy and disclosure. However, we believe that this view need not be an independent, distant alternative to "principlism." Our recommendations will show that an ethics of care

does not exclude the language of patient rights and physician obligations. We argue that rights are part of a larger ethical framework with
four elements. Decisions should be made within a framework of *needs*
(usually patients') and *responsibilities* (usually doctors'), with some reference to the good of society, and, in some cases, responses to the "deserts" of those who have undergone special suffering or discrimination.
Patients' major needs are to receive health benefits and to avoid harm.
Patients also need unbiased information so that they can make their own
decisions. Further, patients in genetics need psychological, social, and
economic support in making their decisions. Doctors have responsibility
for providing for some of these needs and to advance the cause of their
patients within society so that other needs can also be met.

Patients' needs and patients' requests are not synonymous; patients
may need service or support that they do not request and may request
services that they do not need. Assessing the other party's true needs
requires real mutuality, good communication, and sensitivity in the
doctor-patient relationship. The physician must care enough to begin a
relationship that can become deep enough to foster these qualities. Also,
a physician caring for patients should urge them to express their priorities in their own words before making assumptions about what they
need. Ethics in the clinical practice of genetics requires cultivating the
emotions and traits of character appropriate to the mix of interpersonal
relationships in which geneticists and patients find themselves or which
they assume voluntarily.

AN EMPIRICAL STUDY OF MORAL REASONING

An ethics of care more accurately reflects geneticists' decision-
making in actual practice than does an ethical view derived from basic
ethical principles. Our own research on moral reasoning among medical
geneticists supports this statement. In 1985–86 we surveyed medical
geneticists with Ph.D.'s or M.D.'s, including clinicians, counselors, and
researchers, in 19 nations. We asked them about 14 clinical cases and
four screening situations that posed ethical problems.[5] A high response
rate (682 persons, or 62% of those asked to participate) to a questionnaire that took at least two hours to complete suggests a high level of
ethical concern among geneticists.

For each case vignette, respondents were asked to indicate, not only
what they would do (from a list of possible choices of action), but also to
state, in their own words, *why* they had chosen this approach. We did not
ask an even deeper question as to *why* they answered the *why* question
the way they did. If we had asked this, we may have discovered more.
Instead, following tradition, we constructed an initial grid of ethical principles: autonomy, beneficence, justice, and nonmaleficence. We placed

their answers to the principles within this grid. However, we noted that the write-in responses contained few direct references to traditional principles such as autonomy or respect for persons, though some used the term non-maleficence. To compensate for an obvious imposition of our own ethical ideas on to the material we received, and to analyze geneticists' moral reasoning, we then used inductive methods, based on close reading of actual responses, to develop a schema of 93 reasons for action. These reasons fit more closely with an ethical perspective of care than with an approach based on principles.

We include this schema of reasons in Appendix 1. Hopefully, it may be a useful tool for others who study moral reasoning. Most geneticists' responses to the clinical cases fell under the general headings of needs and responsibilities (48%) or rights and obligations (45%), with most of the rest falling under "non-moral answers". Other aspects of geneticists' moral reasoning, including perceptions of conflict and priorities in the welfare of different parties, have been described elsewhere.[6]

Below we focus on the six types of disclosure cases listed in the Introduction, as representative of the range of disclosure problems. For each case, we describe 1) the "rights" approach, derived from traditional ethical principles; 2) the "needs" approach, based on the ethic of care; 3) how our survey respondents would resolve the issue; and 4) what we consider the optimal approach.

APPROACHES TO SIX CASES

1. False Paternity
Our survey presented the following case:

> You are evaluating a child with an autosomal recessive disorder
> for which carrier testing is possible and accurate. In the process
> of testing relatives for genetic counseling, you discover that the
> mother and half the siblings are carriers, whereas the husband
> is not. The husband believes that he is the child's biological
> father.

Using the "rights" approach, one might well argue, on the basis of respect for persons, that the husband has a right to know the truth, because the doctor took his blood for testing and he is therefore as much a "patient" as his wife and child. Even a prestigious President's Commission[7] argued for disclosure, albeit within a "therapeutic privilege" of delayed disclosure, in cases where harm to the other family members might result from immediate disclosure.

An approach based on the insights of Gilligan and others would ask how to fulfill the needs of all persons in the scenario—husband, wife, affected child, other children, biological father, and future siblings, and how to maintain positive human relationships among these people. At least, for future reproductive planning, the husband has no need to know that he is not the father of this particular child. All he *needs* to know is that there is no risk of his fathering another child with this particular disorder. Given that the husband has no medical need to know, the doctor has no *clinical* responsibility to tell him. His needs to know or not know, however, exceed the merely genetic, and must be seen in terms of the overall, ongoing relationships between parents and children. In looking at the husband's needs, an ethics of care finds arguments both for and against disclosure. Arguments in favor of disclosure include possible long-term improvements in relationships between wife and husband (after family therapy) and between the social father and a child who shares none of his own genetic material. Arguments against disclosure include possible deterioration of relationships between husband and wife and husband and child.

In looking at the wife's needs, the doctor will see that she has a clear medical need to know so that she will not risk having another child with a genetic disorder by the first child's biological father. Also, with accurate information she can proceed to have children with her husband (without genetic anxiety), better relate to the existing child, and can decide what to tell her husband. She also needs to know so that she can tell the biological father (who needs to know that he is the carrier of a genetic disorder).

Although the wife needs to know, she and the children need protection, in many contemporary societies, from possible abandonment or physical or psychological abuse by the husband. Unless it is evident that disclosure to the husband would improve relationships or preserve the family, an ethics of care would argue that paternity should be the mother's secret.

In choosing to protect those most in need, this view recognizes the inequality of persons in an imperfect society. Some would consider this recognition a cornerstone of feminist philosophy. According to Sherwin, "By acknowledging the relevance of difference among people as a basis for a difference in sympathy and concern, feminism denies the legitimacy of a central premise of traditional moral theories, namely that all persons should be seen as morally equivalent by us."[8]

An ethical position premised on care recognizes the destructive potential involved in keeping secrets. Some psychoanalysts[9] argue that all secrets are potentially pathological and that therefore the doctor should work with the wife toward disclosure to the husband. Bok opposes this view, arguing that secrets are basic to human identity itself and that sometimes keeping a secret—even a guilty secret—is the course of least harm to all concerned.[10]

An ethics of care must look beyond the needs of the wife, however, and also consider the needs of society itself. On this basis it could be argued that the husband should be told in order to preserve the moral integrity of the health care system. If doctors become known for lying or concealing the truth, patients will not trust them. On the other hand, in existing societies, it is usually considered for the good of society to preserve families even if the flaw of non-paternity exists in a family. The actual rates of non-paternity in society are difficult to ascertain. If these rates are high, it would appear to be for the good of society not to disclose it, lest the divorce and non-support rates climb even higher. However, this judgment must be tentative, because of the lack of data about non-paternity.

The themes of deserts and justice are also important to this perspective (see Appendix 1). In some circumstances, the husband may *deserve* to know, for example if he was forced into marriage under false pretenses, the woman claiming that the child was his when she knew otherwise. (It is unlikely, of course, that a geneticist would have knowledge of the particulars in such a situation.)

A geneticist heeding a responsibility to care would therefore have to consider the needs of all parties concerned, the good of society, and the deserts of wronged parties. Needs, however, are the overriding concern, and the most crucial need is protection of the weaker parties. In this view, one should pay special attention to availability of support systems, such as affordable family therapy. In this sense, this perspective is "situational". Disclosure to all parties might best serve family needs in a society that provided adequate and free access to family therapy, and that also provided supports for women and children (such as well-paying jobs for women, and affordable day care). In contemporary society, however, family needs appear best served by leaving the secret with the woman, offering her referral to psychological help, and letting her decide what to do.

Survey respondents to this case see their responsibilities in terms of an ethics of care rather than in a perspective of rights. Although the husband has the legal right to know, very few geneticists (4%) around the world would tell him the truth. The rest would either tell the mother alone, without the husband present (81%), lie (13%), or tell the couple that there has been a new mutation (2%), a one-in-a-million occurrence.[11]

In giving reasons for their actions in this particular case, respondents shared more concern for avoiding harm to the wife and child than for the husband's legal or moral rights. Their answers were enmeshed in the realities of family life rather than in a hierarchy of abstract principles. Instead of considering whether the husband had a *right* to know, clinicians were primarily concerned about whether he *needed* to know. Most concluded that he had no medical need to know. On the other hand, 58% argued that the family unit needed to be preserved and 30% argued that the mother needed control over this secret.

In our view, the optimal approach in this case has several steps. First is a disclosure of non-paternity to the mother so that she can avoid genetic risks in future pregnancies. Physicians should meet with the woman first, in respect for her privacy, to advise her of the finding. Secondly, they should recommend special care to help her with her choice about disclosure and the process of any future genetic counseling. The choices about disclosure are the woman's and should be safeguarded. Thirdly, she should be urged to tell the biological father about his carrier status or to permit the physician to do so.

When the husband asks specifically about paternity, which would be a very rare occurrence, and the truth must be revealed, the geneticist should tell the mother first, and should tell the husband in a group context with her and a therapist present, after careful arrangements have been made for social supports (e.g., a refuge for battered women) if necessary.

2. Disclosure of Genetic Information to Spouses

Some cases of Down syndrome result from a rearranged chromosome carried by one of the parents. In our survey, we presented the following case:

> You identify a parent of a Down syndrome child as having a balanced translocation. What is your approach to disclosure of this information to the parents?

In a rights framework, both spouses have the right to know because their blood has been drawn. An ethics of rights would require disclosure of the carrier parent to both spouses equally.

An ethics of care recognizes that in this case there is a strong possibility of causing harm, whatever course is chosen. Both parties *need* to know which is the carrier, in order to be able to decide about alternative means of reproduction such as artificial insemination or a donated egg. On the other hand, the woman may also need special protection because in many contemporary societies, women are usually blamed—and also blame themselves—for whatever goes wrong with reproduction.[12] If no disclosure is made to either party, both spouses may blame the woman for causing the genetic defect. Disclosure to both spouses that the woman is the carrier could lead to shame, guilt, recriminations from the husband, her further loss of power in the marriage and perhaps even divorce. On the other hand, disclosure that the man is the carrier will cause him no loss of power and probably little guilt. Typically, men deny their own involvement in infertility and other reproductive problems, and their wives "cover up" for them.

Protection of the weak is central to an ethics of care. As Gilligan explains, "While an ethic of justice proceeds from the premise of equality—that everyone should be treated the same—an ethic of care rests on the premise of nonviolence—that no one should be hurt. In the representation of maturity, both perspectives converge in the realization that just as inequality adversely affects both parties in an unequal relationship, so too violence is destructive for everyone involved".[13]

In this approach, because of a woman's overriding need for protection, doctors might disclose to both spouses in cases where the man was the carrier (thus freeing the woman from guilt) and to the wife alone in cases where she was the carrier (thus enabling her to inform her relatives at risk of being carriers). She might also inform her husband if she wishes. Unequal disclosure may appear contrary to traditional conceptions of justice and may compromise the moral integrity of the physician in the presence of the husband. Nevertheless, in societies where women are given vastly unequal status and value with men, it may be necessary to redress this inequality by publicly disclosing the contributions of men to genetic disorders while downplaying, and if necessary in the face of danger, even concealing the contributions of women.

Survey respondents were divided about disclosure in this case, with 54% saying that they would provide the information to both parties, unasked, and 43% saying that they would tell the couple that the information exists and give them the choice of knowing or not knowing.[14] Many were aware of the potential for damage to family relationships, but the majority (62%) based their reasoning on patients' individual rights. A minority (35%) said the welfare of the extended family was their primary consideration. Few (2%) mentioned a need for protection of the woman in this case.

We believe that full disclosure to both parties—and to relatives in the extended family who may be carriers—is the preferable course of action, both on the basis of rights *and* needs. As the human genome is mapped, the level of knowledge about genetics in most societies will increase, supplanting the old beliefs that blame women for birth defects and reproductive failures. Until that day comes, however, because women have received unequal blame for reproductive problems throughout history, they may deserve special protection in some cases. Unequal disclosure is an interim ethic arising from inadequate education. In the interim, geneticists should work toward raising the family's level of education, with the goal of full disclosure.

3. Disclosure to Relatives at Higher Genetic Risk

The most difficult cases of disclosure involve telling relatives at genetic risk about a patient's diagnosis against the patient's wishes. Suppose that in a case of Huntington disease (HD) the "proband" (the person with the diagnosis) refuses to permit disclosure of the diagnosis to relatives at risk of developing the disorder and/or passing it on to children. HD is a progressive, always fatal, neurological disorder that strikes in middle age, leading to mental and motor deterioration. HD is not treatable, but can now be diagnosed presymptomatically or prenatally in some families, using recombinant DNA techniques. Behavioral changes, especially secretiveness, may be evident while the patient is still legally mentally competent. Therefore, some patients refuse to disclose their diagnosis to siblings or children, despite the geneticist's urging that they do so. The information is important, because the children of persons with HD (a Mendelian dominant) have a 50% chance of developing the disorder themselves. Most of the 25% of grandchildren who will eventually develop the disease will have been born before their parents have developed sufficient symptoms to be diagnosed.

In traditional ethical discussions, the doctor faces a difficult conflict between two time-honored medical duties or obligations: to protect patient confidentiality (or the doctor-patient relationship) and to warn third parties of harm. An ethics of care would consider the patient to be the *family* at genetic risk (rather than the individual). If the family asks, overriding the individual desire for privacy is in the interests of the wider family. However, how should one proceed when the family not only does not ask, but may not even suspect that they are at high risk for a fatal, untreatable disorder that strikes in middle age? Should the geneticist seek them out and tell them? What if they do not wish to know? There is no way for them to exercise the choice of not knowing, because in the very process of asking, "Do you want to know whether you are at risk for HD?" the geneticist has already made the essence of the information known. Whether to seek out and inform the unsuspecting is the stuff of tragic drama; lives may be destroyed in the act of telling. Nevertheless, in the interest of preventing harm to future generations and allowing this generation to plan their lives in the fullest knowledge of their own future, an ethic of caring would require doctors to break confidentiality and opt for disclosure.

Survey respondents were divided in their responses to this question: 32% would preserve the patient's confidentiality, 34% would tell the relatives if they asked, 24% would tell the relatives even if they did not ask, and 10% would refer the matter back to the family physician.[15]

We agree with the family-oriented recommendations of the President's Commission that patient confidentiality may be overridden, provided that four conditions are met: (1) reasonable efforts to elicit voluntary consent to disclosure have failed; (2) there is a high probability both that harm will occur if the information is withheld and that the disclosed information will actually be used to avert harm; (3) the harm that identifiable individuals would suffer would be serious; and (4) appropriate precautions are taken to ensure that only the genetic information needed for diagnosis and/or treatment of the disease in question is disclosed.[16] This moral logic is already being applied to permit disclosure to spouses and partners of HIV-infected patients.

The ethics of disclosure of genetic risks *begin* with intrafamilial duties to warn and protect family members from harm. These duties are not confined to the immediate family. Identified patients or parents of an affected child have an ethical duty to inform relatives in the extended family once they are informed themselves about the condition. A basic function of the family itself is protection from harm for its members. However, those at risk must first *learn* about their risks. Physicians, especially geneticists, are the primary mediators of genetic knowledge in society today. Geneticists are surely entitled to ask assertively, if not to require, that the identified patient or parents help in contacting relatives so that they may be informed about specific risks. Physicians should be prepared to *use* genetic knowledge in a context of cooperation with *families* in the practice of medicine, rather than relying on an overly individualistic standard of patient communication and education.

4. Ambiguous or Conflicting Test Results

A fourth frequent problem in genetics is disclosure of ambiguous test results. Sometimes prenatal diagnosis results are ambiguous (possibly indicating a severe disorder, but possibly a mere laboratory artifact), or are conflicting (one test says the fetus is normal, another indicates a defect).

Our survey described the following two cases:

Case A

Laboratory analysis of amniotic fluid cells suggests that the fetus may be a trisomy 13 mosaic. There is disagreement among the medical geneticists responsible for the analysis as to whether or not the laboratory results are artifacts of culture, in other words, false positives. Given the present state of knowledge, there is no way of resolving this disagreement scientifically within the legal time limit for termination of pregnancy, because the results of repeat tests will not be available until after 24 weeks gestational age. You were not responsible for the laboratory work in this case and have not taken one side or the other. You are, however, the medical geneticist responsible for dealing directly with the prospective mother.

Case B

Maternal serum alpha-fetoprotein has been elevated in your patient on two occasions, but level II ultrasound discloses no abnormality, despite careful examination of the fetal head, spine, abdomen, and kidneys. The fetal karyotype is normal. Amniotic alpha-fetoprotein is elevated and acetylcholinesterase is borderline. These results raise the possibility of a small neural tube defect. What do you tell the parents?

A rights-based approach would require full disclosure. An ethics of care, on the other hand, recognizes the possibilities of harm arising from disclosure. Most women expect to be told that their fetus either does or does not have a severe disorder, such as Down syndrome. They are not prepared for the ambiguities. Given that disclosure of uncertain results can lead to anguish, Rothman suggests that women make contracts with their doctors in advance as to exactly how much they want to know.[17] Some may want to know only about Down syndrome and not about sex chromosome abnormalities. Rothman argues that women have a "right not to know". One problem with this argument, as she acknowledges, is that in order to exercise her right not to know, a woman first *needs* to know, in detail, about all of the disorders that prenatal diagnosis may reveal, and also about the fact that results may be ambiguous or conflicting. Providing this information is such a formidable task that even Rothman doubts its practicality.

Our survey respondents overwhelmingly endorsed full disclosure of ambiguous (97%) or conflicting (98%) results, though fewer (66%) would also disclose colleague disagreement about the meaning of these results. We believe that full disclosure is required under both a rights-based ethic and an ethic of care. However unwelcome the information about uncertain results, the woman *needs* to know in order to make a decision about the fetus, and therefore it is the doctor's responsibility to tell her.

5. Disclosure of Fetal Sex

Moral and social arguments weigh heavily against performing prenatal diagnosis solely for sex selection, in the absence of X-linked disease.[18] Sex selection, whether for boy or girl, reinforces sexual stereotyping and may reinforce sexism. Sex selection may set a precedent for attempts to select other cosmetic characteristics, such as height, thinness, skin color, and straight teeth. Parents could argue that having a child with "undesirable" characteristics—shortness, obesity, nearsightedness, colorblindness, or just an average IQ would make them miserable, make the child miserable, and lower the quality of their family life, especially if they already had several such children. These are many of the same arguments now given in favor of sex selection. Within the next 20 years, or sooner as the human genome is mapped, some of the more exotic choices may be technically possible, especially those related to body size and height. At the extreme, such prenatal tinkering with desired characteristics could lead to a technology-driven positive eugenics. Sex selection is the beginning of a dangerous road.

Most survey respondents outside the United States (74%) would refuse to perform prenatal diagnosis for sex selection. In the United States, however, responses were divided. When presented with a couple with four daughters who desire a son, 38% would refuse to perform prenatal diagnosis for sex selection, 34% would perform it, and 28% would offer a referral. Most of those who refused said either that "sex is not a disease" or that they opposed the abortion of a healthy fetus. Those who would honor the couple's request would do so either out of respect for patient autonomy or because they believed that the uses patients make of medical information are none of the doctor's business. We argue elsewhere that geneticists should not reduce themselves to mere technicians who grant every request of each patient; there are some requests in the name of autonomy that lead to too much harm to a normal fetus and to important social values.[19] Further, the profession should assume a moral stance that prenatal diagnosis be used only for the detection of disease or malformation.

Direct requests for sex selection, however, are likely to be rare in Western nations. Instead, most moral problems will evolve from the knowledge about sex that is incidental to prenatal diagnosis performed for other purposes. The possibility of sex selection presents parents with a moral nightmare. Most would not seek to have prenatal diagnosis solely for sex selection, but their eligibility for the procedure on other grounds, usually age, presents a temptation. The temptation is especially acute for those with unexpected pregnancies, who do not want an additional child, but who have always secretly desired a child of a particular sex. Such parents may decide to wait until they have prenatal diagnosis, find out the fetus' sex, and then make their decision about abortion. Some parents may welcome the possibility of making such decisions, but for many it is an unwanted, agonizing choice. They are faced with a decision that may cause moral agony, not so much because they may make the "wrong" choice, but because the choice exists.

Why not simply withhold information about sex, rather than withholding prenatal diagnosis? This would seem a logical solution to the problem. Sex is not a disease, and it would probably be legal for doctors to withhold the information about gender as it is clinically irrelevant. This alternative has not yet been put to a legal test. Withholding information of any kind, however, is a very sensitive moral and policy issue. Patients in the United States have become used to asking for full disclosure, and ethicists have tried to educate professionals to convey the "whole truth" to competent patients. Withholding information puts control into the hands of doctors, not patients, and sets a precedent for a resurgence of medical paternalism.

Knowledge is power in the doctor-patient interaction. Many patients in Western societies consider it unfair if the doctor knows something that they do not know. The perceived imbalance of power is further aggravated if the patient is a woman and the doctor is a man. Therefore, in an ethics of care, doctors should also remain ignorant of any "incidental" information, such as sex, that is not to be routinely conveyed to patients. The information would remain in the laboratory and would be available if patients request it, but would not be routinely provided in the laboratory report to the patient's doctor. Therefore, the doctor would not know something that the patient did not know. Parents would thereby be spared the temptation to abort on the basis of sex. They would also avoid gender stereotyping their children before birth.[20]

6. Disclosure to Institutions

In the next ten years, the disclosure issue that will affect the greatest number of persons is in the context of insurance and employment. Will insurers and employers have access to genetic information about the person screened? Will these third parties be free to secure their own economic benefit, likely to be detrimental to the person screened? The survey respondents overwhelmingly believed that employers (81%) and insurers (89%) should have no access to such information without the patient's consent. This included 22% and 40%, respectively, who thought that employers and insurers should have no access at all, even with consent.[21] We believe that because this issue will be fought in the courts, a rights-based approach is appropriate. To respect the autonomy of the individual, to protect the patient from harm, and to maintain the confidentiality of the geneticist-patient relationship, genetic information derived from screening in the workplace or from presymptomatic testing (Huntington disease) should not be given to insurers and employers without the consent of the worker or the patient.

Institutions, however, have the power to coerce consent by withholding employment or insurance. Therefore it will be necessary to have laws that either a) protect patient privacy, or b) allow institutional access to information but protect patients' rights to employment and insurance free from discrimination on the basis of genotype.

Conclusions

Considering difficult issues of privacy and disclosure from the perspective discussed above, we come to three conclusions. The first is descriptive. An ethics of care is closer to the actual reasoning process of clinicians in genetics than is the traditional applied "principles" approach. An approach based on principles may complement a care-based approach to ethical problems, especially when reasoning about the largest social situation or institutional issues. In clinical cases, "principlism" seems to leave reasoning suspended in mid-air and does not focus on the needs of parties to the ethical problem.

Second, an ethics of care recommends full disclosure but recognizes the need to protect weaker members of society. Distortions of the ethical imperative of full disclosure, where they occur, may be necessary on account of gender or class inequalities in contemporary society. Wherever we have not recommended disclosure, the recommendation has been based on women's and children's need for protection in a male-dominated society that gives unequal value to women and men. Non-disclosure has drawbacks. Keeping secrets can lead to psychological burdens for both doctor and patient. Non-disclosure can also lead to professional paternalism which puts the patient into a position of inequality with the doctor.

Third, to care means to identify with patients as persons who are members of families and communities rather than as atomistic individuals. Genetic knowledge will gradually transform the practice of medicine. People will come to physicians, not with complaints of illness, but with requests for insight into their destinies. As more is known about the human genome, respect for persons in medicine will translate into respect for families and future generations. An ethics of care is never "case-bound", but looks to the wider network of relationships, which are always growing into the future, in order to provide compassionate guidance.

APPENDIX 1: SCHEMA OF MORAL REASONING

The 93 moral reasons given by geneticists fall under five headings:

I. Rights and Obligations—Reciprocals
II. Needs and Responsibilities—Reciprocals
III. Deserts and Justice—Reciprocals
IV. Good of the Health Care System and Other Institutions
V. Good of Society

Explanation of Headings

I. Rights and Obligations

These terms derive from legal concepts and are reciprocals. If the patient has a right, the doctor has an obligation to respect that right, and vice versa. There are two kinds of rights, both recognized by law: 1) *Rights of noninterference* or freedom from interference (negative rights); and 2) *Rights of entitlement* or access to services even if scarce or expensive (positive rights). Rights of entitlement apply to *all* persons, regardless of deserts or need. Obligations are acts that are the reciprocals of rights (including both negative and positive rights). Obligations differ from Responsibilities in that they are performances of acts. Responsibilities focus on the promotion of some aspects of the other person's well-being.

II. Needs and Responsibilities

These are reciprocals. Patients need psychological support, comfort, protection from physical or moral harm. Doctors have a responsibility to provide for these needs. One of the major patient needs is *avoidance of harm*. Fetuses have needs, but not rights (only *persons* recognized as such by law have rights).

III. Deserts and Justice

Deserts go beyond rights of entitlement of needs. They are what a particular person or special group deserves because of prior suffering or injustice, or because of prior good works or other special qualities. Hiring policies that attempt to redress previous wrongs by giving special preference to groups that have suffered injustice are based on the concept of deserts. Very few reasons given in this survey fall under the concept of deserts. Deserts are something *extra* to be given to people in special circumstances, and are not to be confused with needs.

Justice is the reciprocal of deserts, and includes the concept of fairness and the demand on the doctor to provide what patients deserve.

93 Reasons Given in International Survey

I. Rights of Noninterference (Negative Rights)

A. The ethical conviction that individuals should be treated as autonomous agents, e.g., right to self-determination, choice, autonomy, own decision, right to refuse, right to abortion.
patients;
parents;
spouse;
relatives at risk;
geneticist or physician (right to refuse to perform a procedure or to withhold information).

B. Right to privacy or confidentiality
patients;
parents;
child;
relatives at risk.

C. Other
They have a right to whatever service they can pay for out of pocket.

II. Rights of Entitlement (Positive Rights)

A. Access
equal access;
entitlement to full insurance coverage;
right to medical care that is affordable.

B. Right to know (entitled or deserve to know; reasonable request; includes right *not* to know)
patient;
spouse;
parents;
relatives at risk;
geneticist;
professional colleagues or third parties.

III. Obligations

A. Doctor's obligations
duty to warn third parties;
duty to warn about new or experimental procedures or interpretations;

truth-telling (rule-oriented; use for Kantian arguments);
honesty, obligation to tell the truth;
refusal to lie;
all available services should be provided on request;
gaining acceptance (historical evolution);
law, regulations, supervisor, institution forbids;
counselor should be non-directive, support whatever decision clients make;
patient requests should be respected, whether they're right
or wrong.

B. Patients' obligations
"duty to know", whether they want to or not, and to use
information.

IV. *Needs*

A. Needs for information
Optimal choices or decisions are *based upon use* of medical/
genetic information by patient, relatives, geneticist, or referring physician;
they may change their mind about abortion after receiving
test results.

B. Need to avoid harm
preserve family unity;
truth-telling to avoid harm;
truth-telling as a source of harm;
no benefit gained from truth-telling (no need to know);
benefits outweigh possible harm;
parents' request serves no useful purpose.

C. Psychosocial needs
special mention of position of women in society or family;
removal of guilt or anxiety now;
help with present problem;
family planning;
making informed reproductive choices;
mother's anxiety is predictive of fetal health (she needs the
service).

D. Needs of child/fetus
child will be in normal range, despite genetic diagnosis;
interests of the fetus ought to be treated equally with those of
living persons.

E. Allocation of resources according to patient's needs
use resources wisely, don't waste resources;
appropriate or inappropriate use of technology;
medical indication or no medical indication.

V. *Responsibilities*

A. Ethical conviction that there is a responsibility to protect the autonomy of the person even though it may be diminished (e.g., person is vulnerable, incapacitated, has knowledge that is incommensurate with the geneticist's knowledge, or geneticist has knowledge of patient's secrets or diagnosis)
patient;
child;
relatives at risk;
explicitly acknowledges that autonomy is diminished.

B. Doctor-patient relationship
doctor-patient relationship (trust, confidentiality);
responsibility to give advice, direction, guidance, education.

C. Avoidance of harm
Do no harm (include harm to third parties or relatives);
Prevent or minimize physical or moral harm or risk of harm
(moral harm = deceit)
to patient (includes burden of disease on parents);
to fetus or child;
to future children, including prevention of birth defects (includes helping patient have a normal child).
Prevent harm to fetus
oppose abortion;
oppose abortion of normal fetus.
Potential misuse of information by third parties
avoid social stigmatization, discrimination in the workplace;
harm through regulations or government intervention.
Don't set a precedent that will harm the moral order ("slippery slope" argument).

D. Caring for the welfare of others
the physician's responsibility to provide health care for family, society;
the Golden Rule;
means of truth-telling so as to maximize good (means of telling truth, support, counseling, referrals);

prepare patient for the future, including help cope with stresses of disease or abortion.

VI. *Deserts*

Fairness or unfairness; they deserve or don't deserve the service.

VII. *Good of Society*

A. Improvement of life
   future generations;
   health care;
   social planning;
   insurance coverage;
   workers' health (includes responsibility of factory to worker);
   working conditions;
   social unity;
   protection of persons through regulation or licensing of labs and providers (insure proper level of service, quality control) to prevent misuse.

B. Common good, public health

C. Other
   population limitation;
   maintain balanced sex ratio;
   eugenic arguments;
   harm to society if sex ratio upset.

VIII. *Good of the Health Care System*

efficiency or utility;
cost-benefit analysis;
protection of economic interests of third parties.

IX. *Compromise*

Compromise (stated as such by respondent—includes referral to another center, disclosure to another physician rather than patients).

X. *Non-moral Answers (no ethical principles involved)*

fear of lawsuit;
logistically or technically difficult, accurate or inaccurate, correct or incorrect;

not accepted, controversial;
I do not accept or approve of this;
this is not a geneticist's problem; should be dealt with by another professional;
the Bible (or equivalent in my religion) tells me so;
ethics should not be based on regulations or on legislation;
other non-moral reason;
medicine (or genetics) should not be a business;
not applicable in my country;
I approve of this.

School of Public Health
Boston University

Biomedical Ethics and Religious Studies
University of Virginia

NOTES

1. Office of Technology Assessment, *Mapping Our Genes*, Washington, DC: Superintendent of Documents, U.S. Government Printing Office, 1988, OTA-BA-373.

2. Tom L. Beauchamp and James F. Childress, *Principles of Biomedical Ethics*, 3rd edn. New York: Oxford University Press, 1983.

3. Carol Gilligan, *In a Different Voice: Psychological Theory and Women's Development.* Cambridge, MA: Harvard University Press, 1982; Christine Overall, *Ethics and Human Reproduction: A Feminist Analysis.* Boston: Allen and Unwin, 1987; Margaret S. Farley, "Feminist Theology and Bioethics," in *Theology and Bioethics*, ed. by E. E. Shelp, Dordrecht: D. Reidel, 1985; Virginia Held, "Feminism and Moral Theory", ed. by Eva Feder Kittay and Diana T. Meyers, Totowa, NJ: Rowman and Littlefield, 1987; Sara Ruddick, "Maternal Thinking", in *Women and Values: Readings in Recent Feminist Philosophy*, ed. by Marilyn Pearsall, Belmont, CA: Wadsworth, 1986; Marilyn Friedman, "Care and Context in Moral Reasoning", in *Women and Moral Theory*, ed. by Eva Feder Kittay and Diana T. Meyers, Totowa, NJ: Rowman and Littlefield, 1987; John Ladd, "The Distinction Between Rights and Responsibility: A Defense", *Linacre Quarterly* 49, 1982; 121–142; Susan Sherwin, "A Feminist Approach to Ethics", *Dalhousie Review* 64, 1987: 704–713.

4. Sandra Harding, "The Curious Coincidence of Feminine and African Moralities: Challenges for Feminist Theory", in *Women and Moral Theory*, ed. by Eva Feder Kittay and Diana T. Meyers, Totowa, NJ: Rowman and Littlefield, 1987.

5. Dorothy C. Wertz and John C. Fletcher, *Ethics and Human Genetics: A Cross-Cultural Perspective.* Heidelberg: Springer-Verlag, 1989, pp. 1–79; Dorothy C. Wertz and John C. Fletcher, "Medical Geneticists Confront Ethical Dilemmas: Cross-Cultural Comparisons in 18 Nations". *American Journal of Human Genetics* 46, June, 1990, pp. 1200–1213; Dorothy C. Wertz and John C. Fletcher, "Ethics and Genetics: An International Survey", *Hastings Center Report* 19, Special Supplement, July/August, 1989, pp. 20–24; Dorothy C. Wertz and John C. Fletcher, "Ethical Problems in Prenatal Diagnosis: A Cross-Cultural Survey of Medical Geneticists in 18 Nations", *Prenatal Diagnosis* 9, March, 1989, pp. 145–157; Dorothy C. Wertz and John C. Fletcher, "Attitudes of Genetic Counselors: A Multi-National Survey",

American Journal of Human Genetics 42, April, 1988, pp. 592–600; Dorothy C. Wertz and John C. Fletcher, "An International Survey of Attitudes of Medical Geneticists Toward Mass Screening and Access to Results", *Public Health Reports*, 4 Jan/Feb 1989, pp. 35–44; Dorothy C. Wertz and John C. Fletcher, "Ethics and Medical Genetics in the United States: A National Survey", *American Journal of Medical Genetics* 29, April, 1988, pp. 815–827.

6. Dorothy C. Wertz and John C. Fletcher, "Moral Reasoning Among Medical Geneticists in 18 Nations", *Theoretical Medicine* 10, 1989, pp. 123–138.

7. President's Commission for the Study of Ethical Problems in Medicine and Biomedical and Behavorial Research, *Screening and Counseling for Genetic Conditions*. Washington, DC: U.S. Government Printing Office, 1983, p. 58.

8. Sherwin, "A Feminist Approach to Ethics", p. 709.

9. Theodor Reik, *The Compulsion to Confess*. New York: Farrar, Strauss and Cudahy, 1959; Carl Fullerton Sulzberger, "Why It is Hard to Keep Secrets", *Psychoanalysis* 2, Fall 1953: 37–43; Russell Meares, "The Secret", *Psychiatry* 39, 1976: 258–265.

10. Sissela Bok, *Secrets: On the Ethics of Concealment and Revelation*. New York: Random House, 1984, pp. 25, 81–88, 118–130.

11. Wertz and Fletcher, *Ethics and Human Genetics: A Cross-Cultural Perspective*, pp. 15–16.

12. Judith N. Lasker and Susan Borg, *In Search of Parenthood: Coping with Infertility and High-Tech Conception*, Boston: Beacon Press, 1987, pp. 11–38.

13. Gilligan, *In a Different Voice*, p. 174.

14. Wertz and Fletcher, *Ethics and Human Genetics*, pp. 17–18.

15. Ibid.

16. President's Commission, p. 44.

17. Barbara Katz Rothman, *The Tentative Pregnancy: Prenatal Diagnosis and the Future of Motherhood*. New York: Viking, 1986, pp. 155–176, 245–258.

18. Dorothy C. Wertz and John C. Fletcher, "Fatal Knowledge? Prenatal Diagnosis and Sex Selection", *Hastings Center Report* 19, May/June, 1989, pp. 21–27. See also Overall, *Ethics and Human Reproduction*, pp. 17–39; Helen Bequaert Holmes, "Review of *Gendercide*, by Mary Anne Warren", *Bioethics* Jan. 1987, pp. 100–110; Mary Anne Warren, "A Reply to Holmes on *Gendercide*," *Bioethics*, April, 1987, pp. 189–198.

19. Wertz and Fletcher, "Fatal Knowledge . . .," p. 26.

20. Such a policy of not revealing fetal sex was recently instituted in prenatal diagnostic laboratories in the Birmingham region of England, not because parents were requesting sex selection, but because some parents complained that they wished they had not known the fetus's sex. In 1987–1988, when the information was no longer made available as a matter of course, of 3,883 amniotic fluid analyses there were only 95 (2.4%) parental requests to know fetal sex. (Maj. Hulten, East Birmingham Hospital, Birmingham, U.K., personal communication).

21. Wertz and Fletcher, *Ethics and Human Genetics*, pp. 38–40; Wertz and Fletcher, *Public Health Reports*.

PART FOUR

PUBLIC POLICY ISSUES

Susan Wendell
John La Puma, M.D.
Edward F. Lawlor, Ph.D.
David C. Hadorn
James F. Childress, Ph.D.
Robert M. Veatch, Ph.D.
Leon R. Kass, M.D.
Alexander Morgan Capron
Ronald Bayer, Ph.D.
Nancy S. Jecker, Ph.D.
Robert Pearlman, M.D.

22 Toward a Feminist Theory of Disability

SUSAN WENDELL

Susan Wendell is Associate Professor of Philosophy and Women's Studies at Simon Fraser University in Burnaby, British Columbia.

In 1985, I fell ill overnight with what turned out to be a disabling chronic disease. In the long struggle to come to terms with it, I had to learn to live with a body that felt entirely different to me—weak, tired, painful, nauseated, dizzy, unpredictable. I learned at first by listening to other people with chronic illnesses or disabilities; suddenly able-bodied people seemed to me profoundly ignorant of everything I most needed to know. Although doctors told me there was a good chance I would eventually recover completely, I realized after a year that waiting to get well, hoping to recover my healthy body, was a dangerous strategy. I began slowly to identify with my new, disabled body and to learn to work with it. As I moved back into the world, I also began to experience the world as structured for people who have no weaknesses.[1] The process of encountering the able-bodied world led me gradually to identify myself as a disabled person, and to reflect on the nature of disability.

Some time ago, I decided to delve into what I assumed would be a substantial philosophical literature in medical ethics on the nature and experience of disability. I consulted *The Philosopher's Index*, looking under "Disability," "Handicap," "Illness," and "Disease." This was a depressing experience. At least 90% of philosophical articles on these topics are concerned with two questions: Under what conditions is it morally permissible/right to kill/let die a disabled person and how potentially disabled does a fetus have to be before it is permissible/right to prevent its being born? Thus, what I have to say here about disability is not a response to philosophical literature on the subject. Instead, it reflects what I have learned from the writings of other disabled people

This article appeared in Helen Bequaert Holmes and Laura Purdy (eds.), Feminist Perspectives in Medical Ethics *(Bloomington: Indiana University Press, 1992): 63–81, and* Hypatia 2 (Summer 1989): 104–124.

(especially disabled women), from talking with disabled people who have shared their insights and experiences with me, and from my own experience of disability. It also reflects my commitment to feminist theory, which offers perspectives and categories of analysis that help to illuminate the personal and social realities of disability, and which would, in turn, be enriched by a greater understanding of disability.

We need a theory of disability. It should be a social and political theory, because disability is largely socially-constructed, but it has to be more than that; any deep understanding of disability must include thinking about the ethical, psychological and epistemic issues of living with disability. This theory should be feminist, because more than half of disabled people are women and approximately 16% of women are disabled (Fine and Asch 1988), and because feminist thinkers have raised the most radical issues about cultural attitudes to the body. Some of the same attitudes about the body which contribute to women's oppression generally also contribute to the social and psychological disablement of people who have physical disabilities. In addition, feminists are grappling with issues that disabled people also face in a different context: Whether to stress sameness or difference in relation to the dominant group and in relation to each other; whether to place great value on independence from the help of other people, as the dominant culture does, or to question a value-system which distrusts and de-values dependence on other people and vulnerability in general; whether to take full integration into male dominated/able-bodied society as the goal, seeking equal power with men/able-bodied people in that society, or whether to preserve some degree of separate culture, in which the abilities, knowledge and values of women/the disabled are specifically honoured and developed.[2]

Disabled women struggle with both the oppressions of being women in male-dominated societies and the oppressions of being disabled in societies dominated by the able-bodied. They are bringing the knowledge and concerns of women with disabilities into feminism and feminist perspectives into the disability rights movement. To build a feminist theory of disability that takes adequate account of our differences, we will need to know how experiences of disability and the social oppression of the disabled interact with sexism, racism and class oppression. Michelle Fine and Adrienne Asch and the contributors to their 1988 volume, *Women and Disabilities*, have made a major contribution to our understanding of the complex interactions of gender and disability. Barbara Hillyer Davis has written in depth about the issue of dependency/independence as it relates to disability and feminism (Davis 1984). Other important contributions to theory are scattered throughout the extensive, primarily experiential, writing by disabled women;[3] this work offers vital insights into the nature of embodiment and the experience of oppression.

Unfortunately, feminist perspectives on disability are not yet widely discussed in feminist theory, nor have the insights offered by women writing about disability been integrated into feminist theorizing about the body. My purpose in writing this essay is to persuade feminist theorists, especially feminist philosophers, to turn more attention to constructing a theory of disability and to integrating the experiences and knowledge of disabled people into feminist theory as a whole. Toward this end I will discuss physical disability[4] from a theoretical perspective, including: some problems of defining it (here I will criticize the most widely-used definitions—those of the United Nations); the social construction of disability from biological reality on analogy with the social construction of gender; cultural attitudes toward the body which oppress disabled people while also alienating the able-bodied from their own experiences of embodiment; the "otherness" of disabled people; the knowledge that disabled people could contribute to culture from our diverse experiences and some of the ways this knowledge is silenced and invalidated. Along the way, I will describe briefly three issues discussed in disability theory that have been taken up in different contexts by feminist theory: sameness vs. difference, independence vs. dependency, and integration vs. separatism.

I do not presume to speak for disabled women. Like everyone who is disabled, I have a particular standpoint determined in part by both my physical condition and my social situation. My own disability may be temporary; it could get better or worse. My disability is usually invisible (except when I use a walking stick). I am a white university professor who has adequate medical and long-term disability insurance; that makes me very privileged among the disabled. I write what I can see from my standpoint. Because I do not want simply to describe my own experience but to understand it in a much larger context, I must venture beyond what I know first-hand. I rely on others to correct my mistakes and fill in those parts of the picture I cannot see.

Who Is Physically Disabled?

The United Nations offers the following definitions of and distinctions among impairment, disability and handicap:

> *Impairment:* Any loss or abnormality of psychological, physiological, or anatomical structure or function. *Disability:* Any restriction or lack (resulting from an impairment) of ability to perform an activity in the manner or within the range considered normal for a human being. *Handicap:* A disadvantage for

a given individual, resulting from an impairment or disability, that limits or prevents the fulfillment of a role that is normal, depending on age, sex, social and cultural factors, for that individual.

Handicap is therefore a function of the relationship between disabled persons and their environment. It occurs when they encounter cultural, physical or social barriers which prevent their access to the various systems of society that are available to other citizens. Thus, handicap is the loss or limitation of opportunities to take part in the life of the community on an equal level with others (U.N. 1983:I.c. 6–7)

These definitions may be good enough for the political purposes of the U.N. They have two advantages: First, they clearly include many conditions that are not always recognized by the general public as disabling, for example, debilitating chronic illnesses that limit people's activities but do not necessarily cause any visible disability, such as Crohn's disease. Second, the definition of "handicap" explicitly recognizes the possibility that the primary cause of a disabled person's inability to do certain things may be social—denial of opportunities, lack of accessibility, lack of services, poverty, discrimination—which it often is.

However, by trying to define "impairment" and "disability" in physical terms and "handicap" in cultural, physical and social terms, the U.N. document appears to be making a shaky distinction between the physical and the social aspects of disability. Not only the "normal" roles for one's age, sex, society, and culture, but also "normal" structure and function, and "normal" ability to perform an activity, depend on the society in which the standards of normality are generated. Paradigms of health and ideas about appropriate kinds and levels of performance are culturally dependent. In addition, within each society there is much variation from the norm of any ability; at what point does this variation become disability? The answer depends on such factors as what activities a society values and how it distributes labour and resources. The idea that there is some universal, perhaps biologically or medically describable paradigm of human physical ability is an illusion. Therefore, I prefer to use a single term, "disability," and to emphasize that disability is socially constructed from biological reality.

Another objection I have to the U.N. definitions is that they imply that women can be disabled, but not handicapped, by being unable to do things which are not considered part of the normal role for their sex. For example, if a society does not consider it essential to a woman's normal role that she be able to read, then a blind woman who is not provided with education in Braille is not handicapped, according to these definitions.

In addition, these definitions suggest that we can be disabled, but not handicapped, by the normal process of aging, since although we may lose some ability, we are not handicapped unless we cannot fulfill roles that are normal *for our age.* Yet a society which provides few resources to allow disabled people to participate in it will be likely to marginalize *all* the disabled, including the old, and to define the appropriate roles of old people as very limited, thus handicapping them. Aging is disabling. Recognizing this helps us to see that disabled people are not "other," that they are really "us." Unless we die suddenly, we are all disabled eventually. Most of us will live part of our lives with bodies that hurt, that move with difficulty or not at all, that deprive us of activities we once took for granted or that others take for granted, bodies that make daily life a physical struggle. We need an understanding of disability that does not support a paradigm of humanity as young and healthy. Encouraging everyone to acknowledge, accommodate and identify with a wide range of physical conditions is the road to self-acceptance as well as the road to liberating those who are disabled now.

Ultimately, we might eliminate the category of "the disabled" altogether, and simply talk about individuals' physical abilities in their social context. For the present, although "the disabled" is a category of "the other" to the able-bodied, for that very reason it is also a politically useful and socially meaningful category to those who are in it. Disabled people share forms of social oppression, and the most important measures to relieve that oppression have been initiated by disabled people themselves. Social oppression may be the only thing the disabled have in common;[5] our struggles with our bodies are extremely diverse.

Finally, in thinking about disability we have to keep in mind that a society's labels do not always fit the people to whom they are applied. Thus, some people are perceived as disabled who do not experience themselves as disabled. Although they have physical conditions that disable other people, because of their opportunities and the context of their lives, they do not feel significantly limited in their activities (see Sacks 1988); these people may be surprised or resentful that they are considered disabled. On the other hand, many people whose bodies cause them great physical, psychological and economic struggles are not considered disabled because the public and/or the medical profession do not recognize their disabling conditions. These people often long to be perceived as disabled, because society stubbornly continues to expect them to perform as healthy people when they cannot and refuses to acknowledge and support their struggles.[6] Of course, no one wants the social stigma associated with disability, but social recognition of disability determines the practical help a person receives from doctors, government agencies, insurance companies, charity organizations, and often from family and friends. Thus, how a society defines disability and whom it recognizes as disabled are of enormous psychological, economic and social importance, both to people who are experiencing themselves as disabled and to those who are not but are nevertheless given the label.

There is no definitive answer to the question: Who is physically disabled? Disability has social, experiential and biological components, present and recognized in different measures for different people. Whether a particular physical condition is disabling changes with time and place, depending on such factors as social expectations, the state of technology and its availability to people in that condition, the educational system, architecture, attitudes towards physical appearance, and the pace of life. (If, for example, the pace of life increases without changes in other factors, more people become disabled simply because fewer people can keep up the "normal" pace.)

The Social Construction of Disability

If we ask the questions: Why are so many disabled people unemployed or underemployed, impoverished, lonely, isolated; why do so many find it difficult or impossible to get an education (Davis and Marshall 1987; Fine and Asch 1988, 10–11); why are they victims of violence and coercion; why do able-bodied people ridicule, avoid, pity, stereotype and patronize them?, we may be tempted to see the disabled as victims of nature or accident. Feminists should be, and many are, profoundly suspicious of this answer. We are used to countering claims that insofar as women are oppressed they are oppressed by nature, which puts them at a disadvantage in the competition for power and resources. We know that if being biologically female is a disadvantage, it is because a social context makes it a disadvantage. From the standpoint of a disabled person, one can see how society could minimize the disadvantages of most disabilities, and, in some instances, turn them into advantages.

Consider an extreme case: the situation of physicist Stephen Hawking, who has had Amyotrophic Lateral Sclerosis (Lou Gehrig's disease) for more than twenty-seven years. Professor Hawking can no longer speak and is capable of only the smallest muscle movements. Yet, in his context of social and technological support, he is able to function as a professor of physics at Cambridge University; indeed he says his disability has given him the *advantage* of having more time to think, and he is one of the foremost theoretical physicists of our time. He is a courageous and talented man, but he is able to live the creative life he has only because of the help of his family, three nurses, a graduate student who travels with him to maintain his computer-communications systems, and the fact that his talent had been developed and recognized before he fell seriously ill (*Newsweek* 1988).

Many people consider providing resources for disabled people a form of charity, supererogatory in part because the disabled are perceived as unproductive members of society. Yet most disabled people are placed in a double-bind: they have access to inadequate resources because they are unemployed or underemployed, and they are unemployed or underemployed because they lack the resources that would enable them to make their full contribution to society (Matthews 1983; Hannaford 1985). Often governments and charity organizations will spend far more money to keep disabled people in institutions where they have no chance to be productive than they will spend to enable the same people to live independently and productively. In addition, many of the "special" resources the disabled need merely compensate for bad social planning that is based on the illusion that everyone is young, strong, healthy (and, often, male).

Disability is also frequently regarded as a personal or family problem rather than a matter for social responsibility. Disabled people are often expected to overcome obstacles to participation by their own extraordinary efforts, or their families are expected to provide what they need (sometimes at great personal sacrifice). Helping in personal or family matters is seen as supererogatory for people who are not members of the family.

Many factors contribute to determining whether providing a particular resource is regarded as a social or a personal (or family) responsibility.[7] One such factor is whether the majority can identify with people who need the resource. Most North Americans feel that society should be organized to provide short-term medical care made necessary by illness or accident, I think because they can imagine themselves needing it. Relatively few people can identify with those who cannot be "repaired" by medical intervention. Sue Halpern makes the following observation:

> Physical health is contingent and often short-lived. But this truth eludes us as long as we are able to walk by simply putting one foot in front of the other. As a consequence, empathy for the disabled is unavailable to most able-bodied persons. Sympathy, yes, empathy, no, for every attempt to project oneself into that condition, to feel what it is like not to be ambulatory, for instance, is mediated by an ability to walk (Halpern 1988, 3).

If the able-bodied saw the disabled as potentially themselves or as their future selves, they would be more inclined to feel that society should be organized to provide the resources that would make disabled people fully integrated and contributing members. They would feel that "charity" is as inappropriate a way of thinking about resources for disabled people as it is about emergency medical care or education.

Careful study of the lives of disabled people will reveal how artificial the line is that we draw between the biological and the social. Feminists have already challenged this line in part by showing how processes such as childbirth, menstruation and menopause, which may be represented, treated, and therefore experienced as illnesses or disabilities, are socially constructed from biological reality (Rich 1976; Ehrenreich and English 1979). Disabled people's relations to our bodies involve elements of struggle which perhaps cannot be eliminated, perhaps not even mitigated, by social arrangements. *But,* much of what is *disabling* about our physical conditions is also a consequence of social arrangements (Finger 1983; Browne, Connors, and Stern 1985; Fine and Asch 1988) which could, but do not, either compensate for our physical conditions, or accommodate them so that we can participate fully, or support our struggles and integrate us into the community *and our struggles into the cultural concept of life as it is ordinarily lived.*

Feminists have shown that the world has been designed for men. In North America at least, life and work have been structured as though no one of any importance in the public world, and certainly no one who works outside the home for wages, has to breast-feed a baby or look after a sick child. Common colds can be acknowledged publicly, and allowances made for them, but menstruation cannot. Much of the world is also structured as though everyone is physically strong, as though all bodies are "ideally shaped," as though everyone can walk, hear and see well, as though everyone can work and play at a pace that is not compatible with any kind of illness or pain, as though no one is ever dizzy or incontinent or simply needs to sit or lie down. (For instance, where could you sit down in a supermarket if you needed to?) Not only the architecture, but the entire physical and social organization of life, assumes that we are either strong and healthy and able to do what the average able-bodied person can do, or that we are completely disabled, unable to participate in life.

In the split between the public and the private worlds, women (and children) have been relegated to the private, and so have the disabled, the sick and the old (and mostly women take care of them). The public world is the world of strength, the positive (valued) body, performance and production, the able-bodied and youth. Weakness, illness, rest and recovery, pain, death and the negative (de-valued) body are private, generally hidden, and often neglected. Coming into the public world with illness, pain or a de-valued body, we encounter resistance to mixing the two worlds; the split is vividly revealed. Much of our experience goes underground, because there is no socially acceptable way of expressing it and having our physical and psychological experience acknowledged and shared. A few close friends may share it, but there is a strong impulse to protect them from it too, because it seems so private, so unacceptable. I found that, after a couple of years of illness, even answering the question, "How are you?" became a difficult, conflict-ridden business. I don't want to alienate my friends from my experience, but I don't want to risk their discomfort and rejection by telling them what they don't want to know.[8]

Disabled people learn that many, perhaps most, able-bodied people do not want to know about suffering caused by the body. Visibly disabled women report that curiosity about medical diagnoses, physical appearance and the sexual and other intimate aspects of disability is more common than willingness to listen and trying to understand the experience of disability (Matthews 1983). It is not unusual for people with invisible disabilities to keep them entirely secret from everyone but their closest friends.

Contrary to what Sue Halpern says, it is not simply because they are in able bodies that the able-bodied fail to identify with the disabled. Able-bodied people can often make the imaginative leap into the skins of people physically unlike themselves; women can identify with a male protagonist in a story, for example, and adults can identify with children or with people much older than themselves. Something more powerful than being in a different body is at work. Suffering caused by the body, and the inability to control the body, are despised, pitied, and above all, feared. This fear, experienced individually, is also deeply embedded in our culture.

THE OPPRESSION OF DISABLED PEOPLE IS THE OPPRESSION OF EVERYONE'S REAL BODY.

Our real human bodies are exceedingly diverse—in size, shape, colour, texture, structure, function, range and habits of movement, and development—and they are constantly changing. Yet we do not absorb or reflect this simple fact in our culture. Instead, we idealize the human body. Our physical ideals change from time to time, but we always have ideals. These ideals are not just about appearance; they are also ideals of strength and energy and proper control of the body. We are perpetually bombarded with images of these ideals, demands for them, and offers of consumer products and services to help us achieve them.[9] Idealizing the body prevents everyone, able-bodied and disabled, from identifying with and loving her/his real body. Some people can have the illusion of acceptance that comes from believing that their bodies are "close enough" to the ideal, but this illusion only draws them deeper into identifying with the ideal and into the endless task of reconciling the reality with it. Sooner or later they must fail.

Before I became disabled, I was one of those people who felt "close enough" to cultural ideals to be reasonably accepting of my body. Like most feminists I know, I was aware of some alienation from it, and I worked at liking my body better. Nevertheless, I knew in my heart that too much of my liking still depended on being "close enough." When I was disabled by illness, I experienced a much more profound alienation from my body. After a year spent mostly in bed, I could barely identify my body as my own. I felt that "it" was torturing "me," trapping me in exhaustion, pain and inability to do many of the simplest things I did when I was healthy. The shock of this experience and the effort to identify with a new, disabled body made me realize I had been living a luxury of the able-bodied. The able-bodied can postpone the task of identifying with their *real* bodies. The disabled don't have the luxury of demanding that their bodies fit the physical ideals of their culture. As Barbara Hillyer Davis says: "For all of us the difficult work of finding (one's) self includes the body, but people who live with disability in a society that glorifies fitness and physical conformity are forced to understand more fully what bodily integrity means" (Davis 1984, 3).

In a society which idealizes the body, the physically disabled are marginalized. People learn to identify with their own strengths (by cultural standards) and to hate, fear and neglect their own weaknesses. The disabled are not only de-valued for their de-valued bodies (Hannaford 1985), they are constant reminders to the able-bodied of the negative body—of what the able-bodied are trying to avoid, forget and ignore (Lessing 1981). For example, if someone tells me she is in pain, she reminds me of the existence of pain, the imperfection and fragility of the body, the possibility of my own pain, the *inevitability* of it. The less willing I am to accept all these, the less I want to know about her pain; if I cannot avoid it in her presence, I will avoid her. I may even blame her for it. I may tell myself that she *could have* avoided it, in order to go on believing that I *can* avoid it. I want to believe I am not like her; I cling to the differences. Gradually, I make her "other" because I don't want to confront my real body, which I fear and cannot accept.[10]

Disabled people can participate in marginalizing ourselves. We can wish for bodies we do not have, with frustration, shame, self-hatred. We can feel trapped in the negative body; it is our internalized oppression to feel this. Every (visibly or invisibly) disabled person I have talked to or read has felt this; some never stop feeling it. In addition, disabled women suffer more than disabled men from the demand that people have "ideal" bodies, because in patriarchal culture people judge women more by their bodies than they do men. Disabled women often do not feel seen (because they are often not seen) by others as whole people, especially not as sexual people (Campling 1981; Matthews 1983; Hannaford 1985; Fine and Asch 1988). Thus, part of their struggle against oppression is a much harder version of the struggle able-bodied women have for a realistic *and positive* self-image (Bogle and Shaul 1981; Browne, Connors, and Stern 1985). On the other hand, disabled people who cannot hope to meet the physical ideals of a culture can help reveal that those ideals are not "natural" or "normal" but artificial social creations that oppress everyone.

Feminist theorists have probed the causes of our patriarchal culture's desire for control of the body—fear of death, fear of the strong impulses and feelings the body gives us, fear of nature, fear and resentment of the mother's power over the infant (de Beauvoir 1949; Dinnerstein 1976; Griffin 1981). Idealizing the body and wanting to control it go hand-in-hand; it is impossible to say whether one causes the other. A physical ideal gives us the goal of our efforts to control the body, and the myth that total control is possible deceives us into striving for the ideal. The consequences for women have been widely discussed in the literature of feminism. The consequences for disabled people are less often recognized. In a culture which loves the idea that the body can be controlled, those who cannot control their bodies are seen (and may see themselves) as failures.

When you listen to this culture in a disabled body, you hear how often health and physical vigour are talked about as if they were moral virtues. People constantly praise others for their "energy," their stamina, their ability to work long hours. Of course, acting on behalf of one's health can be a virtue, and undermining one's health can be a vice, but "success" at being healthy, like beauty, is always partly a matter of luck and therefore beyond our control. When health is spoken of as a virtue, people who lack it are made to feel inadequate. I am not suggesting that it is always wrong to praise people's physical strength or accomplishments, any more than it is always wrong to praise their physical beauty. But just as treating cultural standards of beauty as essential virtues for women harms most women, treating health and vigour as moral virtues for everyone harms people with disabilities and illnesses.

The myth that the body can be controlled is not easily dispelled, because it is not very vulnerable to evidence against it. When I became ill, several people wanted to discuss with me what I thought I had done to "make myself" ill or "allow myself" to become sick. At first I fell in with this, generating theories about what I had done wrong; even though I had always taken good care of my health, I was able to find some (rather far-fetched) accounts of my responsibility for my illness. When a few close friends offered hypotheses as to how *they* might be responsible for my being ill, I began to suspect that something was wrong. Gradually, I realized that we were all trying to believe that nothing this important is beyond our control.

Of course, there are sometimes controllable social and psychological forces at work in creating ill health and disability (Kleinman 1988). Nevertheless, our cultural insistence on controlling the body blames the victims of disability for failing and burdens them with self-doubt and self-blame. The search for psychological, moral and spiritual causes of illness, accident and disability is often a harmful expression of this insistence on control (see Sontag 1977).

Modern Western medicine plays into and conforms to our cultural myth that the body can be controlled. Collectively, doctors and medical researchers exhibit very little modesty about their knowledge. They focus their (and our) attention on cures and imminent cures, on successful medical interventions. Research, funding and medical care are more directed toward life-threatening conditions than toward chronic illnesses and disabilities. Even pain was relatively neglected as a medical problem until the second half of this century. Surgery and saving lives bolster the illusion of control much better than does the long, patient process of rehabilitation or the management of long-term illness. These latter, less visible functions of medicine tend to be performed by nurses, physiotherapists and other low-prestige members of the profession. Doctors are trained to do something to control the body, to "make it better" (Kleinman 1988); they are the heroes of medicine. They may like being in the role of hero, but we also like them in that role and try to keep them there, because *we* want to believe that someone can always "make it better."[11] As long as we cling to this belief, the patients who cannot be "repaired"—the chronically ill, the disabled and the dying—will symbolize the failure of medicine and more, the failure of the Western scientific project to control nature. They will carry this stigma in medicine and in the culture as a whole.

When philosophers of medical ethics confine themselves to discussing life-and-death issues of medicine, they help perpetuate the idea that the main purpose of medicine is to control the body. Life-and-death interventions are the ultimate exercise of control. If medical ethicists looked more closely at who needs and who receives medical help, they would discover a host of issues concerning how medicine and society understand, mediate, assist with and integrate experiences of illness, injury and disability.

Because of the heroic approach to medicine, and because disabled people's experience is not integrated into the culture, most people know little or nothing about how to live with long-term or life-threatening illness, how to communicate with doctors and nurses and medical bureaucrats about these matters, how to live with limitation, uncertainty, pain, nausea, and other symptoms when doctors cannot make them go away. Recently, patients' support groups have arisen to fill this gap for people with nearly every type of illness and disability. They are vitally important sources of knowledge and encouragement for many of us, but they do not fill the cultural gulf between the able-bodied and the disabled. The problems of living with a disability are not private problems, separable from the rest of life and the rest of society. They are problems which can and should be shared throughout the culture as much as we share the problems of love, work and family life.

Consider the example of pain. It is difficult for most people who have not lived with prolonged or recurring pain to understand the benefits of accepting it. Yet some people who live with chronic pain speak of "making friends" with it as the road to feeling better and enjoying life. How do they picture their pain and think about it; what kind of attention do they give it and when; how do they live around and through it, and what do they learn from it? We all need to know this as part of our education. Some of the fear of experiencing pain is a consequence of ignorance and lack of guidance. The effort to avoid pain contributes to such widespread problems as drug and alcohol addiction, eating disorders, and sedentary lives. People with painful disabilities can teach us about pain, because they *can't* avoid it and have had to learn how to face it and live with it. The pernicious myth that it is possible to avoid almost all pain by controlling the body gives the fear of pain greater power than it should have and blames the victims of unavoidable pain. The fear of pain is also expressed or displaced as a fear of people in pain, which often isolates those with painful disabilities. All this is unnecessary. People *in* pain and knowledge *of* pain could be fully integrated into our culture, to everyone's benefit.

If we knew more about pain, about physical limitation, about loss of abilities, about what it is like to be "too far" from the cultural ideal of the body, perhaps we would have less fear of the negative body, less fear of our own weaknesses and "imperfections," of our inevitable deterioration and death. Perhaps we could give up our idealizations and relax our desire for control of the body; until we do, we maintain them at the expense of disabled people and at the expense of our ability to accept and love our own real bodies.

DISABLED PEOPLE AS "OTHER"

When we make people "other," we group them together as the objects of *our* experience instead of regarding them as fellow *subjects* of experience with whom we might identify. If you are "other" to me, I see you primarily as symbolic of something else—usually, but not always, something I reject and fear and that I project onto you. We can all do this to each other, but very often the process is not symmetrical, because one group of people may have more power to call itself the paradigm of humanity and to make the world suit its own needs and validate its own experiences.[12] Disabled people are "other" to able-bodied people, and (as I have tried to show) the consequences are socially, economically and psychologically oppressive to the disabled and psychologically oppressive to the able-bodied. Able-bodied people may be "other" to disabled people, but the consequences of this for the able-bodied are minor (most able-bodied people can afford not to notice it). There are, however, several political and philosophical issues that being "other" to a more powerful group raises for disabled people.

I have said that for the able-bodied, the disabled often symbolize failure to control the body and the failure of science and medicine to protect us all. However, some disabled people also become symbols of heroic control against all odds; these are the "disabled heroes," who are comforting to the able-bodied because they reaffirm the possibility of overcoming the body. Disabled heroes are people with visible disabilities who receive public attention because they accomplish things that are unusual even for the able-bodied. It is revealing that, with few exceptions (Helen Keller and, very recently, Stephen Hawking are among them), disabled heroes are recognized for performing feats of physical strength and endurance. While disabled heroes can be inspiring and heartening to the disabled, they may give the able-bodied the false impression that anyone can "overcome" a disability. Disabled heroes usually have extraordinary social, economic and physical resources that are not available to most people with those disabilities. In addition, many disabled people are not capable of performing physical heroics, because many (perhaps most) disabilities reduce or consume the energy and stamina of people who have them and do not just limit them in some particular kind of physical activity. Amputee and wheelchair athletes are exceptional, not because of their ambition, discipline and hard work, but because they are in better health than most disabled people can be. Arthritis, Parkinsonism and stroke cause severe disability in far more people than do spinal cord injuries and amputations (Bury 1979). The image of the disabled hero may reduce the "otherness" of a few disabled people, but because it creates an ideal which most disabled people cannot meet, it *increases* the "otherness" of the majority of disabled people.

One recent attempt to reduce the "otherness" of disabled people is the introduction of the term, "differently-abled." I assume the point of using this term is to suggest that there is nothing *wrong* with being the way we are, just different. Yet to call someone "differently-abled" is much like calling her "differently-coloured" or "differently-gendered." It says: "This person is not the norm or paradigm of humanity." If anything, it increases the "otherness" of disabled people, because it reinforces the paradigm of humanity as young, strong and healthy, with all body parts working "perfectly," from which this person is "different." Using the term "differently-abled" also suggests a (polite? patronizing? protective? self-protective?) disregard of the special difficulties, struggles and suffering disabled people face. We are *dis-abled*. We live with particular social and physical struggles that are partly consequences of the conditions of our bodies and partly consequences of the structures and expectations of our societies, but they are struggles which only people with bodies like ours experience.

The positive side of the term "differently-abled" is that it might remind the able-bodied that to be disabled in some respects is not to be disabled in all respects. It also suggests that a disabled person may have abilities that the able-bodied lack in virtue of being able-bodied. Nevertheless, on the whole, the term "differently-abled" should be abandoned, because it reinforces the able-bodied paradigm of humanity and fails to acknowledge the struggles disabled people face.

The problems of being "the other" to a dominant group are always politically complex. One solution is to emphasize similarities to the dominant group in the hope that they will identify with the oppressed, recognize their rights, gradually give them equal opportunities, and eventually assimilate them. Many disabled people are tired of being symbols to the able-bodied, visible only or primarily for their disabilities, and they want nothing more than to be seen as individuals rather than as members of the group, "the disabled." Emphasizing similarities to the able-bodied, making their disabilities unnoticeable in comparison to their other human qualities may bring about assimilation one-by-one. It does not directly challenge the able-bodied paradigm of humanity, just as women moving into traditionally male arenas of power does not directly challenge the male paradigm of humanity, although both may produce a gradual change in the paradigms. In addition, assimilation may be very difficult for the disabled to achieve. Although the able-bodied like disabled tokens who do not seem very different from themselves, they may *need* someone to carry the burden of the negative body as long as they continue to idealize and try to control the body. They may therefore resist the assimilation of most disabled people.

The reasons in favour of the alternative solution to "otherness"—*emphasizing difference* from the able-bodied—are also reasons for emphasizing similarities among the disabled, especially social and political similarities. Disabled people share positions of social oppression that separate us from the able-bodied, and we share physical, psychological and social experiences of disability. Emphasizing differences from the able-bodied demands that those differences be acknowledged and respected and fosters solidarity among the disabled. It challenges the able-bodied paradigm of humanity and creates the possibility of a deeper challenge to the idealization of the body and the demand for its control. Invisibly disabled people tend to be drawn to solutions that emphasize difference, because our need to have our struggles acknowledged is great, and we have far less experience than those who are visibly disabled of being symbolic to the able-bodied.

Whether one wants to emphasize sameness or difference in dealing with the problem of being "the other" depends in part on how radically one wants to challenge the value-structure of the dominant group. A very important issue in this category for both women and disabled people is the value of independence from the help of others, so highly esteemed in our patriarchal culture and now being questioned in feminist ethics (see, for example, Sherwin 1984, 1987; Kittay and Meyers 1987) and discussed in the writings of disabled women (see, for example, Fisher and Galler 1981; Davis 1984; Frank 1988). Many disabled people who can see the possibility of living as independently as any able-bodied person, or who have achieved this goal after long struggle, value their independence above everything. Dependence on the help of others is humiliating in a society which prizes independence. In addition, this issue holds special complications for disabled women; reading the stories of women who became disabled as adults, I was struck by their struggle with shame and loss of self-esteem at being transformed from people who took physical care of others (husbands and children) to people who were physically dependent. All this suggests that disabled people need every bit of independence we can get. Yet there are disabled people who will always need a lot of help from other individuals just to survive (those who have very little control of movement, for example), and to the extent that everyone considers independence necessary to respect and self-esteem, those people will be condemned to be devalued. In addition, some disabled people spend tremendous energy being independent in ways that might be considered trivial in a culture less insistent on self-reliance; if our culture valued *interdependence* more highly, they could use that energy for more satisfying activities.

In her excellent discussion of the issue of dependency and independence, Barbara Hillyer Davis argues that women with disabilities and those who care for them can work out a model of *reciprocity* for all of us, if we are willing to learn from them. "Reciprocity involves the difficulty of recognizing each other's needs, relying on the other, asking and receiving help, delegating responsibility, giving and receiving empathy, respecting boundaries" (Davis 1984, 4). I hope that disabled and able-bodied feminists will join in questioning our cultural obsession with independence and ultimately replacing it with such a model of reciprocity. If *all* the disabled are to be fully integrated into society without symbolizing failure, then we have to change social values to recognize the value of depending on others and being depended upon. This would also reduce the fear and shame associated with dependency in old age—a condition most of us will reach.

Whether one wants to emphasize sameness or difference in dealing with the problems of being "other" is also related to whether one sees anything valuable to be preserved by maintaining, either temporarily or in the long run, some separateness of the oppressed group. Is there a special culture of the oppressed group or the seeds of a special culture which could be developed in a supportive context of solidarity? Do members of the oppressed group have accumulated knowledge or ways of knowing which might be lost if assimilation takes place without the dominant culture being transformed?

It would be hard to claim that disabled people as a whole have an alternative culture or even the seeds of one. One sub-group, the deaf, has a separate culture from the hearing, and they are fighting for its recognition and preservation, as well as for their right to continue making their own culture (Sacks 1988). Disabled people do have both knowledge and ways of knowing that are not available to the able-bodied. Although ultimately I hope that disabled people's knowledge will be integrated into the culture as a whole, I suspect that a culture which fears and denigrates the real body would rather silence this knowledge than make the changes necessary to absorb it. It may have to be nurtured and cultivated separately while the able-bodied culture is transformed enough to receive and integrate it.

THE KNOWLEDGE OF DISABLED PEOPLE AND HOW IT IS SILENCED

In my second year of illness, I was reading an article about the psychological and philosophical relationship of mind to body. When the author painted a rosy picture of the experience of being embodied, I was outraged at the presumption of the writer to speak for everyone from a healthy body. I decided I didn't want to hear *anything* about the body from anyone who was not physically disabled. Before that moment, it had not occurred to me that there was a world of experience from which I was shut out while I was able-bodied.

Not only do physically disabled people have experiences which are not available to the able-bodied, they are in a better position to transcend cultural mythologies about the body, because they *cannot* do things that the able-bodied feel they *must* do in order to be happy, "normal" and sane. For example, paraplegics and quadriplegics have revolutionary things to teach about the possibilities of sexuality which contradict patriarchal culture's obsession with the genitals (Bullard and Knight 1981). Some people can have orgasms in any part of their bodies where they feel touch. One man said he never knew how good sex could be until he lost the feeling in his genitals. Few able-bodied people know these things, and, to my knowledge, no one has explored their implications for the able-bodied.

If disabled people were truly heard, an explosion of knowledge of the human body and psyche would take place. We have access to realms of experience that our culture has not tapped (even for medical science, which takes relatively little interest in people's *experience* of their bodies). Like women's particular knowledge, which comes from access to experiences most men do not have, disabled people's knowledge is dismissed as trivial, complaining, mundane (or bizarre), *less than* that of the dominant group.

The cognitive authority (Addelson 1983) of medicine plays an important role in distorting and silencing the knowledge of the disabled. Medical professionals have been given the power to describe and validate everyone's experience of the body. If you go to doctors with symptoms they cannot observe directly or verify independently of what you tell them, such as pain or weakness or numbness or dizziness or difficulty concentrating, and if they cannot find an objectively observable cause of those symptoms, you are likely to be told that there is "nothing wrong with you," no matter how you feel. Unless you are very lucky in your doctors, no matter how trustworthy and responsible you were considered to be *before* you started saying you were ill, your experience will be invalidated.[13] *Other* people are the authorities on the reality of your experience of your body.

When you are very ill, you desperately need medical validation of your experience, not only for economic reasons (insurance claims, pensions, welfare and disability benefits all depend upon official diagnosis), but also for social and psychological reasons. People with unrecognized illnesses are often abandoned by their friends and families.[14] Because almost everyone accepts the cognitive authority of medicine, the person whose bodily experience is radically different from medical descriptions of her/his condition is invalidated as a knower. Either you decide to hide your experience, or you are socially isolated with it by being labelled mentally ill[15] or dishonest. In both cases you are silenced.

Even when your experience is recognized by medicine, it is often re-described in ways that are inaccurate from your standpoint. The objectively observable condition of your body may be used to determine the severity of your pain, for instance, regardless of your own reports of it. For example, until recently, relatively few doctors were willing to acknowledge that severe phantom limb pain can persist for months or even years after an amputation. The accumulated experience of doctors who were themselves amputees has begun to legitimize the other patients' reports (Madruga 1979).

When you are forced to realize that other people have more social authority than you do to describe your experience of your own body, your confidence in yourself and your relationship to reality is radically undermined. What can you know if you cannot know that you are experiencing suffering or joy; what can you communicate to people who don't believe you know even this?[16] Most people will censor what they tell or say nothing rather than expose themselves repeatedly to such deeply felt invalidation. They are silenced by fear and confusion. The process is familiar from our understanding of how women are silenced in and by patriarchal culture.

One final caution: As with women's "special knowledge," there is a danger of sentimentalizing disabled people's knowledge and abilities and keeping us "other" by doing so. We need to bring this knowledge into the culture and to transform the culture and society so that everyone can receive and make use of it, so that it can be fully integrated, along with disabled people, into a shared social life.

CONCLUSION

I have tried to introduce the reader to the rich variety of intellectual and political issues that are raised by experiences of physical disability. Confronting these issues has increased my appreciation of the insights that feminist theory already offers into cultural attitudes about the body and the many forms of social oppression. Feminists have been challenging medicine's authority for many years now, but not, I think, as radically as we would if we knew what disabled people have to tell. I look forward to the development of a full feminist theory of disability.[17] We need a theory of disability for the liberation of both disabled and able-bodied people, since the theory of disability is also the theory of the oppression of the body by a society and its culture.

NOTES

Many thanks to Kathy Gose, Joyce Frazee, Mary Barnes, Barbara Beach, Elliott Gose and Gordon Renwick for helping me to think about these questions, and to Maureen Ashfield for helping me to research them.

1. Itzhak Perlman, when asked in a CBC interview about the problems of the disabled, said disabled people have two problems: the fact that the world is not made for people with any weaknesses but for supermen and the attitudes of able-bodied people.

2. An excellent description of this last issue as it confronts the deaf is found in Sacks 1988.

3. See Matthews 1983; Hannaford 1985; Rooney and Israel 1985; Browne, Connors, and Stern 1985; Deegan and Brooks 1985; Saxton and Howe 1987; and, for a doctor's theories, Kleinman 1988.

4. We also need a feminist theory of mental disability, but I will not be discussing mental disability in this essay.

5. In a recent article in *Signs,* Linda Alcoff argues that we should define "woman" thus: "woman is a position from which a feminist politics can emerge rather than a set of attributes that are 'objectively identifiable.' " (Alcoff 1988, 435). I think a similar approach may be the best one for defining "disability."

6. For example, pelvic inflammatory disease causes severe prolonged disability in some women. These women often have to endure medical diagnoses of psychological illness and the skepticism of family and friends, in addition to having to live with chronic severe pain. See Moore 1985.

7. Feminism has challenged the distribution of responsibility for providing such resources as childcare and protection from family violence. Increasingly many people who once thought of these as family or personal concerns now think of them as social responsibilities.

8. Some people save me that trouble by *telling me* I am fine and walking away. Of course, people also encounter difficulties with answering "How are you?" during and after crises, such as separation from a partner, death of a loved one, or a nervous breakdown. There is a temporary alienation from what is considered ordinary shared experience. In disability, the alienation lasts longer, often for a lifetime, and, in my experience, it is more profound.

9. The idealization of the body is clearly related in complex ways to the economic processes of a consumer society. Since it pre-dated capitalism, we know that capitalism did not cause it, but it is undeniable that idealization now generates tremendous profits and that the quest for profit demands the reinforcement of idealization and the constant development of new ideals.

10. Susan Griffin, in a characteristically honest and insightful passage, describes an encounter with the fear that makes it hard to identify with disabled people. See Griffin 1982, 648–649.

11. Thanks to Joyce Frazee for pointing this out to me.

12. When Simone de Beauvoir uses this term to elucidate men's view of women (and women's view of ourselves), she emphasizes that Man is considered essential, Woman inessential; Man is the Subject, Woman the Other (de Beauvoir 1952, xvi). Susan Griffin

expands upon this idea by showing how we project rejected aspects of ourselves onto groups of people who are designated the Other (Griffin 1981).

13. Many women with M. S. have lived through this nightmare in the early stages of their illness. Although this happens to men too, women's experience of the body, like women's experience generally, is more likely to be invalidated (Hannaford 1985).

14. Accounts of the experience of relatively unknown, newly discovered, or hard-to-diagnose diseases and conditions confirm this. See, for example, Jeffreys 1982, for the story of an experience of chronic fatigue immune dysfunction syndrome, which is more common in women than in men.

15. Frequently people with undiagnosed illnesses are sent by their doctors to psychiatrists, who cannot help and may send them back to their doctors saying they must be physically ill. This can leave patients in a dangerous medical and social limbo. Sometimes they commit suicide because of it (Ramsay 1986). Psychiatrists who know enough about living with physical illness or disability to help someone cope with it are rare.

16. For more discussion of this subject, see Zaner 1983 and Rawlinson 1983.

17. At this stage of the disability rights movement, it is impossible to anticipate everything that a full feminist theory will include, just as it would have been impossible to predict in 1970 the present state of feminist theory of mothering. Nevertheless, we can see that besides dealing more fully with the issues I have raised here, an adequate feminist theory of disability will examine all the ways in which disability is socially constructed; it will explain the interaction of disability with gender, race and class position; it will examine every aspect of the cognitive authority of medicine and science over our experiences of our bodies; it will discuss the relationship of technology to disability; it will question the belief that disabled lives are not worth living or preserving when it is implied in our theorizing about abortion and euthanasia; it will give us a detailed vision of the full integration of disabled people in society, and it will propose practical political strategies for the liberation of disabled people and the liberation of the able-bodied from the social oppression of their bodies.

REFERENCES

Addelson, Kathryn P. 1983. The man of professional wisdom. In *Discovering reality*. Sandra Harding and Merrill B. Hintikka, eds. Boston: D. Reidel.

Alcoff, Linda. 1988. Cultural feminism versus poststructuralism: The identity crisis in feminist theory. *Signs: Journal of Women in Culture and Society* 13(3):405–436.

Beauvoir, Simone de. 1952. *The second sex.* New York: Alfred A. Knopf.

Browne, Susan E., Debra Connors, and Nanci Stern, eds. 1985. *With the power of each breath—A disabled women's anthology.* Pittsburgh: Cleis Press.

Bullard, David G., and Susan E. Knight, eds. 1981. *Sexuality and physical disability.* St. Louis: C. V. Mosby.

Bury, M. R. 1979. Disablement in society: Towards an integrated perspective. *International Journal of Rehabilitation Research* 2(1):33–40.

Campling, Jo, ed. 1981. *Images of ourselves—Women with disabilities talking.* London: Routledge and Kegan Paul.

Davis, Barbara Hillyer. 1984. Women, disability and feminism: Notes toward a new theory. *Frontiers: A Journal of Women Studies* VIII(1):1–5.

Davis, Melanie, and Catherine Marshall. 1987. Female and disabled: Challenged women in education. *National Women's Studies Association Perspectives* 5:39–41.

Deegan, Mary Jo, and Nancy A. Brooks, eds. 1985. *Women and disability—The double handicap.* New Brunswick: Transaction Books.

Dinnerstein, Dorothy. 1976. *The mermaid and the minotaur: Sexual arrangements and human malaise.* New York: Harper and Row.

Ehrenreich, Barbara, and Dierdre English. 1979. *For her own good: 150 years of the experts' advice to women.* New York: Anchor.

Fine, Michelle, and Adrienne Asch, eds. 1988. *Women with disabilities: Essays in psychology, culture and politics.* Philadelphia: Temple University Press.

Finger, Anne. 1983. Disability and reproductive rights. *off our backs* 13(9):18–19.

Fisher, Bernice, and Roberta Galler. 1981. Conversation between two friends about feminism and disability. *off our backs* 11(5):14–15.

Frank, Gelya. 1988. On embodiment: A case study of congenital limb deficiency in American culture. In *Women with disabilities.* Michelle Fine and Adrienne Asch, eds. Philadelphia: Temple University Press.

Griffin, Susan. 1981. *Pornography and silence: Culture's revenge against nature.* New York: Harper and Row.

Griffin, Susan. 1982. The way of all ideology. *Signs: Journal of Women in Culture and Society* 8(3):641–660.

Halpern, Sue M. 1988. Portrait of the artist. Review of *Under the eye of the clock* by Christopher Nolan. *The New York Review of Books,* June 30:3–4.

Hannaford, Susan. 1985. *Living outside inside. A disabled woman's experience. Towards a social and political perspective.* Berkeley: Canterbury Press.

Jeffreys, Toni. 1982. *The mile-high staircase.* Sydney: Hodder and Stoughton Ltd.

Kittay, Eva Feder, and Diana T. Meyers, eds. 1987. *Women and moral theory.* Totowa, NJ: Rowman and Littlefield.

Kleinman, Arthur. 1988. *The illness narratives: Suffering, healing, and the human condition.* New York: Basic Books.

Lessing, Jill. 1981. Denial and disability. *off our backs* 11(5):21.

Madruga, Lenor. 1979. *One step at a time.* Toronto: McGraw-Hill.

Matthews, Gwyneth Ferguson. 1983. *Voices from the shadows: Women with disabilities speak out.* Toronto: Women's Educational Press.

Moore, Maureen. 1985. Coping with pelvic inflammatory disease. In *Women and Disability.* Frances Rooney and Pat Israel, eds. *Resources for Feminist Research* 14(1).

Newsweek. 1988. Reading God's mind. June 13:56–59.

Ramsay, A. Melvin. 1986. *Postviral fatigue syndrome, the saga of Royal Free disease.* London: Gower Medical Publishing.

Rawlinson, Mary C. 1983. The facticity of illness and the appropriation of health. In *Phenomenology in a pluralistic context.* William L. McBride and Calvin O. Schrag, eds. Albany: SUNY Press.

Rich, Adrienne. 1976. *Of woman born: Motherhood as experience and institution.* New York: W. W. Norton.

Rooney, Frances, and Pat Israel, eds. 1985. *Women and disability. Resources for Feminist Research* 14(1).

Sacks, Oliver. 1988. The revolution of the deaf. *The New York Review of Books,* June 2:23–28.

Saxton, Marsha, and Florence Howe, eds. 1987. *With wings: An anthology of literature by and about women with disabilities.* New York: The Feminist Press.

Shaul, Susan L., and Jane Elder Bogle. 1981. Body image and the woman with a disability. In *Sexuality and physical disability.* David G. Bullard and Susan E. Knight, eds. St. Louis: C. V. Mosby.

Sherwin, Susan. 1984. A feminist approach to ethics. *Dalhousie Review* 64(4):704–713.

Sherwin, Susan. 1987. Feminist ethics and in vitro fertilization. In *Science, morality and feminist theory.* Marsha Hanen and Kai Nielsen, eds. Calgary: The University of Calgary Press.

Sontag, Susan. 1977. *Illness as metaphor.* New York: Random House.

U.N. Decade of Disabled Persons 1983–1992. 1983. *World programme of action concerning disabled persons.* New York: United Nations.

Whitbeck, Caroline. 1983. Afterword to the maternal instinct. In *Mothering: Essays in feminist theory.* Joyce Trebilcot, ed. Totowa: Rowman and Allanheld.

Zaner, Richard M. 1983. Flirtations or engagement? Prolegomenon to a philosophy of medicine. In *Phenomenology in a pluralistic context.* William L. McBride and Calvin O. Schrag, eds. Albany: SUNY Press.

23 Quality-Adjusted Life-Years: Ethical Implications for Physicians and Policymakers

JOHN LA PUMA, M.D. AND EDWARD F. LAWLOR, PH.D.

Dr. John La Puma is at the Center for Clinical Ethics, Lutheran General Hospital, Park Ridge, Illinois. Dr. Edward Lawlor is at the School of Social Service Administration, University of Chicago.

A quality-adjusted life-year (QALY) is a numerical description of the value that a medical procedure or service can provide to groups of patients with similar medical conditions. Quality-adjusted life-years attempt to combine expected survival with expected quality of life in a single metric: if an additional year of healthy life is worth a value of 1 (year), then a year of less healthy life is worth less than 1 (year).[1]

Quality-adjusted life-years represent a progression in the cost-effectiveness analysis of health care, as concepts of health, quality of life, and utility are inherently amorphous and elusive. Albert Mulley, MD, calls this "the stuff of poets and philosophers," but in QALY assessment they are also the stuff of economists and psychometricians. Health economists have struggled for decades to estimate the value of life and many have been uncomfortable with life-years gained as an outcome, but have had little more to offer.[2]

Serious clinical ethical questions, however, have been raised about QALYs.[3-9] We review herein QALY methods and historical development and attempt to identify the ethical issues they present.

This article first appeared in the Journal of the American Medical Association *263 (6 June 1990): 2917–2921.*

QALY Methods

Calculations of QALYs are based on measurements of the value that individuals place on expected years of life. Measurements can be made in several ways: by simulating gambles about preferences for alternative states of health, by inferring willingness to pay for alternative states of health, or through "trading off" some or all likely survival time that a medical intervention might provide to gain less survival time of higher quality.

A reference gamble reveals preference by asking the respondent to choose the consequences of a hypothetical game (such as choosing balls out of an urn) with known probabilities. Willingness-to-pay estimates rely either on statements of the sacrifice an individual is willing to make to obtain alternative outcomes or on the analysis of actual observed behavior. Estimates of QALYs can also be derived by asking respondents to explicitly trade years of life for different presentations of quality of life.

In theory, these techniques could be employed to elicit QALYs for an individual patient who faces a choice between alternative therapies that yield different probabilities for pain reduction, abilities to engage in activities of daily living, and life expectancies. A patient with severe angina and triple-vessel disease will likely generate different QALYs with bypass surgery, without surgery, and with medications; a patient with severe angina and single-vessel disease would generate still different QALYs than the former patient.

How much survival time groups of patients would trade off for what degree of quality may change as more is learned about disease. New data may be folded into the analysis as they become available, eg, cyclosporine has improved survival after organ transplantation, requiring QALY recalculations to higher, more accurate values. In effect, QALYs "discount" years of life saved by a health care intervention by how much patients' subjective well-being is diminished by discomfort or distress.

The methods used to calculate QALYs are still under development.[10] Quality-adjusted life-year assessments have been shown to vary by how health states are described, how outcomes are reported, how scales are generated, and how surveys are administered.[11] We will not belabor the technical issues involved in utility measurement[12] and quality-of-life assessment,[13] but they are controversial and variable.

Cost-Effectiveness Analysis in Health Policy

Cost-effectiveness analyses attempt to assess how efficiently interventions are being used, given how much they cost. When divided by cost, QALYs can yield a measure of cost-effectiveness[14] and help establish priorities for funding. Interventions of highest priority (yielding the most QALYs per unit of cost) would receive the most resources: the more QALYs per dollar, the more resources and the greater development of that intervention. In theory, QALYs can help provide for an efficient use of those resources that already exist and for the allocation of new resources.

Quality-adjusted life-years are also a potential result of community medical ethics: the public identification, prioritization, and implementation of an equitable, virtuous distribution of health care resources. Accurate, detailed knowledge of community preferences is essential to allocate resources fairly. At least 10 state programs in community clinical ethics now exist.[15] Oregon Health Decisions, for example, helped persuade the state legislature not to fund organ transplantation because it received a lower community priority than preventive programs.[16] Although coverage for transplantation was reinstated after a public outcry,[17] the concept of small town meetings to allocate resources has broad appeal.

QALYs as a Rationing Tool

Most QALY proponents expect QALYs to inform resource allocation decisions, especially large-scale decisions that deploy resources across disease states and population groups. In theory, a QALY analysis compares the merits of devoting resources to an intervention likely to extend the lives of a population for a specific period, but with high levels of disability and distress, with another intervention, which may not yield as many years of life saved, but generates higher levels of subjective well-being.

Cost-per-QALY analyses are motivated by scarcity: if resources were unlimited, rationing would be unnecessary. In the United Kingdom, there is explicit rationing of some health care services, requiring physicians to be both caretakers and resource agents. In the United States, rationing is accomplished through patients' differential ability to pay: 37 million uninsured people do not have equal access to health care.[18] Aaron and Schwartz[19] found that British physicians most often find medical reasons to deny a needed treatment (eg, dialysis) to a patient. Such patients are said to be too old, too sick, or too unlikely to benefit; physicians generally do not say that the resource is relatively scarce and unavailable.

Explicit health care rationing, with selected priorities for funding, has been proposed in Oregon[20] and by scholars.[21] Oregon state officials hope to ration Medicaid services by July 1, 1990, using the "Quality of Well-Being Scale" and "Well-Years" very similar to QALYs.[22] These plans call on physicians to ration care at the bedside and could benefit from a clear explication of how QALYs have developed.

Historical Development

Technical Development

Derived from operations research in engineering and mathematics, QALYs were first introduced by decision analysts and researchers in the United States.[23,24] Weinstein and Stason[25] described QALYs as a way of elucidating the trade-offs between quality of life and additional survival, representing "the net health effectiveness of the program or practice in question."

In 1978 in Britain, Rosser and Kind[26] reported the results of psychometric testing of 70 selected patients, volunteers, physicians, and nurses. The authors devised a scale that assigned a numerical value to 29 hypothetical states of disability and distress. The resulting Rosser index has been the foundation of most British work on QALYs, pioneered by health economist Alan Williams.

Clinical Decision Making

Quantitative analytic techniques such as those of economic analysis can make the components of clinical decision making more clear; these techniques are most effective when their underlying value assumptions are made explicit. The algorithms and decision trees of health status assessment are not readily accepted as clinical tools,[27] however, as they miss the complexity and subtlety necessary for many clinical decisions. Still, Jennett and Buxton[28] have suggested that QALYs can and should be part of clinical considerations about quality of life and should be used at the bedside.

The process of clinical decision making, itself an outcome, is not taken into account by measures such as QALYs. The significance of this criticism is undervalued. Many interactions between physician and patient do not result in a tangible intervention or easily measurable data. Patients often seek physicians for attention, information, reassurance, encouragement, and permission, not just prescriptions and procedures. In QALYs, there is no attempt to integrate the therapeutic value and outcome of talking with patients[29] or their families: patient care is evidenced by the boxes checked on the office encounter sheet.

Health Policy Proposals

Calculations for numerous interventions have been reported. Weinstein and Stason[25] applied QALYs to the resources allocated to manage hypertension and proposed a threshold value of blood pressure below which it would not be cost-effective to treat patients. It costs less than £200 ($350) to gain 1 year of quality-adjusted life for general practitioners to counsel patients not to smoke, £1000 ($1500) for coronary artery bypass grafting for left main disease with severe angina, more than £2000 ($3000) for coronary artery bypass grafting for left main disease with mild angina, and £15,000 ($22,500) for hospital hemodialysis.[30] Policy implications of these findings are that treatments with costs-per-day QALY above £5000 ($7500) "should be taken off the . . . budget completely and financed only as research and development activities."[30] More recently in America, QALYs and quality-adjusted life-months have been calculated for estrogen use in postmenopausal women,[31] neonatal intensive care,[32] dialysis,[33] coronary artery bypass grafting,[34] and prostatectomy.[35]

In 1985, Williams[36] compared the QALY costs and benefits of coronary artery bypass grafting with renal transplantation, concluding that bypass grafting for left main disease with severe or moderate angina and for triple-vessel disease should be funded before renal transplantation.

In 1986, Gudex[37,38] reported the results of the preliminary use of QALYs in the North Western Regional Health Authority in Britain, which, like other health authorities, receives monies from the National Health Service to fund its health care activities. Gudex compared the QALY efficiency of several unrelated interventions, using life-expectancy data from current literature and a revised Rosser index.[39] Surgery for a "neuromuscular" patient had the lowest cost per QALY (£194 [$291]), corrective surgery for an adolescent scoliotic patient had a higher cost per QALY (£2619 [$3929]), and chronic ambulatory peritoneal dialysis lasting 4 years had the highest cost per QALY (£13,434 [$20,151]). The North Western Regional Health Authority has not continued the studies and the Department of Health and Social Services has not made a formal statement about QALYs, although it continues to fund the work of Williams, Rosser, and Gudex.

The need for outcome management in American and British health care is increasingly newsworthy; the brief, efficient, accurate measurement of quality of life is an important part of that management. Ellwood[40] has encouraged the Health Care Financing Administration to define the quality-of-life data set, and more than 100 scales can be used to measure quality of life. Despite continuing uncertainty about how to deploy these measurements in health policy,[41,42] we can identify the ethical assumptions that underlie QALYs.

QALYs AND MEDICAL ETHICS

The debate about QALYs occurs on at least four levels. First, there are methodological problems of theory, measurement, and interpretation. Second, practical questions of implementation arise, assuming the technical properties of QALY-based policy guidance are clarified and agreed on. Third, QALYs present moral and professional challenges to the fundamental values and assumed prerogatives of physicians. Fourth, QALYs hold an uneasy, conspicuous, critical place in the recent evolution of health policy, an evolution preoccupied with the agenda of cost containment.

QALYs' Ethical Assumptions

The formal use of QALYs and QALY-like scales makes six ethical assumptions. First, quality of life can be accurately measured and should have "standing" in determining resource allocation. Second, utilitarianism ("the greatest good for the greatest number") is the appropriate ethical theory for resolving resource allocation dilemmas. Third, equity and efficiency are compatible and should be balanced in QALY construction. Fourth, projections of community preferences for interventions can ethically substitute for the preferences of individual patients when allocating and rationing resources. Fifth, older and sicker patients have less "capacity to benefit" from interventions than those who are younger and healthier. Sixth, physicians will be able to differentiate between a patient's medical need and a resource's availability and between being a patient advocate and a public agent, will favor the measurable outcome of clinical decision making over its process, and will not use QALYs as clinical maxims.

Quality of Life

The President's Commission for the Study of Ethical Problems in Medicine and Biomedical and Behavioral Research noted that "quality of life [is] an ethically essential concept that focuses on the good of the individual, what kind of life is possible given the person's condition, and whether that condition will allow the individual to have *a life that he or she views as worth living* [italics added]." One prominent philosopher has recently suggested that quality-based societal limits are needed and are morally correct.[43] In a recent national survey, nearly three fourths of Americans felt that an unconscious, terminally ill patient should be removed from life-support systems because of his or her quality of life and that of his or her family.[44]

Quality-adjusted life-years assume that quality of life can be measured well enough to make policy judgments about it. They also assume that at some point—the same point for all persons—life becomes so miserable that it is worse than death.[45] Incalculables such as freedom from the fear of dependency on a ventilator or the value of time spent awake, alert, and participatory are part of quality of life.

We do not say that such incalculables render impossible the useful measurement of quality of life. Some patients, though, would rather live no matter what their disability/distress score. Other patients cannot or will not decide and have no one to speak for them. The lives of these patients—the demented, the mentally ill, and the "old-old"—QALYs judge to be of inadequate worth; for these patients, quality-of-life assessments cannot be made accurately.

The Greatest Good for the Greatest Number

Consider the estimation of QALYs generated by a zidovudinelike therapy for patients infected with the human immunodeficiency virus. Whose utility assessments count? Should a representative sample of the public be interviewed? Or should potential candidates for the therapy be interviewed? Should some form of weighing be developed for respondents with knowledge of or experience with the relevant health states? How should the valuation of outcomes in the distant future be treated?[46] How should individual preferences and attitudes about risk taking be accommodated?[47] How should resources for individuals with impaired decision making be handled? How should these assessments be summed or interpreted, particularly if there are major differences in assessments among respondents?

These questions are not new or unfamiliar to health planners and analysts, but the answers may be contained within the ideology of cost containment and the moral perspective of utilitarianism. As Caplan[48] has said, "The quantification of value . . . often is ideology masquerading as a moral point of view."

Equity and Efficiency

Legitimate concerns arise about how QALYs may influence the conduct and direction of health policy. Our society continues to evolve toward a utilitarian ethic, one that appreciates medicine for what it can measurably produce, rather than for humanistic care. Quality-adjusted life-years are controversial not only for what they are, but also for the new financial ethos they represent. They symbolize a movement to make health a commodity and to shift the balance of power in and philosophy of clinical practice from highly discretionary physician-patient encounters to more standardized, quantified, and regulated protocols.[49] Thus, many critics of QALYs are fundamentally concerned with the problems of integrating explicit economic guidance and formulas with clinical decision making, fearing that policymakers will conflate efficiency and equity[50] and that physicians will be forced to choose between being a patient advocate or a public agent,[51] to the disadvantaged patient's disadvantage.[14]

Whose Autonomy? Whose Justice?

Quality-adjusted life-years risk projecting community preferences over those of individual patients. The ethical principle of autonomy or self-determination, generally most important for individual patients, would be trumped by that of justice or fairness, generally most important for a community. The preferences of a selected population sample or the preferences of a representative sample of patients in hypothetical medical situations would be used as if they were individual patient preferences. For example, Williams, Rosser, and Gudex use an assessment of community values in QALY calculations. Their assessment for an individual patient would come from the preferences of the average member of the public, not the average patient and not the patient himself.

This departure from codes of medical ethics and from clinical ethics reflects underlying QALY assumptions—that the projections of healthy others can be generalized to any patient with a particular medical condition. If all members of the public were reliably asked how many years of life they would trade off for different conditions and their verified responses were analyzed, a sound public policy statement on health care resources could be made. Using such a policy to allocate resources at a high level could be tenable, but does not obviate the physician's professional responsibility to work at the bedside for a patient's medical interests. In the current era of cost containment, the physician should not be in the position of defending public policy: patient advocate or public agent should be an easy choice.

Finally, individual patient preferences cannot always be accurately assessed by others. One study has suggested that chronically ill elderly outpatients believe their quality of life is better than their physicians believe it is.[52] Another study found that quality of life is a poor predictor of individual patient preferences for intensive care.[53] Although the preferences of family members and others can be included in technology evaluation, even family preferences may not represent those of the patient. Spouses may overestimate patient preferences for many intensive therapies, including cardiopulmonary resuscitation, and physicians both underestimate and overestimate patients' preferences.[54,55] Given the variability and difficulty of assessing individual preferences[53] and the potential for misuse when grouped, implementation of QALY-like standards in clinical practice would present significant risks to patients.

What Is "Capacity to Benefit"?
Several studies of QALYs assume that patients' "capacity to benefit" from an intervention is a relevant measure of QALYs. Researchers define "capacity to benefit" as the ability of an intervention to provide more life-years of adjusted quality. This definition would likely direct care away from patients who have a poor quality of life and little or no "capacity to benefit" (eg, terminally ill, locked-in, and comatose patients),[56,57] because their care would yield few QALYs at a relatively high cost. While

the care of the terminally ill and the neurologically impaired may not be QALY efficient, it is part of the traditional role of health professionals. Attending to time-consuming patients and their families is part of this compassionate, although QALY-inefficient ethos of medicine.

Although straight counting of life-years undervalues the lives of the elderly,[3] they have less "capacity to benefit" than the young. If QALYs are calculated with patients' families in mind, reducing the disability or distress of patients with dependents will be preferable to reducing the disability or distress of patients without dependents. Patients who are more critically ill or whose quality of life is poorer would probably receive treatments *after* those who were less critically ill or whose quality of life was better.

QALYs as Clinical Maxims: The New Diagnosis Related Groups?

Much of the concern about QALY implementation appears to have less to do with their technical properties than with how they might be abused. Clinician reaction to a 1977 *Hastings Center Report* article, for example, is instructive.[58] A simple didactic quality-of-life equation (not a QALY) was presented; the equation was intended to aid decision making for incompetent individuals. It was misinterpreted by many as a decision-making rule—an algorithm to be interpreted strictly and applied uncritically to individual cases. Neither the author nor critics envisioned any such use for this formulation.

Diagnosis related groups were similarly conceived to provide guidance about use for relatively large numbers of cases,[59] but instead of simply guiding prospective payment they have been employed directly in clinical decision making about individual cases.[60,61] The overall effect of diagnosis related groups has been to force hospitals to economize, accepting fewer uninsured patients, reducing patients' length of stay, and increasing the acuity of illness at discharge. While there is nothing wrong with encouraging physicians to be efficient, the point is that both QALYs and diagnosis related groups try to combine efficiency with equity to yield a blunt, economically driven tool. Whether QALYs will be used as clinical maxims remains to be seen.

QALYs and Clinical Practice

Quality-adjusted life-years attempt to clarify judgments about quality of life. Clinicians make quality, cost, and survival judgments implicitly and individually, based on their experience with different patients and on the particular needs of an individual patient. These judgments are often subjective and always difficult to quantify. By identifying specific quality states, survival estimates, and societal preferences, QALYs may improve the efficiency and objectivity of medical decision making, reducing the subjectivity of judgments about quality of life.[62]

Quality-adjusted life-years are intended to be a "macro" tool. Quality-adjusted life-years use aggregate community preferences and trade-offs to determine what is best for an individual patient, regardless of whether societal preferences and an individual's preferences are the same. Using QALYs as a "micro" clinical decision-making tool has health system–wide implications that may promote decision making not by the numbers from physical examination and laboratory measurement, but by single metrics, eg, QALYs, diagnosis related groups, and age. Such decision making impoverishes medicine as a science of numbers and robs it of the richness of clinical detail.

Quality-adjusted life-years assume that the duration and quality of an individual patient's life are not different from most other commodities that can be purchased. While utilitarianism may be an acceptable ethical theory with which to make health policy at the macro level, at present, clinical practice is not primarily conducted to benefit society as a whole, the public interest, or the common good. The physician's primary duty is to meet the patient's medical needs as they together find them, the physician with technical knowledge and expertise and the patient with his or her personal history and values. Conserving society's resources is secondary or tertiary; if such conservation is brought about by considering some patients expendable or by serving opposing masters of patient and society,[63-66] the seemingly imminent role of public agent must be acknowledged, appealed, and refuted.

Using resources in response to patient need, however, as assessed by health professionals and as differentiated from patient or physician want, and in proportion to the expected benefit, should be the objective of clinical encounters. If rational, reasonable health policies are constructed and physicians are constrained from offering expensive technologies of marginal benefit,[67] then can we keep straight the difference between what is medically needed and medically available? Civil suits, licensure actions, courts of public opinion,[68,69] ethics consultants,[70] and the media have already appealed these constraints, but the real question is whether the physician's role must be redefined to include "negotiator" and "advocate" at the policy level. Understanding QALYs will help physicians influence policy in a way that preserves a level of choice within the reality of increasing fiscal constraints on patient care.

CONCLUSION

Quality-adjusted life-years are a new health measurement tool that many health care economists and decision analysts believe has promise to provide health care to those who have the greatest capacity to benefit.

Despite interest in the deployment of QALYs, there are significant computational problems of utility theory, instrumentation, measurement, and interpretation and ethical dilemmas of equity, justice, autonomy, beneficence, and discrimination.

Policymakers who wish to use QALYs to allocate resources must fully identify and disclose QALYs' ethical assumptions, so that they can be debated. How to reconcile variability in individual medical values and preferences with cost-per-QALY calculations is still uncertain. What is certain is that QALY analyses have bedside implications for patients and physicians.

If physicians use community-derived QALYs to determine which of their patients will receive treatment, full disclosure to patients will not help. Medical treatments are not like other commodities that can be proffered and purchased. Patients' preferences and needs for health care may be replaced by an economic analysis that relies on selected community opinions, giving insufficient weight to the patient's preferences or the clinician's judgment. Physicians' social responsibility to use resources carefully may supplant our professional responsibility to care for our patients medically.

It is unclear whether resources available for research should be directed toward cost-effectiveness analyses such as QALYs or toward superior outcome measures. The improper or overzealous deployment of QALYs may mask a simpler and more arbitrary cost-containment agenda. Policymakers should consider quality-of-life factors in decision making, but must do so with better data and great compassion. Excluding needy patients must be an anathema to both policymakers and physicians. The tension between selected societal and individual interests will continue and heighten; guarding against economic analyses' imposition of selected societal interests on individual patients will increasingly become the physician's duty and charge, one that physicians must seize and defend.

This work was supported in part by the American College of Physicians in Philadelphia, through an American College of Physicians A. Blaine Brower Traveling Scholarship for 1988 through 1989 (Dr La Puma).

REFERENCES

1. Williams A. The importance of quality of life in policy decisions. In: Walker SR, Rosser RM, eds. *Quality of Life: Assessment and Application.* Lancaster, England: MTP Press Ltd; 1988:279–290.

2. Avorn J. Benefit and cost analysis in geriatric care. *N Engl J Med.* 1984;310:310–322.

3. Menzel PT. *Medical Costs, Moral Choices*. New Haven, Conn: Yale University Press; 1983:185–195.

4. Maynard A, Devlin JB. Economists v clinicians: the crucial debate. *Health Soc Service J.* July 18, 1985:7–8.

5. Jarret RJ. Economics or coronary artery bypass grafting. *Br Med J.* 1985;291:600.

6. Smith A. Qualms about QALYs. *Lancet.* 1987;1:1134–1136.

7. Harris J. QALYfying the value of life. *J Med Ethics.* 1987;13:117–123.

8. *The Ian Ramsey Centre Working Party Report on Decision-Making and Quality of Life.* Oxford, England: The Ian Ramsey Centre; 1989.

9. Rawles J. Castigating QALYs. *J Med Ethics.* 1989;15:143–147.

10. Smith GT, ed. *Measuring Health: A Practical Approach.* New York, NY: John Wiley & Sons Inc; 1988.

11. Mulley AG. Assessing patient utilities: can the ends justify the means? *Med Care.* 1989;27(suppl): S269–S281.

12. Eisenberg JM. Clinical economics: a guide to the economic analysis of clinical practices. *JAMA.* 1989;262:2879–2886.

13. Guyatt GH. Measuring quality of life in clinical trials. *Can Med Assoc J.* 1989;140:1441–1448.

14. Emery DD, Schneiderman LJ. Cost-effectiveness analysis in health care. *Hastings Cent Rep.* 1989;19(4):8–13.

15. Jennings B. A grassroots movement in bioethics. *Hastings Cent Rep.* 1988;18(suppl to No. 3):1–16.

16. Garland MJ, Crawshaw R. Oregon's decision to curtail funding for organ transplantation. *N Engl J Med.* 1988;319:1420.

17. Welch HG, Larson EB. Dealing with limited resources: the Oregon decision to curtail funding for organ transplantation. *N Engl J Med.* 1988;319:171–173.

18. Todd J. It is time for universal access, not universal insurance. *N Engl J Med.* 1989;321: 46–47.

19. Aaron HJ, Schwartz WB. *The Painful Prescription: Rationing Health Care.* Washington, DC: The Brookings Institute; 1984.

20. Lund DS. Health care rationing plan OK'd in Oregon, stymied in California. *Am Med News.* July 21, 1989:1.

21. Churchill LR. *Rationing Health Care in America: Perceptions and Principles of Justice.* University of Notre Dame (Ind) Press; 1987.

22. Meyer H. Oregon Medicaid plan gets boost from health care executives' poll. *Am Med News.* March 16, 1990:2.

23. Patrick DL, Bush HW, Chen MM. Toward an operational definition of health. *J Health Soc Behav.* 1973;14:6–23.

24. Torrance GW, Sackett DL, Thomas WH. Utility maximization model for program evaluation: a demonstration application, Health Status Indexes. In: Berg RL, ed. *Proceedings of a Conference Conducted by Health Services Research Tucson, Arizona, 1972.* Chicago, Ill: Hospital Research and Educational Trust; 1973.

25. Weinstein MC, Stason WB. Foundations of cost-effectiveness analysis for health and medical practices. *N Engl J Med.* 1977;296:716–721.

26. Rosser R, Kind P. A scale of valuations of states of illness: is there a social consensus? *Int J Epidemiol.* 1978;7:347–358.

27. Deyo R, Patrick DL. Barriers to the use of health status measures in clinical investigation, patient care and policy research. *Med Care.* 1989;27(suppl):S254–S268.

28. Jennett B, Buxton M. Economics and the management of cancer: placing a value on human life. In: Stoll B, ed. *Social Impact of Cancer.* London, England: Macmillan Publishers Ltd; 1989.

29. Cassell EJ. *Talking With Patients: Clinical Technique.* Cambridge, Mass: MIT Press; 1985:2.

30. Williams A. The cost-effectiveness approach to the treatment of angina. In: Patterson DLH, ed. *The Management of Angina Pectoris.* Dobbs Ferry, NY: Castle House Publications; 1987:131–146.

31. Weinstein MC. Estrogen use in postmenopausal women. *N Engl J Med.* 1980;303:308–316.

32. Boyle MS, Torrance GW, Sinclair JC, Horwood SP. Economic evaluation of neonatal intensive care of very-low-birth-weight infants. *N Engl J Med.* 1983;308:1330–1337.

33. Churchill DN, Lemon BC, Torrance GW. A cost-effectiveness analysis of continuous ambulatory peritoneal dialysis and hospital hemodialysis. *Med Decis Making.* 1984;4:489–500.

34. Weinstein MC, Stason WB. Cost-effectiveness of coronary artery bypass surgery. *Circulation.* 1982;66(suppl III):III-56–III-66.

35. Barry MJ, Mulley AG, Fowler FJ, Wennberg JW. Watchful waiting vs immediate transurethral resection for symptomatic prostatism. *JAMA.* 1988;259:3010–3017.

36. Williams A. Economics of coronary artery bypass grafting. *Br Med J.* 1985;291:326–329.

37. Gudex C. *QALYs and Their Use by the Health Service.* University of York (England) Centre for Health Economics; 1986. Discussion Paper 20.

38. Gudex C. QALYs: an explicit outcome measure for today's NHS. *Public Finance Accountancy.* November 13, 1987:13–15.

39. Kind P, Rosser R, Williams A. Valuation of quality of life: some psychometric evidence. In: Jones-Lee MW, ed. *The Value of Life and Safety.* Amsterdam, the Netherlands: Elsevier/North Holland; 1982.

40. Ellwood PM. Shattuck Lecture: outcomes management: a technology of patient experience. *N Engl J Med.* 1988;318:1549–1556.

41. Drummond MF. Resource allocation decisions in health care: a role for quality of life assessments? *J Chronic Dis.* 1987;40:605–616.

42. Sisk JE. Discussion: Drummond's 'Resource Allocation Decisions in Health Care: A Role for Quality of Life Assessments?' *J Chronic Dis.* 1987;40:617–619.

43. Callahan D. *Setting Limits.* New York, NY: Simon & Schuster Inc Publishers; 1987.

44. Blendon RJ. The public's view of the future of health care. *JAMA.* 1988;259:3587–3593.

45. McNeil BJ, Pauker SG, Sox HC, Tversky A. On the elicitation of preferences for alternative therapies. *N Engl J Med.* 1982;306:1259–1262.

46. Lipscomb J. Time preference for health in cost-effectiveness analysis. *Med Care.* 1989; 27(suppl):S233–S248.

47. Piliskin JS, Shepard DS, Weinstein MC. Utility functions for life years and health status. *Operations Res.* 1980;28:206–224.

48. Caplan AL. How should values count in the allocation of new technologies in health care? In: Bayer R, Caplan AL, Daniels N, eds. *In Search of Equity: Health Care Needs and the Health Care System.* New York, NY: Plenum Press; 1983:95–124.

49. Siegler M. The progression of medicine: from physician paternalism to patient autonomy to bureaucratic parsimony. *Arch Intern Med.* 1985;145:713–715.

50. Mendeloff J. Measuring elusive benefits: on the value of health. *J Health Politics Policy Law.* 1983;8:554–580.

51. Abrams FR. Patient advocate or secret agent. *JAMA.* 1986;256:1784–1785.

52. Pearlman RA, Uhlmann RF, Cain KC. Quality of life in chronic diseases: perceptions of elderly patients. *J Gerontol.* 1988;43(2):M25–M30.

53. Danis M, Patrick DL, Southerland LI, Green ML. Patients' and families' preferences for medical intensive care. *JAMA.* 1988;260:797–802.

54. Uhlmann RF, Pearlman RA, Cain KC. Physicians' and spouses' predictions of elderly patients' resuscitation preferences. *J Gerontol.* 1988;43(5):M115–M121.

55. Zweibel NR, Cassel CK. Treatment choices at the end of life: a comparison of decisions by older patients and their physician-selected proxies. *Gerontologist.* 1989;29:615–621.

56. La Puma J, Schiedermayer DL, Gulyas AE, Siegler M. Talking to comatose patients. *Arch Neurol.* 1988;45:20–22.

57. Wolf SM. The persistent problem of PVS. *Hastings Cent Rep.* 1988;18(1):26.

58. Shaw A. QL revisited. *Hastings Cent Rep.* 1988;18(2):10–12.

59. Vladeck BC. Medicare hospital payment by diagnosis-related groups. *Ann Intern Med.* 1984;100:576–591.

60. Hsiao WC, Dunn DL. The impact of DRG payment on New Jersey hospitals. *Inquiry.* 1987;24:2120.

61. Greer EG, Kronenfeld JJ, Baker SL, Amidon RL. An appraisal of organizational response to fiscally constraining regulation: the case of hospitals and DRGs. *J Health Soc Behav.* 1989;30:41–55.

62. Kruse JA, Thill-Baharozian MC, Carlson RW. Comparison of clinical assessment with APACHE II for predicting mortality risk in patients admitted to a medical intensive care unit. *JAMA.* 1988;260:1739–1742.

63. Levinson DF. Toward full disclosure of referral restrictions and financial incentives by prepaid health plans. *N Engl J Med.* 1987;317:1729–1731.

64. Reagan MD. Physicians as gatekeepers: a complex challenge. *N Engl J Med.* 1987;317:1731–1734.

65. Hillman AL. Financial incentives for physicians in HMOs: is there a conflict of interest? *N Engl J Med.* 1987;317:1743–1748.

66. La Puma J, Cassel CK, Humphrey H. Ethics, economics, and endocarditis: the physician's role in resource allocation. *Arch Intern Med.* 1988;148:1809–1811.

67. Morreim EH. Fiscal scarcity and the inevitability of bedside budget balancing. *Arch Intern Med.* 1989;149:1012–1015.

68. In the courts. *Hastings Cent Rep.* 1986;16(6):32.

69. *Wickline v California,* 2nd Appellate District, Division 5, No. B010156, July 30, 1986.

70. Schiedermayer DL, La Puma J, Miles SH. Ethics consultations masking economic dilemmas in patient care. *Arch Intern Med.* 1989;149:1303–1305.

24 The Oregon Priority-Setting Exercise: Quality of Life and Public Policy

David C. Hadorn

David C. Hadorn is Senior Research Associate at the Center for Health Ethics and Policy, University of Colorado, Denver, Colorado, and a postdoctoral fellow in health services research at The RAND Corporation, Santa Monica, California.

I n 1989 the Oregon State legislature passed the Oregon Basic Health Services Act, which created a Health Services Commission charged with "developing a priority list of health services, ranging from the most important to the least important for the entire population to be served."[1] The goal of this legislation was to permit the expansion of Medicaid to 100 percent of all Oregonians living in poverty by covering only services deemed to be of sufficient importance or priority.

The Oregon Health Services Commission (OHSC) initially interpreted "for the entire population to be served" as suggesting the use of cost-effectiveness principles for developing the priority list. These principles are based on the utilitarian quest for "the greatest good for the greatest number" and tend to de-value adverse effects of a policy on specific individuals.[2] By the lights of cost-effectiveness, the "importance" of a health service depends not only on the expected outcomes of treatment (such as prolongation of life, reduction of pain), but also on the cost of that service and on the number of patients who can benefit from

This article first appeared in Hastings Center Report 20 *(May/June 1991): 11–16.*

it. Thus, even very beneficial treatments might not be considered important if the costs of providing those treatments are high or if only a few people benefit from them.

In keeping with their interpretation of the statute, the OHSC initially conducted a cost-effectiveness analysis of over 1,600 health services ranging from appendectomies to treatment of colds and flu. Predictably, the resulting draft list rated outpatient office visits for minor problems as the "most important" services; the cost of these visits was estimated at $98.51. Indeed, the first 94 items on Oregon's initial list were for office visits, for often self-limiting conditions such as thumb-sucking and low back pain. By contrast, certain life-saving surgeries, such as appendectomies, were rated relatively low because of their higher associated costs.

This counterintuitive priority order (and negative public reaction to it[3]) led the OHSC to abandon cost-effectiveness analysis for purposes of developing its final priority list.[4] Instead, the OHSC developed a set of seventeen health service "categories," which described either a specific type of service (for example, maternity care, preventive services) or, more generically, the expected outcomes of care (for example, "treatment of life-threatening illness where treatment restores life-expectancy and return to previous health"). Commissioners formally ranked these seventeen categories in order of importance according to three subjective criteria: value to the individual, value to society, and whether the category seemed "necessary."

Each treatment was then assigned to the single most appropriate category, based on Commissioners' judgment. Services were ranked within categories according to the degree of benefit expected from treatment. Finally, the OHSC rearranged apparently misplaced services "by hand," for example, moving obviously important services rated low by the method higher on the final list.

This alternate methodology produced a much more intuitively sensible final priority list than the earlier draft list, although more work may be needed before the "final" list can serve as the basis for public policy, particularly with respect to better specifying treatments and indications for treatment.[5]

At the time of this writing, independent actuaries are estimating the costs of providing services on the final list. The Oregon legislature will then decide whether to accept the list as the basis for expanding the State's Medicaid program, as per the Oregon Basic Health Services Act. If so, the legislature will draw a line somewhere on the list to separate the services that will be covered under Medicaid from those that will not. Finally, if this step is taken, Oregon will appeal to the federal government for a Medicaid waiver, which must be granted if the plan is to proceed.

ROLE OF QUALITY OF LIFE

The Oregon priority-setting process is significant in many ways, particularly with respect to its implications for social policy. Some of the most important of these implications relate to questions of distributive justice, including Rawlsian attempts to identify the least advantaged members of society and to assess how the Oregon process affects them. (For my money, the uninsured poor are the worst off and the Oregon process improves their lot.) In addition, the fact that cost-effectiveness analysis failed to produce a reasonable priority list has significant implications for future efforts to set health care priorities.[6]

Another important story concerning the Oregon priority-setting exercise remains to be told, however. This story concerns the critical role played by quality of life judgments in constructing Oregon's final priority list. Estimates of how treatments affect quality of life were by far the single most important factor in determining the priority order on that list. Most of the service categories that constituted the principal method of prioritization were explicitly defined in terms of quality of life or, in what was generally treated as an equivalent term, "health status." Furthermore, the secondary (within-category) rank-ordering was performed by reference to the "net benefit" from treatment, which, as we shall see, was an explicit *numerical* estimate of the impacts of treatment on quality of life.

Lack of understanding about the role of quality of life in formulating the final priority list has already led to erroneous interpretations of the list. For example, a spokesperson for Children's Defense Fund in Washington, D.C., criticized the fact that treatment for extremely premature infants (less than 500 grams and less than 23 weeks' gestation) was rated next to last on the list (just prior to treatment for infants born without a brain), saying, "If you're looking at it from a purely economic view, it makes sense not to cover those infants. Of course, we think it's completely unethical to do that."[7]

In fact, however, economic considerations had little or nothing to do with placement of this (or any other) treatment on the *final* list; rather, like most items near the bottom of the list, treatment of extremely premature infants was rated low because it had been assigned to the lowest-ranked service category: treatments offering "minimal or no improvement in QWB," or Quality of Well-Being, the OHSC's term for quality of life. It was a consideration of the *outcomes* (in this case, severe retardation and cerebral palsy) of treating extremely premature infants that led the OHSC to make this category assignment—and in turn determined placement on the final list.

Similarly, active medical or surgical treatments for terminally ill patients were rated near the bottom of the list by virtue of having been assigned to the same poor-outcome category just described. Terminally ill patients were defined (problematically, perhaps) as those with less than a 10 percent chance of surviving five years, even with treatment, and included patients suffering from "cancer with distant metastases" or "terminal HIV disease." Comfort care for these patients, including hospice programs and pain medication, was ranked relatively high, however—at 164 out of 709 total items—as was the longevity- and quality-of-life-enhancing drug AZT for patients with HIV disease, at 158.

BACKGROUND

Before describing the method used by the OHSC to obtain explicit estimates of quality-of-life outcomes (the basis for within-category ranking of services) a little background is required, both historical and philosophical. The focus on quality of life as a principal factor in health care resource allocation has a long history in Oregon, most of which concerns the activity of a community grassroots bioethics project known as Oregon Health Decisions (OHD).[8] For several years preceding creation of the OHSC, OHD had held hundreds of citizen meetings around the state to discuss health care and resource allocation issues. In September 1988 a Citizens Health Care Parliament was held in Portland in which fifty delegates met for a day and a half to develop "a set of public policy principles which are intended to be guideposts for the state legislature and other policy-makers concerned with health care resource allocation."[9] The principles developed by the parliament focused on quality of life to a remarkable extent. Indeed, the first six (of fifteen) principles contained explicit references to the importance of quality of life in making health care allocation decisions. Of particular interest are these:

1. The responsibility of government in providing health care resources is to improve the overall quality of life of people by acting within the limits of available financial and other resources.

4. Health care activities should be undertaken to increase the length of life and/or the health-related quality of life during one's life span.

5. Quality of life should be used as one of the ethical standards when allocating health care expenditures with insurance or government funds.

6. Health-related quality of life includes physical, mental, social, cognitive, and self-care functions, as well as a perception of pain and sense of well-being.

As part of the process of developing its priority list, the OHSC commissioned OHD to hold a series of public meetings to discuss people's values concerning the outcomes of care. OHD used a set of service categories similar to those ultimately adopted by the OHSC to elicit relative preferences for different treatments. Quality of life again emerged as a major priority.

ETHICAL CONSIDERATIONS

One final, critical clarification is required before describing the OHSC's approach to measuring quality of life. The use of quality of life information to develop public policy is potentially problematic from a couple of perspectives. First, the use of purely objective measures of quality of life, such as the degree of assistance required to walk or level of independence in self-care activities, does not correlate well with *perceived* quality of life. For example, Najman and Levine reviewed an extensive literature in which quality of life reports were obtained from patients who were "objectively" living restricted lives. Almost invariably, perceived quality of life was higher than might have been predicted.[10]

Second, judging others' quality of life may place us on a slippery slope. In the *Encyclopedia of Bioethics*, Reich notes that judgments of "unacceptable quality of life" are often determined by the "social acceptability" of various diseases or conditions.[11] Similarly, Harris worries about the use of quality of life for resource allocation policy:

> If for example some people were given life-saving treatment in preference to others because they had a better quality of life than those others, or more dependents and friends, or because they were considered more useful, this would amount to regarding such people as more valuable than others on that account. Indeed it would be tantamount, literally, to sacrificing the lives of others so that they might continue to live. . . . To discriminate between people on the grounds of quality of life . . . is as unwarranted as it would be to discriminate on the grounds of race or gender.[12]

There is, however, a key distinction between underestimating quality of life or using the concept to bring about invidious discrimination, on the one hand, and Oregon's use of it on the other. Specifically, the concerns expressed in the previous paragraphs involve judgments made about a person's quality of life at a given point in time—independent of any medical or surgical treatments. Such judgments are *inappropriate* bases upon which to ground resource allocation policy.

By contrast, the *appropriate*, non-discriminatory way to deal with quality-of-life information (and the approach adopted by the OHSC) is to focus on the *change* in quality of life expected with the use of a specific treatment or procedure. How much *better* or *worse* (if at all) is a patient's quality of life likely to be with application of a particular health service? This focus permits appropriate consideration to be given to the important impacts of treatments on quality of life which, as described earlier, are of considerable importance to the public in determining fair and rational systems of resource allocation. At the same time, the potential for discrimination is eliminated because treatments for handicapped or "poor quality of life" patients are evaluated on the same basis as are treatments for everyone else. It is the *change* in quality of life, or net benefit, realized from a *treatment* that matters, not the *point-in-time* quality of life of a *patient*.

Quality-Adjusted Life Years

After consulting with advisors at Oregon Health Decisions, the OHSC decided to incorporate quality of life considerations into the priority-setting process using the "quality-adjusted life year" (QALY) approach.[13] This method permits integration of the quality-of-life effects of treatment with its associated impacts on life expectancy. Some treatments, such as appendectomies, are valued not for any improvements in quality of life, but rather for their substantial positive effects in life expectancy: in the case of appendicitis, going from perhaps two weeks to normal. Other treatments have significant impact on quality of life, but little or no effect on life expectancy—such as medication or surgery for arthritis, or prostatectomy for benign obstruction. Still other treatments involve trade-offs between quality and quantity of life, where a longer life expectancy may come at the expense of various side effects from treatment, resulting in a possible decrease in quality of life.

Use of the QALY approach requires the explicit estimation of "percentage of normal quality of life." One year of "normal" quality of life is considered equivalent in value to two years of "one-half normal" quality of life: moreover, two treatments offering these respective outcomes would be valued equally (other things being equal). The QALY concept is useful primarily because it reminds us of a few key principles:

> *Necessity.* We have no choice but to consider both quality and quantity of life in some integrative fashion to properly evaluate health care services.

> *Common Sense.* Other things being equal, treatments offering fewer net benefits in terms of either quality of life, longevity, or both, should be valued less highly than treatments offering more such benefits. Thus, if two treatments each offer about a

year of additional life, the one that offers greater benefits in terms of quality of life should be favored.

Proportionate Value. Building on the last concept, treatments should be valued *roughly in proportion to the degree of benefit they offer to patients.* Thus, we should be able to distinguish between treatments that offer highly valued outcomes, such as comfort and the relief of pain that is characteristic of hospice programs, from treatments that provide less-valued outcomes, such as the marginal prolongation of life with severe side effects characteristic of many aggressive treatments for terminally ill patients. The QALY approach in theory permits this sort of distinction to be made.

Several problems with the QALY concept have so far caused it to remain merely a heuristic device, by limiting real-world application:

Questionable Assumption. The QALY method assumes that people see no difference between, say, one year of normal-quality life and ten years of life at one-tenth quality (whatever *that* is). The QALY approach assumes that a short, good life is of equal value to a long, ailing one. This assumption seems unlikely to be valid.

Equity Problems. The QALY approach suffers from a limitation common to any purely utilitarian construct: our intuitive rejection of conclusions to the effect that one person should be treated rather than many. In particular, QALY logic supposes that if a choice comes down to treating one person who stands to gain ten QALYs, or nine people who each stand to gain one QALY, then the single person should be treated.

Measurement Problems. What does it mean to speak of someone having a "one-tenth normal" quality of life? How could we come up with such an overall numerical estimate? Anyway, how can we quantify a *quality,* especially one so amorphous and ill-defined as quality of life?

The first two of these problems speak to the fact that QALYs cannot be used as the sole basis for resource allocation decisionmaking. This conclusion is hardly new; even the staunchest advocates of the QALY concept realize that the conflict between individual and societal preferences and issues of justice and equity must also be entered into the resource allocation equation.

It is the measurement problem that is responsible for the fact that QALYs have had so little impact on the health care system since their introduction almost twenty years ago. And it is here that the OHSC made its greatest methodological contribution to the goal of setting health care priorities. As such, the Oregon process represents the first large-scale effort in the United States to operationalize the QALY concept for purposes of resource allocation policy.

THE OHSC METHOD FOR QUALITY OF LIFE MEASUREMENT

The methodology adopted by the OHSC for estimating QALYs was based on a set of descriptions of poor health or impaired quality of life borrowed (after slight modification) from a set of generic quality-of-life states developed by Kaplan and Bush.[14] These states consist of descriptions of physical or emotional symptoms and of different degrees of limitations or impairment in mobility, physical activity, and social activity. The OHSC assigned each quality-of-life problem a decrement value, based on the results of a telephone survey of 1,000 randomly selected Oregonians (see below), estimating the degree to which each problem would reduce overall quality of life. Figure 1 shows some of the quality-of-life states used by the OHSC, as well as their associated decrement values. For example, "moderate limitation in physical activity" and "seizure, fainting, or coma" were estimated to reduce overall quality of life by about 37 percent and 11 percent, respectively.

To derive a numerical estimate of the quality-of-life benefit from treatments, local physicians predicted which problems, if any, patients would experience *five years* after diagnosis, both *with* and *without* treatment. (The five-year window was selected as a reasonable yardstick against which to standardize the expected benefit of different treatments and procedures.) The numerical difference between the aggregate values of the treated compared to untreated health states was considered to be the *net benefit* from treatment.

An example of this process is shown in Figure 2; analogous calculations were performed for each service on the priority list. In this case, the evaluated treatment was surgery for bleeding into the brain. Consultant physicians estimated that without surgery 95 percent of patients with this condition would die within five years, and that the five-year mortality rate would drop to 20 percent if surgery was performed. Furthermore, physicians predicted that all untreated survivors would experience severe disability, including difficulty with cognition, whereas "only" 40 percent of treated patients would experience such a disability. On the other hand, 20 percent of the patients who undergo surgery for this

Figure 1. Descriptions of Limitations and Symptoms Used to Calculate Net Benefit from Treatment
(Partial List)

Limitation or Symptom	Decrement Value
Moderate mobility limitation (e.g., unable to use transportation outside the home)	−.046
Major mobility limitation (e.g., hospitalized)	−.049
Moderate physical activity limitation (e.g., wheelchair)	−.373
Major physical activity limitation (e.g., bedbound)	−.560
Moderate social activity limitation (e.g., unable to work)	−.062
Major social activity limitation (e.g., unable to perform self-care activities)	−.106
Loss of consciousness such as seizure, fainting, or coma	−.114
Burn over large areas of face, body, arms, or legs	−.372
Trouble learning, remembering, or thinking clearly	−.367
Any combination of one or more hands, feet, arms, or legs either missing, deformed, paralyzed, or broken—includes wearing artificial limbs or braces	−.277
Sick or upset stomach, vomiting or loose bowel movement, with or without fever, chills, or aching all over	−.370
General tiredness, weakness, or weight loss	−.275
Coughing, wheezing, or shortness of breath, with or without fever, chills, or aching all over	−.318
Spells of feeling upset, being depressed, or of crying	−.326
Trouble talking, such as lisp, stuttering, hoarseness, or being unable to talk	−.188

Descriptions were slightly modified by the OHSC from Kaplan's QWB scale (Robert Kaplan and John Anderson, "A General Health Policy Model: Update and Applications," *Health Services Research* 23 [1988]: 203–35).

Decrement values were obtained as described in the text.

Figure 2. Example of Net Benefit Calculation

Problem: Subarachnoid and Intracerebral Hemorrhage/Hematoma

Without Treatment

(Outcomes expected in five years)	Percent of Patients	Decrement Value	Percentage x Value
1. Dead	95%	−1.00	−.950
2. Moderate mobility limitation		−.046	−.002
+			
Major physical activity limitation		−.560	−.028
+	5%		
Major social activity limitation		−.106	−.005
+			
Trouble learning, remembering, or thinking clearly		−.367	−.018
3. Asymptomatic	0%	0	0
	100%		−1.003

Value of Expected Untreated Health Status = 1.00 (good health) − 1.003 = −.003

LEGEND: Percentage of patients expected to experience specified health states with and without treatment. Decrement values are from Figure 1.

Treatment: Burr Holes, Craniectomy/Craniotomy

With Treatment

(Outcomes expected in five years)	Percent of Patients	Decrement Value	Percentage x Value
1. Dead	20%	−1.00	−.200
2. Moderate mobility limitation		−.046	−.016
+			
Major physical activity limitation		−.560	−.224
+	40%		
Major social activity limitation		−.106	−.040
+			
Trouble learning, remembering, or thinking clearly		−.367	−.146
3. Loss of consciousness such as seizure, fainting, or coma	10%	−.114	−.011
4. Trouble talking, such as lisp, stuttering, hoarseness, or being unable to talk	10%	−.188	−.018
5. Asymptomatic	20%	0	0
	100%		−.655

Value of Expected Treated Health Status = 1.00 (good health) − .655 = .345

The difference in value between untreated vs. treated states in this example is [.345 − (−.003)] = .348, equivalent to about a third of the "distance" between being alive and being dead.

condition were predicted to suffer from residual side effects (loss of consciousness and difficulty speaking) that were not predicted to occur in untreated patients. Thus, the expected risks and side-effects of treatment were "deducted" from any expected benefits in estimating overall impacts on quality of life.

As shown in Figure 2, the predicted aggregate health status of *untreated* patients figured to a little less than zero—a little worse, that is, than being dead. *Treated* patients, on average, were expected to be restored to about 35 percent of normal quality of life (i.e., 0.348), which is a substantial improvement over a "worse-than-death" state. This example also demonstrates the lack of discrimination against handicapped people that occurs when only *changes* in quality of life *with treatment* are considered. Thus, even though most survivors of this condition are expected to be significantly handicapped, even with treatment, the large improvement in expected quality of life resulted in a relatively high priority ranking for this treatment (no. 86).

The impact of treatment on *life-expectancy*—the other component of the QALY measure—was integrated in two ways. First, life-expectancy was factored into the equation by virtue of the "zero quality of life" status assigned to the percentage of patients estimated to die in each group. Second, the net-benefit component was multiplied by the expected duration of that benefit for computation of cost-effectiveness ratios, although the "net-benefit" component alone—without multiplication by expected duration of benefit—was used to prioritize services within categories for creating the final priority list.

ANALYSIS OF THE OREGON PROCESS

Several features of the described method for setting priorities are of interest. Most fundamentally, perhaps, the QALY approach to priority setting was a systematic alternative to more traditional methods of involving the public in health care resource allocation. More typically, citizens are asked which *programs* they prefer: neonatal intensive care units, transplant surgery programs, screening for high blood pressure, hospice care, and so on. This approach is limited by the fact that most people know very little about the expected health outcomes associated with these programs, or about associated costs and other important factors that should shape public policy. By contrast, the method adopted by the OHSC asked people about their preferences for the *outcomes* of care, including various states of ill health and disability. Everyone has been ill at one time or another and has experienced at least temporary periods of disability. Most people are in a position to recall what care can do, and therefore can offer opinions about various states of health that are better informed than their opinions about programs.

Several questions arise, however, regarding (1) the process of asking people to imagine a state of poor health and to apply a rating to that state and (2) the subsequent process of aggregating individual ratings. I take up these problems more fully elsewhere,[15] but a couple of issues deserve brief mention here. First, I believe that Oregon was correct in surveying generally healthy citizens, rather than actively ill patients, because the inevitable biases of the latter group would hopelessly confound the rating process. True, people may have difficulty imagining states of poor health or of impaired quality of life, but by surveying enough people (and 1,000 randomly selected individuals is more than enough) an adequate indication of public preferences can probably be obtained. Moreover, in related work we have found that the task of imagining and rating health states can be substantially facilitated by using visual representations of the various states, and by using paired comparisons in addition to simple ratings of individual health states.[16]

But what about the prototypical problem of the "happy quadriplegic"? How can we account for the fact that many patients with chronic illnesses or disabilities adjust emotionally to those states? This is a common enough finding. Might it be a mistake, therefore, to label a severely impaired or painful health state as less desirable than one without impairment or pain? Surely no, for although people in wheelchairs may adjust to their situation, it does not follow that they would not value a procedure that enabled them to walk again. This consideration relates again to the importance of focusing on *changes* in quality of life brought about by health services.

Another important observation is that OHSC's use of *generic health states* (those that can be applied to any illness or condition, rather than illness- or treatment-specific outcomes) enabled all types of health services to be denominated in terms of a "common currency" of benefits and harms. This is a critical consideration from the perspective of health care resource allocation,[17] since it is necessary to compare directly the outcomes of, say, coronary bypass surgery with those of chemotherapy to assess the relative value of these two procedures.

Thus, Oregon's process—explicitly estimating generic treatment outcomes, weighted according to empirically derived public values for those outcomes—was a sophisticated exercise in priority setting, congruent with contemporary thinking. Just this sort of approach is required if public values are to be meaningfully incorporated into the priority-setting process.

Inevitably, however, the Oregon effort to implement a preference-for-outcomes approach was limited by imperfections in available methods. A couple of examples will suffice. The described health states are very broad, often encompassing a wide variety of problems and conditions. For example, the "trouble talking" state incorporates everything from a slight lisp to total mutism. Moreover, the decrement values assigned to the states often do not make sense; "unable to use transportation outside the home" was rated the same as "bed-bound," while "burn over large areas of the body" was rated the same as an "upset stomach."

The rating problem may be due in part to the simplified telephone rating task used to obtain decrement values. Raters were asked to assign a numerical rating between 0 and 100 (0=death, 100=good health) to each of 10 health states. A typical scenario was: "You can go anywhere and have no limitations on physical or other activity but have stomach aches, vomiting, or diarrhea." (Ratings were then rescaled to a decrement value between 0 and 1, with higher numbers associated with more serious, lower-rated problems.) Thus, only one problem at a time was stipulated to be present in each scenario; everything else was assumed to be normal. Obviously, this assumption is problematic, since illness and disability tend to occur together. It is difficult to imagine a patient with a large burn, for example, who is not limited in mobility and social activity. In related work, we have observed that the use of a similar one-dimensional, direct rating approach failed to produce valid preference ratings.[18]

A related potential problem with OHSC's quality-of-life measurement method is that the decrement values of the various problems and conditions are assumed to be cumulative in their effect on overall quality of life. There is evidence, however, that the interactions among quality of life problems is more complicated than simple addition would suggest.[19]

These methodological limitations notwithstanding, the Oregon priority-setting exercise was a remarkably far-sighted and sophisticated effort to incorporate quality of life measurement into resource allocation policy. The OHSC correctly focused on the *change* in quality of life afforded by *treatments*, rather than on *point-in-time* quality of life assessments of *patients* or on people's feelings about health care *programs*. The method selected by the OHSC properly included the explicit estimation of (generic) outcomes of treatment and empirically derived preferences for those outcomes.

Only the details of this process—among them, better specification of health states—need change in subsequent iterations of the Oregon process. In the meantime, can Oregon's final list serve as a legitimate basis for public policy? The answer to this question is unclear, and may depend on whether and how Oregon better specifies treatments and indications for treatment.[20] Much more will be known in a few months, after the Oregon legislature has considered the list and federal action is taken on a Medicaid waiver. The events in Oregon are critically important for American health and social policy; they will bear close watching over the coming months and years.

ACKNOWLEDGMENT

Preparation of this article was supported by a grant from the Pew Charitable Trusts.

REFERENCES

1. Oregon Senate Bill 27.

2. Milton Weinstein and William Stason, "Foundations of Cost-effectiveness Analysis for Health and Medical Practices," *NEJM* 296 (1976): 716–21.

3. T. Egan, "Problems Could Delay Proposal by Oregon to Ration Health Care," *New York Times*, 30 July 1990.

4. David Hadorn, "Setting Health Care Priorities in Oregon: Cost-effectiveness Meets the Rule of Rescue," *JAMA* 265 (1991): 2218–25.

5. Hadorn, "Setting Health Care Priorities."

6. Hadorn, "Setting Health Care Priorities."

7. Dean Mayer and Merit Kimball, "Oregon Commission OKs Medicaid Pecking Order," *Healthweek*, 25 February 1991, pp. 1, 36.

8. Brian Hines, "Health Policy on the Town Meeting Agenda," *Hastings Center Report* 16, no. 2 (1986): 5–7; Bruce Jennings, "Community Health Decisions: A Grassroots Movement in Bioethics," *Hastings Center Report* 18, no. 5, Special Supplement (1988).

9. "Quality of Life in Allocating Health Care Resources," adopted by the Citizens Health Care Parliament, 23–24 September 1988, Portland, Oregon.

10. Jackob Najman and Sol Levine, "Evaluating the Impact of Medical Care and Technologies on the Quality of Life: A Review and Critique," *Social Science and Medicine* 15 (1981): 107–15.

11. Warren Reich, "Life: Quality of Life," *Encyclopedia of Bioethics* (New York: The Free Press, 1978), pp. 829–40, at 837.

12. John Harris, "QALYifying the Value of Life," *Journal of Medical Ethics* 13 (1987): 117–23, at 121.

13. Graham Loomes and Lynda McKenzie, "The Use of QALYs in Health Care Decision Making," *Social Science and Medicine* 28 (1989): 299–308.

14. Robert Kaplan and James Bush, "Health-Related Quality of Life Measurement for Evaluation Research and Policy Analysis," *Health Psychology* 1 (1982): 61–80.

15. David Hadorn, "The Role of Public Values in Setting Health Care Priorities," *Social Science and Medicine* 52 (1991): 773–81.

16. David Hadorn, T. Hauber, and Ron Hays, "Improving Task Comprehension in the Measurement of Health State Preferences: A Trial of Informational Cartoon Figures and a Paired-Comparison Task." Unpublished.

17. Hadorn, "The Role of Public Values."

18. David Hadorn and Ron Hays, "Multitrait-multimethod Analysis of Health-related Quality of Life Measures," *Medical Care* 1991, forthcoming.

19. G. Torrance, M. Boyle, and S. Horwood, "Application of Multi-Attribute Utility Theory to Measure Social Preferences for Health States," *Operations Research* 30 (1982): 1043–69.

20. Hadorn, "Setting Health Care Priorities."

25 *Ethics, Public Policy, and Human Fetal Tissue Transplantation Research*

JAMES F. CHILDRESS, PH.D.

James F. Childress, Ph.D. is Edwin B. Kyle Professor of Religious Ethics and Professor of Medical Education at the University of Virginia where he also chairs the Department of Religious Studies.

Controversy about the use of human fetal tissue following elective abortions has raged in the United States over the last few years. The debate centers on transplantation research, especially research that might benefit patients suffering from Parkinson's disease. Ethical arguments have been hurled back and forth about public policies—primarily about whether the federal government should fund such research. In this article I want to analyze and assess various arguments in the debate. I will focus on the deliberations of the Human Fetal Tissue Transplantation Research (HFTTR) Panel, on which I served as a member from September to December 1988.[1]

BACKGROUND

It is important to distinguish fetal research, i.e., research on the living (viable or nonviable) fetus, in utero or ex utero, from the use of tissue from dead fetuses in research. Fetal research is subject to careful scrutiny; federal regulations permit it only under very stringent conditions (Levine 1986, chap. 13). However, fetal tissue has been used in research for many years; one major, widely noted example of its use was in the development of the polio vaccine.[2] In 1987, the National Institutes of Health (NIH) provided more than $11 million in 116 grants and contracts that directly or indirectly used human fetal tissue (OSPL-OD-NIH 1988).

Transplantation research uses fetal tissue *as* therapy rather than to develop therapy (Nolan 1988). On the basis of animal research in the

This article first appeared in the Kennedy Institute of Ethics Journal 1 *(June 1991): 93–121.*

434

United States and elsewhere, several researchers outside the United States experimentally transplanted human fetal neural tissue into patients with Parkinson's disease (Vawter et al. 1990, pp. 57–82; Hoffer 1988). It may have some advantages in treating Parkinson's disease because it is immunologically more naive than developed tissue, and grows and differentiates rapidly. Another experimental procedure is the transplantation of fetal pancreatic tissue into patients with diabetes (Vawter et al. 1990, pp. 57–82; Hoffer 1988). Transplantation of human fetal thymus is now an established therapy for DiGeorge's syndrome, a rare condition of varying degrees of severity (Buckley 1988; Vawter et al. 1990, pp. 21–56).

However, in October 1987, when researchers at the NIH asked for permission to conduct research using tissue from electively aborted fetuses, NIH Director James Wyngaarden chose not to exercise his legal authority to approve that research. Instead, he sought approval from the office of the secretary of the Department of Health and Human Services (DHHS) because of the politically sensitive nature of the research (Wyngaarden 1987). The director's request focused on potential public controversy, but the staff of the Assistant Secretary for Health Robert Windom, which responded to his query, stressed the ethical issues. In March 1988, the assistant secretary declared a moratorium on the use of federal funds in human fetal tissue transplantation research involving tissue from induced abortions until the NIH could convene "special outside advisory committees" to hear testimony, deliberate, and offer recommendations. He wanted the committees to address ten questions, focusing mainly on the connection or linkage between abortion and the use of human fetal tissue in research (see box).

During the summer of 1988, the NIH appointed the Human Fetal Tissue Transplantation Research Panel consisting of twenty-one ethicists, lawyers, biomedical researchers, clinical physicians, public policy experts, and religious leaders. They had been recommended by various sources, including members of Congress, members of the Executive Branch, and organizations interested in this research. While defenders of HFTTR worried about the role on the Panel of strong opponents of abortion, critics of HFTTR objected to what they viewed as the Panel's overall bias in favor of such research.

Before the HFTTR Panel's first meeting a draft executive order that proposed banning HFTTR with tissue from electively aborted fetuses was leaked from the White House. However, Dr. Otis Bowen, the secretary of the Department of Health and Human Services, decided not to impose new restrictions on HFTTR until the advisory committees reported or until the president issued a direct order. The next several weeks saw vigorous efforts to persuade the president to promulgate

Questions Posed by the Assistant Secretary for Health

1. Is an induced abortion of moral relevance to the decision to use human fetal tissue for research? Would the answer to this question provide any insight on whether and how this research should proceed?

2. Does the use of fetal tissue in research encourage women to have an abortion that they might otherwise not undertake? If so, are there ways to minimize such encouragement?

3. As a legal matter, does the very process of obtaining informed consent from the pregnant woman constitute a prohibited "inducement" to terminate the pregnancy for the purposes of the research—thus precluding research of this sort, under HHS regulations?

4. Is maternal consent a sufficient condition for the use of the tissue, or should additional consent be obtained? If so, what should be the substance and who should be the source(s) of the consent, and what procedures should be implemented to obtain it?

5. Should there be and could there be a prohibition on the donation of fetal tissue between family members, or friends and acquaintances? Would a prohibition on donation between family members jeopardize the likelihood of clinical success?

6. If transplantation using fetal tissue from induced abortions becomes more common, what impact is likely to occur on activities and procedures employed by abortion clinics? In particular, is the optimal or safest way to perform an abortion likely to be in conflict with preservation of the fetal tissue? Is there any way to ensure that induced abortions are not intentionally delayed in order to have a second trimester fetus for research and transplantation?

7. What actual steps are involved in procuring the tissue from the source to the researcher? Are there any payments involved? What types of payments in this situation, if any, would fall inside or outside the scope of the Hyde Amendment?

8. According to HHS regulations, research on dead fetuses must be conducted in compliance with State and local laws. A few States' enacted version of the Uniform Anatomical Gift Act contains restrictions on the research applications of dead fetal tissue after induced abortion. In those States, do these restrictions apply to therapeutic transplantation of dead fetal tissue after an induced abortion? If so, what are the consequences for NIH-funded researchers in those States?

9. For those diseases for which transplantation using fetal tissue has been proposed, have enough animal studies been performed to justify proceeding to human transplants? Because induced abortions during the first trimester are less risky to the woman, have there been enough animal studies for each of those diseases to justify the reliance on the equivalent of the second trimester human fetus?

10. What is the likelihood that transplantation using fetal cell cultures will be successful? Will this obviate the need for fresh fetal tissue? In what time frame might this occur?

the executive order. In separate letters, fifty members of Congress and several hundred physicians and others strongly supported the executive order. However, the president took no action.

Then in three public meetings in 1988 (September 14–16, October 20–21, and December 5) the HFTTR Panel heard scientific, legal, and ethical testimony from more than fifty invited speakers and more than fifteen representatives of public interest groups. The panel subsequently drafted "responses" to the assistant secretary's questions, and offered "considerations" for those responses. The Panel concluded that it is "acceptable public policy" for HFTTR to proceed, with federal funds, as long as several guidelines or safeguards are put into place. The safeguards would separate as much as possible the pregnant woman's decision to abort from her decision to donate fetal tissue following the abortion. Four of the twenty-one members of the Panel filed dissents to the report.

On December 14, 1988, the report was submitted to the NIH Director's Advisory Committee. The Committee concluded that:

> the consensus of the Panel reflected the consensus of the country itself, where widely divergent views are held about the morality of elective abortions and about the use of fetal materials derived from such abortions for the purposes of research. (NIH 1988, p. 4)

The Committee unanimously recommended: (1) acceptance of the report and its recommendations; (2) lifting of the moratorium on federal funding of HFTTR; and (3) acceptance of current laws and regulations governing human fetal tissue research along with the development of "additional policy guidance as appropriate, to be prepared by NIH staff, to implement the recommendations of the Human Fetal Tissue Transplantation Research Panel" (NIH 1988, p. 1). No action was taken for almost a year—until November 2, 1989—when the Secretary of the Department of Health and Human Services Louis Sullivan indefinitely extended the moratorium in a letter to William F. Raub, acting director of the NIH.

THE MORAL STATUS OF THE FETUS
AND THE MORALITY OF ABORTION

More than 1.5 million legal abortions occur each year in the United States, some of which most moral and religious traditions would view as ethically justified. For example, there were approximately 75,000 ectopic pregnancies in 1985; about half of these end early in spontaneous abortions and the others in induced abortions to save the pregnant woman

(Vawter et al. 1990, pp. 135–36). Protestants, Catholics (through the rule of double effect), and Jews (through the primacy of maternal health), generally accept abortions in such cases as ethically justified. However, abortions that are generally viewed as ethically justifiable would not provide sufficient fetal tissue. Spontaneous abortions are often marked by fetal conditions that preclude the use of the tissue. Thus, fetal tissue for transplantation would sometimes probably come from abortions that many would not consider ethically justifiable. Moral opposition to many abortions is the main source of the controversy about HFTTR.

There are three major views about the status of fetal life. The fetus may be viewed as (1) mere tissue, (2) potential human life, or (3) full human life. Abortions pose no serious moral problems for those embracing the first view. For those who accept either the second or the third view of fetal life, the fetus has some independent moral standing. In the second view, abortions are not absolutely wrong but they are prima facie or presumptively wrong and thus stand in need of moral justification. Proponents of this view disagree about which reasons are adequate to justify abortions. According to the third view, abortions are generally wrong, except perhaps to protect maternal life.

The moral framework for HFTTR based on the first view is that of tissue donation by a living donor; the fetal tissue belongs to the pregnant woman who may dispose of it as she chooses, just as she may dispose of other products of conception, such as the placenta. For those who defend the second or third view of the fetus, acceptance of HFTTR depends on whether they believe it is possible to separate—morally and practically—the use of fetal tissue from the (immoral) abortions that produce the tissue. Proponents of the third view tend to oppose HFTTR more strongly than those who defend the second view, but even some proponents of the third view can accept HFTTR because it uses tissue from dead fetuses. For example, Judge Arlin Adams, who chaired the HFTTR Panel, strongly opposes abortion except in very limited circumstances, but he believes that HFTTR can be separated from abortion decisions. Such separation can be more readily secured, he argues, through regulations associated with federal funding of the research (Adams 1988, pp. 25–26).

For those who defend the third view of fetal life, the fundamental issue is what *equal respect* entails. The HFTTR Panel insisted on procedures that would accord dead human fetuses "the same respect accorded other cadaveric human tissue entitled to respect" (*Report of the HFTTR Panel* 1988, I:1). Although the Panel did not develop its implications, this requirement of equal respect precludes subjecting the dead human fetus to procedures that would be considered inappropriate because undignified or disrespectful toward cadaveric human tissue. Acceptance of the requirement of equal respect does not necessarily presuppose a conviction that the fetus is a full human being. Rather it may rest on the conviction (1) that the fetus is a potential human being and that the dead fetus has symbolic significance, or (2) that respect for human fetal tissue is appropriate to avoid giving offense to those who view the fetus as full (or potential) human life.

This principle of equal respect implies that if it is justifiable to use any cadaveric human tissue in transplantation research—for example, that obtained after accidents or homicides—then it is justifiable to use cadaveric fetal tissue after abortions. However, opponents of HFTTR distinguish fetal tissue obtained after elective abortions from other cadaveric human tissue in part because they link use of fetal tissue to the abortion that produced it. That is the argument I will explore in the remainder of this article.

Just as it is possible for people with differing views on the status of the fetus and the morality of abortion to accept HFTTR, so it is possible to advocate guidelines that would separate decisions to abort from decisions to donate fetal tissue without implying a single view on the morality of abortion. The Panel proposed such guidelines to reduce the possibility that a pregnant woman's decision to abort would be influenced by the opportunity to donate fetal tissue. Some panelists supported them not because they believed abortion is immoral, but to reduce the chance of exploitation and coercion of pregnant women as sources of fetal tissue, and to avoid fanning the flames of moral controversy about abortion.

The Report notes that:

> a decisive majority of the panel found that it was acceptable public policy to support transplant research with fetal tissue either because the source of the tissue posed no moral problem or because the immorality of its source could be ethically isolated from the morality of its use in research. (*Report of the HFTTR Panel* 1988, I:2)

In short, the majority rejected the view that HFTTR should not receive federal funds because it is, morally speaking, inextricably linked to, or would lead to, immoral abortions.

COMPLICITY, COLLABORATION, AND ASSOCIATION IN MORAL EVIL

Roman Catholic moral theology has a long tradition of reflection on degrees of complicity in moral evil, i.e., complicity in the moral wrongdoing of others. James Burtchaell, a theologian at Notre Dame University, invoked this tradition to stress the impossibility of separating, at least in practice, the use of fetal tissue from the (immoral) abortions that produce the tissue. He raised it in the Panel's deliberations, in a dissent (with James Bopp), and in separate articles. (The language of complicity also appears in Rabbi J. David Bleich's dissent.)

Many of Burtchaell's statements are heavily metaphorical and require careful scrutiny to determine exactly how agents who are involved in the use of fetal tissue following elective abortions may be complicitous in the abortions themselves. For example, he uses such phrases as "supportive alliance," "acquiescent partnership," "silent but unmistakable alliance," "accomplices," "confederates," and "ally" (see Burtchaell 1988, 1989; Bopp and Burtchaell 1988).[3] From his perspective, nothing may be intrinsically wrong with using fetal tissue, just as nothing may be intrinsically wrong about using the tissue of other dead human beings. It is the connection with acts and practices of abortion that is morally problematic.

In a very careful analysis of the issues of complicity in the context of HFTTR, a report from the University of Minnesota's Center for Biomedical Ethics identifies four major types of involvement that may be alleged to render an agent complicit in the wrongdoing of others (Vawter et al. 1990, pp. 251–67). The first two involve causal responsibility—for particular immoral abortions, or for the practice of abortion. According to these HFTTR would (1) lead some women to abort when they would not otherwise have aborted, and (2) would provide societal legitimation of abortion practices, thus rendering society less willing to restrict abortion practices.

In order to identify what is distinctive about the complicity arguments offered by Burtchaell, among others, I want to focus on two other versions of complicity identified in the Minnesota report, which imply approval of immoral abortions, and acceptance of benefits from immoral abortions. In both versions the agents are not causally and morally responsible for the evil actions of others (i.e., immoral abortions), but through their own actions they are complicitous with those evil actions, even after those actions have occurred. All complicity need not be causative. Thus, it is important to distinguish various forms of cooperation that involve causal actions, links in a chain of actions, or parts of a composite action—for example, driving the getaway car after a robbery—from actions that only symbolize, convey, or express approval of the wrong actions of others, without materially contributing to the wrongdoing. Particularly important for Burtchaell is a form of indirect association that implies moral approval: "It is the sort of association which implies and engenders approval that creates moral complicity" (Burtchaell 1988, p. 9).

Burtchaell has invoked various analogies to establish moral complicity. In one analogy, "the Florida banker who accepts for deposit large sums of money from drug transactions that are already completed becomes complicit in the drug trade: after the sales, after the fact," even though it was complete before his subsequent involvement (Burtchaell 1989, p. 10).[4] The banker differs little from the researcher who visits the abortionist each week to obtain fetal tissue, expressing each time his disapproval of abortion, noting that it will continue whatever he does, and making plans to return the following week. Burtchaell's claim is that even though the wrongdoing occurs apart from the complicitous agent's actions, his or her actions involve an association that both yields benefits and conveys approval. Even if the agent expressly condemns the wrong actions, his or her association symbolically eviscerates those condemnations. The agents' actions involve complicity in the moral wrongdoing of others, whether drug trafficking or abortion, whatever the agents say. The agents become accessories after the fact.

Sometimes, as his examples suggest, Burtchaell stresses the institutionalization of the relationship with the wrongdoer and the wrongdoing. For example, he and Bopp write in their dissent from the Panel's report:

> Our argument, then, is that whatever the researcher's intentions may be, by entering into an institutionalized partnership with the abortion industry as a supplier of preference, he or she becomes complicit, though after the fact, with the abortions that have expropriated the tissue for his or her purposes. (Bopp and Burtchaell 1988, p. 70)

Similarly, in written testimony to the Panel, the Bishops' Committee for Pro-Life Activities of the National Conference of Catholic Bishops observed:

> It may not be wrong *in principle* for someone unconnected with an abortion to make use of a fetal organ from an unborn child who died as a result of an abortion; but it is difficult to see how this *practice can be institutionalized* (including arrangements to ensure informed consent) without threatening a morally unacceptable collaboration with the abortion industry. (*Report of the HFTTR Panel* 1988, II:E14, emphasis added)

Which agents are complicitous with the wrongdoing of abortion in HFTTR? Presumably all agents who have this symbolic association—patients who receive transplants, physicians, nurses, and others performing the transplants, and those involved in tissue procurement. In addition, the use of federal funds to support HFTTR would involve the federal government (and ultimately each taxpayer) in complicity as sponsors.

There are at least two responses to the charge of moral complicity in the wrongdoing of others. One is to deny that the primary action, in this case abortion, is morally wrong; another is to deny that the use of fetal tissue implies approval or acquiescence. The Panel did not try to resolve the debate about the morality of abortion, although that issue hovered over the proceedings. The majority took the second approach and insisted that it is at least possible to draw a moral line between the use of fetal tissue and the abortions that make the tissue available, so that unacceptable moral cooperation does not occur (*Report of the HFTTR Panel* 1988, I:2). For example, it is possible to use organs and tissues from homicide and accident victims—and thus to accept benefits from those tragedies and moral evils—without implying approval of homicides and accidents and without diminishing efforts to reduce their occurrence. Even if abortion is viewed as immoral, it does not follow that using fetal remains involves moral complicity in the "abortions that occur prior to or independent of later uses of fetal remains" (Robertson 1988a, p. 31).[5] Agents involved in the use of fetal tissue may deny that they have "dirty hands," and insist that, even in HFTTR, they are sufficiently disassociated from acts of abortion.[6] Numerous abortions are already being performed, and fetal tissue that could benefit others is being destroyed rather than used.

Opponents of HFTTR invoke the analogy with Nazi research to show complicity in the wrongdoing of others. Presented in many different ways, this analogy focuses on Nazi research on living subjects who were destined to die, on researchers' use of dead bodies and parts, and on subsequent uses of research data (Bopp and Burtchaell 1988, pp. 63–71). Critics of the analogy stress several morally relevant differences between the use of tissue from dead fetuses following debatably immoral (but legal) abortions and the clearly immoral actions of the Nazi investigators in experimenting on living subjects against their will (Robertson 1988a, see also Moscona 1988). Still there are questions about whether individuals and society should renounce the benefits (if any) that might be gained from the Nazi experiments in order to avoid the moral taint of those experiments.[7]

A majority of the panelists noted in a concurring statement that the complicity claim "is considerably weakened when the act making the benefit possible is legal and its immorality is vigorously debated, as is the case with abortion" (Robertson 1988a, p. 33). Thus, there are reasons to be cautious about basing public policy regarding HFTTR on perceptions of complicity, apart from establishing that using human fetal tissue in transplantation research would actually lead to (immoral) abortions that would not otherwise have occurred. As Burtchaell concedes, it is "a human estimate how close and operative complicity actually is" (Burtchaell 1988, p. 9). The Panel recognized that individuals, whether patients or professionals, might feel that their participation in HFTTR would involve moral complicity in abortion, and thus recommended disclosure of information that the tissue came from aborted fetuses (*Report of the HFTTR Panel* 1988, I:1).

The charge of complicity in the moral wrongdoing of others could actually be directed against those who invoke it to oppose HFTTR. For example, failure to provide sex education, contraceptives, and social support for pregnant women could be construed as modes of complicity in the act of abortion (*Transcript of the HFTTR Panel* 1988, pp. 688–704, 723). Here the alleged complicity also involves causal responsibility through acts of omission.

I have analyzed complicity mainly in terms of symbolic connections and associations that morally taint the agent. Many critics of HFTTR see the charge of complicity as distinctive in that it focuses on the corruption of the agent apart from any further consequences, in this case, additional abortions (Burtchaell 1988, p. 9). The remaining two major arguments against HFTTR focus on other negative consequences of the research (or developed therapy): societal legitimation of abortion practices, and provision of additional incentives for individual abortions.

Societal Legitimation of Abortion Practices

To some extent, the analytical categories used in this discussion tend to collapse into one another; in particular, societal legitimation of abortion practices can be partially reduced to issues of complicity in, and encouragement of, abortions. However, it is useful to consider societal legitimation separately, apart from the charges of moral complicity and actual causal responsibility for individual abortion decisions. According to Dorothy Vawter et al., "to legitimate an act or practice is to justify or promote it in such a manner that others will become more inclined to regard it as acceptable and to engage in it" (Vawter et al. 1990, p. 259).[8] Here I want to focus on societal legitimation (rather than individual approval) of abortion practices (rather than individual decisions).

In one version of the societal legitimation argument, critics contend that federally funded HFTTR following elective abortions would tend to legitimate abortion practices because in expending federal funds it is difficult—if not impossible—to separate approval of the use of fetal tissue following elective abortions, from approval of the elective abortions that produced the fetal tissue. Rabbi J. David Bleich (1988, p. 40, n. 2) argues that "federal funding conveys an unintended message of moral approval for every aspect of the research program." In response, defenders of the research could argue that the provision of federal funds for kidney transplants to treat end-stage kidney disease does not constitute approval of the homicides, suicides, and accidents that provide the occasions for organ donations (Robertson 1988a, p. 35, n. 23). Furthermore, there is simply no evidence of an abatement of efforts to reduce such tragedies in order to maintain or increase the supply of needed organs in the face of scarcity. Thus, it is important to consider all of society's actions that bear upon such matters as the use of fetal tissue following elective abortions. In addition, symbolic societal legitimation can be reduced, at least in part, by the kinds of separation measures discussed elsewhere in this article.

A second version of the societal legitimation argument focuses on societal acceptance of the benefits of human fetal tissue provided through elective abortions, rather than on governmental funding. It is difficult, perhaps even impossible, critics argue, for society to accept the benefits of HFTTR without becoming increasingly inclined to accept as legitimate the abortions that make the benefits possible. Particularly if HFTTR is successful, society might be less willing to restrict it, even if future Supreme Court decisions made that possible. In this version of the argument, societal legitimation cannot be avoided by the proposed separation measures, since the major impact occurs through acceptance of the positive results of HFTTR following elective abortions; hence it can be avoided only by renouncing the benefits.

It is important to note that the distinction between private and public funding of HFTTR is not adequate to avoid the second version of societal legitimation, however much it may help avoid the first version. Dr. Louis Sullivan, secretary of the Department of Health and Human Services, indefinitely extended the moratorium on the use of federal funds for HFTTR on the grounds that it would encourage or promote abortion. But in a November 2, 1989 letter to the acting director of the NIH he also noted that the private sector can continue HFTTR to generate "whatever biomedical knowledge" might emerge. However, as John Fletcher suggests, it is odd for DHHS officials to hold that it would be wrong for the federal government to fund HFTTR without condemning (and even apparently accepting) privately funded HFTTR and its benefits (Fletcher 1990). Societal acceptance of any benefits from HFTTR would provide societal (though not necessarily governmental) legitimation of abortion practices. And there are potential moral costs in the separation of private and public sectors when the federal government sits on the sidelines. The proposed measures to separate decisions to abort and decisions to provide fetal tissue can best be implemented under the requirements and sanctions attached to federal funding of HFTTR (Adams 1988).

A final criticism of societal legitimation of abortion through HFTTR appears in a dissenting letter by Daniel Robinson, who argues that:

> induced abortion is a moral wrong and that it cannot be redeemed by any actual or potential "good" secured by it. Thus, the possible medical benefits held out by research on tissues obtained by such measures cannot be exculpatory. (Robinson 1988)

Defenders of HFTTR can respond that it in no way "redeems" or "exculpates" the abortions themselves, however much it may reduce feelings of guilt and tragedy. Bringing some good out of evil or tragedy does not cancel the evil or tragedy. HFTTR only involves the use of tissue that would otherwise be discarded or incinerated, without implying either approval or disapproval of abortion practices. And whatever their rationale, the separation measures set a symbolic gulf between abortion practices and the use of fetal tissue.

INCENTIVES FOR ABORTIONS

Despite the importance of these complicity and legitimation arguments, the main criticism of federal funding of HFTTR is that it would lead to abortions that would not otherwise have occurred. (This argument may also extend to private funding especially if HFTTR becomes routine.) Proponents of this causal responsibility argument need not contend that there would be a net increase in the number of abortions; they could contend only that some women who would not otherwise have had some abortions will choose to do so in part because of the possibility of providing tissue to benefit others through transplantation. Both this argument and the societal legitimation argument probably carry greater weight in the context of therapy than research, but they are also offered in regard to HFTTR.

The argument that HFTTR would lead to additional abortions hinges in part on matters that empirical data should resolve—the reasons women choose to have abortions. The Panel's report noted that "the reasons for terminating a pregnancy are complex, varied, and deeply personal" and regarded it as "highly unlikely that a woman would be encouraged to make this decision [to abort] because of the knowledge that the fetal remains might be used in research" (*Report of the HFTTR Panel* 1988, I:3). In addition, the Panel underlined the lack of any evidence that over the last thirty years the possibility of donating fetal tissue for research purposes has resulted in an increase in the number of abortions (*Report of the HFTTR Panel* 1988, I:3). Still, as noted earlier, opponents of HFTTR might contend that there is an important difference between using fetal tissue to develop treatments and using fetal tissue as treatments (Nolan 1988), and that so far the latter has been rare.

Defenders of the causal responsibility argument identify three potential incentives for abortion provided by HFTTR. At least two of these incentives may be largely avoided by the guidelines and safeguards proposed by supporters of the research, while the third remains speculative.

Incentives for Financial Gain

HFTTR could provide a motive for women to have an abortion through financial incentives for the provision of fetal tissue. During the deliberations of the HFTTR Panel, the National Organ Transplant Act was amended to include as part of the human organs that may not be bought or sold "any other human organ (or any subpart thereof, including that derived from a fetus) specified by the Secretary of Health and Human Services by regulation" (42 USC 274e). There is some debate about whether this prohibition covers fetal neural tissue, which may not be an organ or a subpart of an organ. There is also some uncertainty about whether an abortion clinic that receives reimbursement for its expenses in procuring fetal tissue, as is permitted by the National Organ Transplant Act, can then reduce the price of the abortion, thereby passing the earnings on to the pregnant women (Vawter et al. 1990, p. 175). The HFTTR Panel held that "it is essential . . . that no fees be paid to the woman to donate, or to the clinic for its efforts in procuring fetal tissue (other than expenses incurred in retrieving fetal tissue)" (*Report of the HFTTR Panel* 1988, 1:9). There is general agreement on the prohibition of the sale or purchase of fetal tissue. It can be justified on several grounds—to protect fetuses from abortion, to protect women from exploitation and coercion, to reduce moral controversy about abortion, and to prevent society from treating human body parts as a commodity.

Specific Benevolence or Altruism

Already some women have volunteered to become pregnant in order to abort and donate fetal tissue to help a beloved family member (Thompson 1987). This motivation can be called "specific benevolence" or "specific altruism," as distinguished from "general benevolence" or "general altruism," which will be considered below. Specific benevolence or altruism is beneficence directed toward specific, known individuals, usually (but not necessarily) in a loving relationship.

The Panel held that it is both desirable and feasible to prevent such motives from leading to abortions that would not otherwise have occurred. In contrast to the directed donations now permitted by the Uniform Anatomical Gift Act (UAGA), the woman donating the fetal tissue for federally funded HFTTR should not be permitted to designate the beneficiary/recipient. This requirement of anonymity between the donor (the woman donating fetal tissue) and the recipient should protect both parties—the donor should not know who will receive the tissue and the donor's identity should be concealed from the recipient and from the transplant team (*Report of the HFTTR Panel* 1988, I:4). Here, as elsewhere, the rationale may involve maternal welfare and freedom from coercion and exploitation, as well as concerns about the morality of abortion. Furthermore, questions can be raised about the unfairness of the distribution pattern that results from directed donations.

The Panel also noted that there is no evidence that the anonymity requirement would have a negative impact on transplantation, which often involves matching donors and recipients. However, because of the uncertainty about the possible future value of matching donor and recipient, the Panel proposed a procedural solution and urged the secretary for health and human services to "review these recommendations at regular intervals" (*Report of the HFTTR Panel* 1988, I:8) In a concurring statement, several panelists even noted that the ban on donor designation of recipients—and even "aborting for transplant purposes"—should be reexamined if the supply of fetal tissue from elective abortions proves to be inadequate: "The ethical and legal arguments in favor of and against such a policy [i.e., the ban] would then need careful scrutiny to determine whether such a policy remains justified" (Robertson 1988a, p. 38).

General Benevolence or Altruism

This third possible motivation for pregnant women to terminate their pregnancies because of the possibility of HFTTR is the most controversial. It is both the most speculative and the least subject to control. The question is whether the possibility of donating fetal tissue to benefit unrelated and unknown patients would encourage women to obtain an abortion. Neither the defenders nor the critics of HFTTR can find strong evidence to support their claims about the potential impact that the knowledge of the possibility of donating fetal tissue might have on individual abortion decisions (*Report of the HFTTR Panel* 1988, I:3). Thus the debate hinges on speculation, often shaped by sexist perspectives, about women's abortion decisions, and on answers to the moral question about which way society should err in such a situation of doubt.

Critics of HFTTR emphasize that women are often ambivalent and therefore vacillate about abortion, and that this additional motive of general benevolence may lead to some abortions that would not otherwise have occurred. For example, in his November 2, 1989 letter to the acting director of NIH, HHS Secretary Sullivan insisted that providing pregnant women, who "arrive at the abortion decision after much soul searching and uncertainty," with "the additional rationalization of directly advancing the cause of human therapeutics cannot help but tilt some already vulnerable women toward a decision to have an abortion" (see also Bleich 1988, p. 40).

By contrast, I tend to downplay the potential role of general altruism or benevolence in a pregnant woman's decision to abort; it appears that pregnant women usually choose to abort because of their perception of the burdens of the pregnancy or of the future child, and that altruism toward others is mainly directed toward identifiable persons in a relationship rather than anonymous beneficiaries (Vawter et al. 1990, p. 261). However, I was brought up short by a telephone call from a professor who had heard that I had defended HFTTR on a national television program. He indicated that after his wife had delivered their second child, he had had a vasectomy that was unsuccessful and his wife was pregnant for the third time. They wanted to have an abortion but they also wanted to donate fetal tissue in order "to reduce their troublesome thought about abortion." I referred him (and his wife) to others who could help, but I do not know whether his wife chose to have an abortion and, if she did, whether the possibility of donating fetal tissue to help others was significant in her decision.

Even if it helped to relieve her (and his) guilt, it may not have been a necessary or sufficient motive in her decision to abort. That is, she may have had sufficient motivation to abort without this consideration. As C. D. Broad (1970) has reminded us, it is very difficult to determine whether any motive is necessary and/or sufficient in our (or others') decisions. It is important not to confuse primary considerations and secondary considerations, where they can be distinguished, and evidence presented to the Panel indicated that the primary reasons for termination of pregnancy would leave little room for a significant role for general altruism or benevolence (*Transcript of the HFTTR Panel* 1988, pp. 420, 478, 780–81, 791–95, 800–802, et passim).[9]

In contrast to efforts to eliminate motives of financial gain and specific altruism, it is not possible to develop guidelines and safeguards to completely eliminate the possibility that the opportunity to donate fetal tissue, based on general altruism, will play a role in some abortion decisions. However, with the majority of the Panel, I believe that this risk is worth taking in view of the possible benefits of HFTTR. I disagree with the assistant secretary for health that the risk of even one additional abortion would be too high a price to pay for these benefits. He has stated: "If just one additional fetus were lost because of the allure of directly benefiting another life by the donation of fetal tissue, our department would still be against federal funding . . ." (Mason 1990). It is difficult to attribute full moral seriousness to such claims, when the agents fail to perceive that other policies contribute more predictably to abortions that would not otherwise have occurred—the failure to provide sex education, contraception, and psychosocial support for pregnant women.

It is also important to distinguish means, ends, and consequences. Additional elective abortions do not constitute a *means* to the *end* of HFTTR. At most they are a possible *consequence* of the use of HFTTR. Hence, risk-benefit analysis and assessment are required. Risk involves both the probability of a negative outcome and its magnitude. The risk of additional fetal deaths—that is, ones that would not otherwise have occurred—is comparable to other losses of life in the pursuit of important societal goals, such as automobile design, highway engineering, and bridge building. As noted in John Robertson's concurring statement, joined by ten other panelists: "The risk that *some* lives will be lost, however, is not sufficient to stop those projects when the number of deaths is not substantial, when the activity serves worthy goals and when reasonable steps to minimize the loss have been taken" (Robertson 1988a, p. 34). And it is not justifiable to adopt a more stringent policy for HFTTR "just because the risk is to prenatal life from *some* increase in the number of legal abortions" (Robertson 1988a, pp. 34–35).

The concurring statement notes that the risk of additional fetal deaths is speculative, and stresses that it is possible to identify similar speculative risks that society might encourage or legitimate deaths from homicide, suicide, and accidents in order to gain organs for transplantation. However, these speculative risks are not viewed as a sufficient reason to stop using organs from such sources (Robertson 1988a, p. 35, n. 23). The current Assistant Secretary for Health James Mason contends that this argument simply throws out moral and ethical considerations (Mason 1990). However, those of us who signed the concurring statement view it as offering a different balance of moral and ethical considerations, not a denial of those considerations. When there is no evidence to support the claim of a high probability of a large number of additional fetal deaths, and those deaths, if they occur, are the indirect (and unintended) result of legitimate and promising medical research, the rule of multiple effects would appear to justify proceeding with HFTTR. In addition, the Panel held that its recommended guidelines and safeguards would reduce the probability of any increase in the number of abortions.

A different risk-benefit calculation appears in the dissent by Rabbi J. David Bleich. He holds that the safeguards proposed by the Panel will not prevent "an increment in the total number of abortions performed" (Bleich 1988, p. 39). And he argues that the duty to rescue human life through fetal tissue transplants is weakened because current research protocols offer only undetermined and remote benefits for future patients (as opposed to high probabilities of immediate benefits for current patients), and because the "moral harm" of the increase in the number of abortions is virtually certain and immediate. Hence, "on balance, the duty to refrain from a course of action that will have the effect of increasing instances of feticide must be regarded as the more compelling moral imperative" (Bleich 1988, pp. 42–43). Rabbi Bleich's formulation, which closely follows the Jewish tradition's reasoning about the duty to rescue, appears to leave open the possibility of a different balance if the transplantation procedure reaches the point, without federally funded research, of providing an immediate and certain benefit to current patients. By contrast, the majority of the Panel held that the increase in the number of abortions is not certain and immediate and that the probability and the number of additional abortions can be greatly reduced by the proposed guidelines or safeguards.

DONORS AND DONATIONS: AUTHORITY OVER FETAL REMAINS

As noted earlier, one of the difficult questions surrounding HFTTR is the mode of transfer or acquisition of human fetal tissue following induced abortions. A society could adopt one of several possible modes of transfer or acquisition of fetal tissue: express donation, presumed donation, abandonment, expropriation, or sales.[10] Donation is the dominant mode of transfer or acquisition of cadaveric organs and tissue in the United States. *Express donation* by the decedent or by the decedent's next of kin is the main version of donation, but *presumed donation* also exists— about a dozen states authorize procurement teams to remove corneas without express consent unless the decedent or the next of kin has dissented or opted out. (I use the term "donor" to refer to the decision maker, that is, the one who makes the gift, rather than to the source of the organs if that source could not or did not make a decision to give.)

There is some evidence that fetal tissue has occasionally been viewed as abandoned or unclaimed and used without explicit maternal consent (*Report of the HFTTR Panel* 1988, I:11); the ethical justification for such a practice depends in part on expectations about disposition following removal. While such uses of fetal tissue could have been based on presumed consent or donation, it is difficult to justify presumed donation ethically unless there is good reason to believe that silence actually reflects understanding and choice. The Panel heard no evidence that fetal tissue has been expropriated (i.e., taken against the wishes of the next of kin). The reasons for opposing transfer by sales were discussed above, and the Panel heard no evidence to indicate that it is being practiced. By and large then, express donation of fetal tissue prevails. And studies indicate that when asked, more than 90 percent of the pregnant women agree to donate fetal tissue for research (Vawter et al. 1990, p. 199).

The HFTTR Panel held that, in general, the framework of express donation provided by the Uniform Anatomical Gift Act (as revised in 1987) should also apply to the transfer/acquisition of fetal tissue:

> express donation by the pregnant woman after the abortion decision is the most appropriate mode of transfer of fetal tissues because it is the most congruent with our society's traditions, laws, policies, and practices, including the Uniform Anatomical Gift Act and current Federal research regulations. (*Report of the HFTTR Panel* 1988, I:6)[11]

This response in favor of the sufficiency (within certain limits) of maternal consent/donation attracted the smallest majority of any answer to any of the assistant secretary's ten questions—17 yes, 3 no, 1 abstention.

Much of the debate hinges on what donation of tissue presupposes about the relationship between the donor and the cadaveric source of the tissue. Critics of HFTTR contend that when the pregnant woman "resolves to destroy her offspring, she has abdicated her office and duty as the guardian of her offspring, and thereby forfeits her tutelary powers" (Bopp and Burtchaell 1988, p. 47). From this perspective, the abortion decision deprives the pregnant woman of any subsequent authority over the disposition of the fetal remains. This perspective appears to require an absolute separation between the decision to abort and the decision to use fetal tissue by disqualifying the woman who decides to abort from making a decision about use, but that also would disqualify others on the grounds of their failure to exercise their protective powers and their complicity in the moral wrongdoing of others (Burtchaell 1988, pp. 8–9).

By contrast, the Panel argued that a woman's choice of a legal abortion does not disqualify her legally and should not disqualify her morally from serving "as the primary decisionmaker about the disposition of fetal remains, including the donation of fetal tissue for research" (*Report of the HFTTR Panel* 1988, I:6). The Panel rejected arguments that the decision to abort leaves only biological kinship, with no moral authority:

> Disputes about the morality of her decision to have an abortion should not deprive the woman of the legal authority to dispose of fetal remains. She still has a special connection with the fetus and she has a legitimate interest in its disposition and use. Furthermore, the dead fetus has no interests that the pregnant

woman's donation would violate. In the final analysis, any mode of transfer other than maternal donation appears to raise more serious ethical problems. (*Report of the HFTTR Panel* 1988, I:6)

A concurring statement (written by John Robertson and signed by a majority of the panelists) argues that the guardianship model

mistakenly assumes that a person who disposes of cadaveric remains acts as a guardian proxy for the deceased, who has no interests, rather than as a protector of their own interests in what happens to those remains. (Robertson 1988a, p. 36)

Of course, where the decedent has expressed his or her wishes, the situation is different.

It may also be instructive to consider societal practices where parental abuse resulting in a child's death is suspected or admitted. According to one study, "There is no automatic legal disqualification of parents as proxy agents for organ donation when they are suspected of or have admitted playing a role in the death of their child" (Vawter et al. 1990, p. 217). Whatever moral queasiness may exist, organ procurement teams still ask these parents for organ donation. Of course, decisions about the cadaver should be distinguished from decisions about withholding or withdrawing life-support systems from a living person in order to avoid conflicts of interest in life-and-death decisions. However, after the determination of death, there are no cadaveric interests to be protected. Respectful and dignified treatment and disposal of cadaveric remains is required, in part to prevent offense to the living. This requirement is consistent with use of the cadaver in education, transplantation, and research, including, for example, crash tests. And there is no reason on grounds of equal respect to disqualify the woman having a legal abortion from making a decision about donation.

While accepting the structure of the UAGA as generally adequate, the Panel did recommend a modification in policy for the donation of fetal tissue in federally funded research. As applied to fetal tissue, the UAGA allows either parent to donate unless the other parent is known to object. However, the Panel concluded that:

The pregnant woman's consent should be *necessary* for donation—that is, the father should not be able to authorize the donation by himself, and the mother should always be asked before fetal tissue is used. In addition, her consent or donation should be *sufficient*, except where the procurement team knows of the father's objection to such donation. (*Report of the HFTTR Panel* 1988, I:7)

Noting that there is no legal or ethical obligation to seek the father's permission, the Panel held that there is "a legal and ethical obligation not to use the tissue if it is known that he objects (unless the pregnancy resulted from rape or incest)" (*Report of the HFTTR Panel* 1988, I:7).

In its recommendations of guidelines for federal funding of HFTTR, the Panel also stressed compliance with state laws and noted that at least eight states have statutes that prohibit the experimental use of cadaveric fetal tissue from induced abortions (*Report of the HFTTR Panel* 1988, I:13).[12] Another important and unresolved issue is whether state required request laws apply to fetal remains. More than forty states now have such a law which requires institutions to set up mechanisms and procedures to ensure that each family of a decedent who is a possible source of organs and tissues for transplantation is asked about donation.

The argument surrounding this question also focused on ways to separate the abortion decision made by the pregnant woman from the decision about the use of fetal tissue. For various reasons already identified—the desire not to provide incentives for abortions, the desire to protect pregnant women from exploitation and coercion, and the desire not to fan the flames of the abortion controversy—the Panel supported some limits on the pregnant woman's autonomy, without restricting the abortion decision itself. Under the UAGA there is no obligation to accept donated tissue or organs; hence the woman's right to donate fetal tissue does not create an obligation on anyone else to accept the gift. Furthermore, the Panel recommended that directed donations not be accepted and supported the prohibition on the sale of fetal tissue.

Stressing the express donation model embodied in the UAGA, the Panel's recommendations would allow the pregnant woman to choose whether to donate fetal tissue for research or some other purpose and to receive as much information as she requests regarding donation, without allowing her to know or to designate the recipient of the fetal tissue. By contrast, the Polkinghorne report (1989) in the United Kingdom recommended indeterminate donation to the extent of providing the pregnant woman "no knowledge of what will actually happen to the fetus or fetal tissue" and not allowing her "to make any direction regarding the use of her fetus or fetal tissue." This is intended to make it even less likely that her decision to have an abortion will be influenced by the possibility of beneficial use of the tissue.

Regarding potential pressures to modify the timing and method of abortion to secure more viable fetal tissue, the U.S. Report underlined the current absence of pressure for later abortions but insisted that

> to the extent that Federal sponsorship or funding is involved, no abortion should be put off to a later date nor should any abortion be performed by an alternate method entailing greater risk to the pregnant woman in order to supply more useful fetal materials for research. (*Report of the HFTTR Panel* 1988, I:14)

However, the Report did not address what should be permitted and done if the pregnant woman requests information about the advantages of changes in timing and methods of abortion for the later use of donated fetal tissue and then requests those changes.

In general, the level of information disclosure that would be expected in informed consent for therapy or research is not required for fetal tissue donation, although the pregnant woman may request any information prior to making a decision about donation. The pregnant woman who is contemplating donation should receive information about any tests that will be conducted on her to determine the quality of the fetal tissue—e.g., HIV antibody tests—and any modifications of the abortion procedure being considered because of the anticipated donation. Both of these matters may have an impact on her well-being (Vawter et al. 1990, pp. 239f). Since she is donating for transplantation research, she may also have an interest in knowing any plans for commercialization.

When should there be an inquiry about donation? The HFTTR Panel held that "ideally, permission to use tissues from the aborted fetus would not even be sought until the abortion itself had been performed" (*Report of the HFTTR Panel* 1988, I:10). However, because post-mortem tissue deteriorates quickly and cryogenic storage is not fully developed— and may require permission as a departure from the normal expectations regarding disposition—"the pregnant woman must be consulted before the abortion is actually performed" (*Report of the HFTTR Panel* 1988, I:10).[13] However, the Report held that no information about the donation and use of fetal tissue in research should be provided prior to the pregnant woman's decision to abort, unless she specifically requests that information (*Report of the HFTTR Panel* 1988, I:3–4). Separate consent forms for the abortion and for the donation may also reduce the chance that the latter will influence the former and will be simply one part of a single decision. Similarly, in determining who should make the inquiry about donation, there should be a separation of parties to make sure that there is no conflict of interest, and that the woman experiences no pressure to donate.

Regarding disclosure of information to other parties, the U.S. Panel recommends disclosing that the tissue came from a fetus or fetuses, so that the potential recipient of the transplant could choose not to participate; the British report recommends against such disclosure. However, both reports recommend disclosure of information about the source to health care professionals.

CONCLUSION

Despite the moral and political perplexities associated with HFTTR following induced abortions, I believe that such research should go forward, with federal funding, as long as the guidelines and safeguards identified above are in place. They should prevent unacceptable complicity in abortion (or at least allow those who perceive such complicity to opt out, except for the payment of taxes), and they should reduce the likelihood, in conjunction with other policies and practices, of societal legitimation of abortion practices and of providing incentives to pregnant women to have abortions they would not otherwise have had. To be sure, there are no guarantees that these consequences can be prevented, but a reasonable risk analysis/assessment indicates these risks are largely speculative. On the benefit side, the animal studies are promising and may justify human clinical trials, at least for Parkinson's disease and juvenile diabetes (*Report of the HFTTR Panel* 1988, I:14, 19–22). However, my justification is couched in general terms, and it addresses the risks that critics identify as moral obstacles to proceeding with HFTTR, whatever the prospective benefits.[14] The justification of any particular human clinical trials must look more carefully at the scientific evidence for probable benefits and other risks.

This justification and the guidelines proposed by the Panel are in line with the international consensus (Walters 1988; 1990).[15] Indeed, the current U.S. moratorium is a remarkable exception to the international consensus. Of course, an international consensus is no guarantee of moral validity, but it is somewhat reassuring. Nevertheless, certain features of the U.S. context—most notably the political strength of various groups that march under the banner of the right to life—may be relevant. In addition, a couple of concerns about HFTTR may be more appropriate in the United States than in some other countries. First, many European countries have more restrictive abortion laws and may thus have less reason to fear the impact of HFTTR on abortion decisions and on societal legitimation of abortion practices (Glendon 1989). Second, there may be important differences in the commercialization and regulation of abortion clinics and of tissue procurement. For example, it could be argued that the NIH HFTTR Panel did not pay sufficient attention to actual institutional pressures (Annas and Elias 1989). By contrast, in addition to recommending the separation of *decisions* regarding abortion and donation of fetal tissue, the U.K. Polkinghorne report called for an "intermediary" as a mechanism to separate the *practice* of abortion from the use of fetal tissue.

It is reasonable to suggest that U.S. public policy regarding HFTTR is now held hostage to the societal uneasiness about abortion. Our continuing societal debate about HFTTR in part turns on which side has the moral and political burden of proof when irrefutable evidence is lacking that abortion decisions and practices can be separated from decisions and practices about the use of fetal tissue following abortion. In such a context the debate is to a great extent about which analogies from current, justifiable practices should govern decision making. The U.S. Panel chose the analogy with organ and tissue donation as the most defensible one for approaching the use of human fetal tissue following elective abortions, but then argued for some special guidelines and safeguards because of societal concern about abortion.

NOTES

1. References to the *Report of the Human Fetal Tissue Transplantation Research Panel* (1988), including concurring and dissenting statements, will appear throughout the text. This essay draws on my experiences as a member of that Panel, as a member of the Office of Technology Assessment Advisory Panel on New Developments in Neuroscience, and on some materials I developed in preparing a case study for the Institute of Medicine, from which I have drawn some ideas and formulations. That case study contains new information about the context, process, and procedures of the HFTTR Panel.

2. For an excellent discussion of the use of fetal tissue in various contexts see Dorothy E. Vawter et al. (1990) and Dorothy Lehrman (1988).

3. For responses on complicity, see John A. Robertson (1988c, 1988b) Benjamin Freedman (1988). For excellent analyses of issues surrounding complicity see Dorothy E. Vawter et al. (1990, esp. pp. 251–67), and Richard C. Sparks (1990). See also James F. Childress (1990).

4. See also Bopp and Burtchaell (1988, p. 68) and the discussion of this analogy and others in *Transcript of the Meeting of the Human Fetal Tissue Transplantation Research Panel* (1988, pp. 374–403).

5. This statement was signed by ten additional panelists.

6. For a discussion of "association" and "disassociation," see James F. Childress (1990); see also Daniel C. Maguire (1986), Leslie Griffin (1989), and Thomas E. Hill, Jr. (1979).

7. For the debate about the use of Nazi data, see, for example, Michael Weisskopf (1988) and Mark Weitzman (1990).

8. This also provides a good analysis of legitimation charges.

9. Also see Robin Duke's presentation in *Report of the Human Fetal Tissue Transplantation Research Panel* (1988, II:D113–D121). For an analysis see Vawter et al. (1990, esp. pp. 261–67).

10. For a fuller analysis, see James F. Childress (1989).

11. Also see James F. Childress (1988) and contrast Kathleen Nolan's warning about the dangers of viewing fetal material in terms of gift and donation and her argument for the language of contribution (Nolan 1988).

12. For summaries of state laws and federal regulations, see Lori Andrews (1988), Judith Areen (1988), and David H. Smith et al. (1988). See also Patricia King and Judith Areen (1988) and Vawter et al. (1990, pp. 169–87).

13. For other arguments, see Vawter et al. (1990, pp. 244f).

14. For criticism of Parkinson's research, including its animal base, see William M. Landau (1990). For more positive reports of human trials, see Olle Lindvall (1990) and Curt Freed et al. (1990).

15. In the United States similar proposals, with minor variations, have emerged in the last two years from other groups. See the report from the Stanford Medical Center Committee on Ethics in Henry T. Greely et al. (1989) and the Council on Ethical and Judicial Affairs of the American Medical Association (1990).

REFERENCES

Adams, Arlin B. 1988. Concurring Statement. In *Report of the Human Fetal Tissue Transplantation Research Panel,* vol. I, pp. 25–28. Bethesda, MD: National Institutes of Health.

Andrews, Lori. 1988. State Regulation of Human Fetal Tissue Transplantation. In *Report of the Human Fetal Tissue Transplantation Research Panel,* vol. II, pp. D1–D20. Bethesda, MD: National Institutes of Health.

Annas, George, and Elias, Sherman. 1989. The Politics of Transplantation of Human Fetal Tissue. *New England Journal of Medicine* 320 (April 20):1079–82.

Areen, Judith. 1988. Statement on Legal Regulation of Fetal Tissue Transplantation. In *Report of the Human Fetal Tissue Transplantation Research Panel,* vol. II, pp. D21–D26. Bethesda, MD: National Institutes of Health.

Bleich, J. David. Dissenting Statement, Fetal Tissue Research and Public Policy. In *Report of the Human Fetal Tissue Transplantation Research Panel,* vol. I, pp. 39–43. Bethesda, MD: National Institutes of Health.

Bopp, James, and Burtchaell, James Tunstead. 1988. Human Fetal Tissue Transplantation Research Panel: Statement of Dissent. In *Report of the Human Fetal Tissue Transplantation Research Panel,* vol. I, pp. 45–71. Bethesda, MD: National Institutes of Health.

458   JAMES F. CHILDRESS

Broad, C. D. 1970. Conscience and Conscientious Action. In *Moral Concepts,* ed. Joel Feinberg, pp. 74–79. New York: Oxford University Press.

Buckley, Rebecca H. 1988. Fetal Thymus Transplantation for the Correction of Congenital Absence of the Thymus (DiGeorge's Syndrome). In *Report of the Human Fetal Tissue Transplantation Research Panel,* vol. II, pp. D50–D57. Bethesda, MD: National Institutes of Health.

Burtchaell, James Tunstead. 1988. University Policy on Experimental Use of Aborted Fetal Tissue. *IRB: A Review of Human Subjects Research* 10 (July–August):7–11.

———. 1989. The Use of Aborted Fetal Tissue in Research: A Rebuttal. *IRB: A Review of Human Subjects Research* 11 (March–April):9–12.

Childress, James F. 1988. Statement to the Advisory Committee to the Director, NIH. In *Human Fetal Tissue Transplantation Research,* Report of the Advisory Committee to the Director, National Institutes of Health, pp. C7–C8. Bethesda, MD: National Institutes of Health.

———. 1989. Ethical Criteria for Procuring and Distributing Organs for Transplantation. *Journal of Health Politics, Policy and Law* 14 (Spring):87–113.

———. 1990. Disassociation from Evil: The Case of Human Fetal Tissue Transplantation Research. In *Social Responsibility: Business, Journalism, Law, Medicine,* vol. XVI, ed. Louis W. Hodges, pp. 32–49. Lexington, VA: Washington and Lee University.

Committee to Review the Guidance on the Research Use of Fetuses and Fetal Material. 1989. *Review of the Guidance on the Research Use of Fetuses and Fetal Material.* London: Her Majesty's Stationery Office.

Council on Ethical and Judicial Affairs of the American Medical Association. 1990. Medical Applications of Fetal Tissue Transplantation. *Journal of the American Medical Association* 263 (January 26):565–70.

Fletcher, John. 1990. Moratorium on Federal Support for Fetal Tissue Transplant Research. Testimony before the Subcommittee on Health and the Environment, Committee on Energy and Commerce, U.S. House of Representatives, 2 April.

Freed, Curt, et al. 1990. Transplantation of Human Fetal Dopamine Cells for Parkinson's Disease. *Archives of Neurology* 47 (May):505–12.

Freedman, Benjamin. 1988. The Ethics of Using Human Fetal Tissue. *IRB: A Review of Human Subjects Research* 10 (November–December):1–4.

Glendon, Mary Ann. 1989. A World Without Roe: How Different Would It Be? *Hastings Center Report* 19 (July/August):22–37.

Greely, Henry T., et al. 1989. The Ethical Use of Fetal Tissue in Medicine. *New England Journal of Medicine* 320 (April 20):1093–96.

Griffin, Leslie. 1989. The Problem of Dirty Hands. *Journal of Religious Ethics* 17 (Fall): 31–61.

Hill, Jr., Thomas E. 1979. Symbolic Protest and Calculated Silence. *Philosophy and Public Affairs* 9:83–102.

Hoffer, Barry J. 1988. Summary of Current Literature. In *Report of the Human Fetal Tissue Transplantation Research Panel*, vol. I, pp. 19–22. Bethesda, MD: National Institutes of Health.

King, Patricia, and Areen, Judith. 1988. Legal Regulation of Fetal Tissue Transplantation. *Clinical Research* 36:205–8.

Landau, William M. 1990. Artificial Intelligence: The Brain Transplant Cure for Parkinsonism. *Neurology* 40:733–40.

Lehrman, Dorothy. 1988. *Summary: Fetal Research and Fetal Tissue Research*. Washington, D.C.: Association of American Medical Colleges.

Levine, Robert J. 1986. *Ethics and the Regulation of Clinical Research*. 2d ed. Baltimore, MD: Urban and Schwarzenberg.

Lindvall, Olle. 1990. Grafts of Dopamine Neurons Survive and Improve Motor Function in Parkinson's Disease. *Science* 247 (February 2):574–77.

Maguire, Daniel C. 1986. Cooperation with Evil. In *The Westminster Dictionary of Christian Ethics*. 2nd ed. Eds. James F. Childress and John Maquarrie. Philadelphia, PA: The Westminster Press.

Mason, James O. 1990. Should the Fetal Tissue Research Ban Be Lifted? *The Journal of NIH Research* 2 (January–February):17–18.

Moscona, Aaron A. 1988. Concurring Statement. In *Report of the Human Fetal Tissue Transplantation Research Panel*, vol. I, pp. 27–28. Bethesda, MD: National Institutes of Health.

National Institutes of Health, Advisory Committee to the Director. 1988. *Human Fetal Transplantation Research*. Bethesda, MD: National Institutes of Health, 14 December.

Nolan, Kathleen. 1988. Genug ist Genug: A Fetus is Not a Kidney. *Hastings Center Report* 18 (December):13–19.

OSPL-OD-NIH. 1988. Fact Sheet: NIH Fetal Tissue Research, 22 July.

Polkinghorne Report. *See* Committee to Review. . . .

Report of the Human Fetal Tissue Transplantation Research Panel, II vols. 1988. Bethesda, MD: National Institutes of Health.

Robertson, John A. 1988a. Concurring Statement. In *Report of the Human Fetal Tissue Transplantation Research Panel*, vol. I, pp. 29–38. Bethesda, MD: National Institutes of Health.

———. 1988b. Fetal Tissue Transplant Research is Ethical. *IRB: A Review of Human Subjects Research* 10 (November–December):5–8.

———. 1988c. Rights, Symbolism, and Public Policy in Fetal Tissue Transplants. *Hastings Center Report* 18 (December):5–12.

Robinson, Daniel N. 1988. Letter to Dr. Jay Moskowitz. In *Report of the Human Fetal Tissue Transplantation Research Panel*, vol. I, p. 73. Bethesda, MD: National Institutes of Health.

Smith, David H., et al. 1988. Using Human Fetal Tissue for Transplantation and Research: Selected Issues. In *Report of the Human Fetal Tissue Transplantation Research Panel*, vol. II, pp. F1–F43. Bethesda, MD: National Institutes of Health.

Sparks, Richard C. 1990. Ethical Issues of Fetal Tissue Transplantation Research, Procurement, and Complicity with Abortion. Paper read at the annual meeting of the Society of Christian Ethics, 20 January 1990, Arlington, VA.

Thompson, Larry. 1987. Fetal Cells Hold the Most Promise—and Raise Ethical Questions. *Washington Post Health* (14 July).

Transcript of the Meeting of the Human Fetal Tissue Transplantation Research Panel. 1988. 14–16 September 1988. Bethesda, MD: National Institutes of Health.

Vawter, Dorothy E., et al. 1990. *The Use of Human Fetal Tissue: Scientific, Ethical, and Policy Concerns*. A Report of Phase I of an Interdisciplinary Research Project conducted by the Center for Biomedical Ethics, January 1990, University of Minnesota.

Walters, LeRoy. 1988. Statement to the Advisory Committee to the Director, NIH. In *Human Fetal Tissue Transplantation Research*, Report of the Advisory Committee to the Director, p. C5. Bethesda, MD: National Institutes of Health.

———. 1990. Testimony on Human Fetal Tissue Research. Before the Subcommittee on Health and the Environment, Committee on Energy and Commerce, U.S. House of Representatives, 2 April 1990.

Weisskopf, Michael. 1988. EPA Bars Use of Nazis' Human Test Data After Scientists Object. *Washington Post* (March 24):A10.

Weitzman, Mark. 1990. The Ethics of Using Nazi Medical Data: A Jewish Perspective. *Second Opinion: Health, Faith, and Ethics* 14 (July):26–38.

Wyngaarden, James. 1987. Memorandum to Robert E. Windom on "Approval to Perform Experimental Surgical Procedure at NIH Clinical Center—ACTION," 23 October.

26 Routine Inquiry About Organ Donation: An Alternative to Presumed Consent

ROBERT M. VEATCH, PH.D.

Dr. Robert Veatch is a research scholar at the Kennedy Institute of Ethics at Georgetown University, Washington, D.C.

A s of April 1991, there were 22,842 people in the United States on the waiting lists for organs for transplantation.[1] The list is getting longer each year. Many patients die waiting for organs. Others must be maintained on dialysis for want of a transplantable kidney. It is understandable that some people are growing impatient with the system of voluntary donation embodied in the Uniform Anatomical Gift Act—a law that requires specific consent for donation and that has been in place now for two decades.[2] The idea of presuming that the deceased person would consent to the use of his or her organs for lifesaving transplantation is now receiving renewed, more serious attention. Such a change in policy would require specific refusal rather than specific consent for the use of an organ. Although the sentiment favoring the change is understandable, there are good moral and practical reasons why presumed consent is an idea whose time has not come and why other approaches, including a truly systematic effort to ask about donation while patients are still alive and competent, are better, morally more defensible, and more effective. In order to see why, it is necessary to explore both the moral logic behind presumed consent and the alternatives available.

This article first appeared in The New England Journal of Medicine *325 (24 October 1991): 1246–1249.*

Presumed Consent: The Moral Logic

Since the late 1960s, public policy in the United States regarding the procurement of organs for transplantation has rested on a model of consent. The organs and tissues of deceased humans do not belong to the state, the hospital, or any other entity, to be used for its own purposes without permission. The possibility of routinely retrieving organs has long since been rejected.[3] Although neither the living person nor the next of kin technically owns the body parts, they can be thought of as having "quasi-property rights." This right is perhaps better thought of as a duty: the duty to dispose of body parts in a responsible manner, with the discretion to choose among reasonable courses of action. For the past two decades, in the United States and many other countries, this privilege has included the right to donate organs and tissues for transplantation and other uses (education, research, and therapeutic uses other than transplantation), as well as the right to decide not to donate.

This right of refusal has rested, first, with the individual person while he or she is competent. In Western culture, it is the individual himself or herself who is most responsible for choosing a life plan. This commitment has included both the right and the responsibility to determine the disposal of assets after death through a legally binding will. It now also recognizes the priority of the individual's wishes regarding disposal of the body and the use of body parts for medical purposes. Unless instructions about the disposal of body parts have been expressed by the person while competent, the next of kin may decide to donate or to refuse donation after death.

Now, however, some are proposing that consent simply be presumed.[4-8] Often such proposals include a provision for "opting out," so that competent persons (and perhaps their next of kin as well) would have the right to object to the use of organs. Unless such an objection was recorded, however, the consent of the person to the use of his or her organs would be presumed. Such a presumption, it is argued, would greatly increase the number of organs available for transplantation and other medical uses.[8]

Presumed consent is a legal and moral doctrine that has existed in medicine in other contexts. In particular, it applies to treatment of unconscious or incompetent patients in emergencies. The emergency presumption of consent permits persons to receive obviously necessary medical care without their explicit permission. To do anything else would lead to foolish suffering, injury, and the waste of life.

Now the presumption of consent is being applied with renewed vigor to the issue of organ procurement.[9] Since many people have no objection in principle to having their organs used for lifesaving purposes after their deaths but have not made a formal declaration donating their organs, one might at first believe that this legal innovation would substantially increase the number of organs available. There are serious moral and pragmatic problems with this assumption, however.

Consent Cannot Be Presumed

The most serious problem is that the presumption of consent is demonstrably false in many cases. When we presume consent in the emergency room, we rest the presumption on the well-founded belief that, in fact, the person lying unconscious and in need of medical attention would consent if he or she were able to do so. If we surveyed the population asking whether people would want such care, the results would be almost unanimous. Moreover, if people were asked to endorse a public policy of presuming consent on the basis of the demonstrable support for such care, agreement would again be almost unanimous. In fact, courts and legislatures have formally endorsed such a presumption, and the population recognizes its wisdom, given the alternatives.

By contrast, empirical data make it clear that, whatever the reason, a substantial fraction of the American population would not consent to having their organs and tissues used for transplantation. A 1990 Gallup poll found that 85 percent of those polled would donate a loved one's organs.[10] That fact in itself suggests that a presumption of consent would be wrong 15 percent of the time. However, according to the same poll, only 60 percent said they would donate their own organs, suggesting that if the moral goal is to follow the wishes of the individual person, the error rate in presuming consent could be as high as 40 percent. Moreover, we know that the actual consent rate in the hospital setting is even lower than 60 percent—by some reports as low as 25 to 30 percent.[10] One organ-procurement group had an actual consent rate of 46 percent in 1990. In other words, if we presumed the consent of the decision maker, we have reason to believe that we would be making an error at least half the time. It is simply false to say that we can presume the consent of the decision maker in the same way that we can say emergency room patients would consent to treatment.

The Supply of Organs May Not Increase

It may also be false that more organs would be obtained if consent were presumed. Unless presumed consent is used purposely to avoid conversations with the next of kin, the same family members who object to transplantation when asked will still object under a presumed-consent law. The only increase in available organs is likely to come from a particularly vulnerable group: those who are found dead without any family members who can be reached during the time it takes to confirm the diagnosis of death. (Normally, candidates for organ retrieval will be pronounced dead according to brain-based criteria, a condition that takes at least several hours to diagnose; family members are usually sought during this time.) In fact, some people may be so offended by the state's presumption of their consent to organ procurement that, although they did not previously object to donation, they would now place an objection on record. There is simply no good basis for assuming that organ yields would increase substantially if a rule of presumed consent were adopted. The reports from countries with presumed-consent policies are ambiguous about whether such a presumption produces a substantial change.[11,12]

At their best, the proposals for presuming consent are misguided; at their worst, they are deceitful attempts to circumvent the refusal of consent by a substantial percentage of people. Ethically, it is simply wrong to presume that the deceased person or his or her next of kin would consent to use of the organs. As a practical matter, presumed consent will not work and could jeopardize an already fragile system.

THE ALTERNATIVES

The case against presumed consent is strengthened when we examine the alternatives.

Maximizing Actual Consent

First, and most obviously, many things could and should be done to maximize the likelihood of actual consent of persons while they are competent or, if necessary, their next of kin. We are learning a great deal about who should ask about procuring organs and how the request should be made. Some organ-procurement organizations report that inexperienced clinicians frame the request inappropriately, thus inadvertently discouraging donation. We are just beginning to understand why people might resist donation. Some reasons are invalid; others require serious attention. Some resistance comes from the fact that patients and families lack adequate trust in the institution making the request. The way to deal with such problems is to have the representatives of the institution act in such a way as to warrant trust. Other persons may decline to donate out of mistaken beliefs. No major Western religious tradition objects in principle to organ procurement. Some religions— for example, Judaism—consider donation one's moral duty when the donation can save an identifiable life. We have not invested adequately in efforts to encourage the execution of donation cards under the Uniform Anatomical Gift Act by individuals or donation by next of kin.

Required Requests of Next of Kin

Almost all states now have laws requiring that the next of kin be asked for permission for donation in cases in which usable organs may be obtained. Although the results have not been encouraging yet, a great deal could be done to improve the effectiveness of such requests.

Nevertheless, there are problems with requiring requests for consent from the next of kin, rather than the individual patient while he or she is alive and competent. The moral premise of current American public policy (as well as of the proposals for presumed consent) is that the person himself or herself has the primary right and responsibility to determine, within reason, how his or her body should be used after death. Only when that information is unavailable, because the person has never been a mentally competent adult or is not known to have expressed wishes while competent, do we revert to the secondary authority for decisions about the disposal of the body—that is, to the next of kin. The flaw with the current required-request laws is that they ignore the responsibility of the person himself or herself and focus attention instead on the surrogate decision maker.

Routine Requests of Competent Persons

A more defensible alternative is to systematize inquiries to competent adults as to how they would want their bodies used after death.[13] Under such arrangements, required requests of next of kin would be a fallback position, used only when the deceased person had never made a formal decision while competent to do so.

It is not too much to say that morally one should at least make the effort to think enough about this difficult subject to decide whether to participate in the lifesaving process of organ donation. I believe the time has come to adopt as social policy procedures to ask people whether they are willing to donate their organs and tissues after their deaths. Some of these requests should be informal, in settings in which the inquiry is not required legally. Many could occur in medical settings. For example, it seems only reasonable that a question about one's wishes about organ donation should become a routine part of every history and physical examination. Physicians are learning that they cannot provide good and proper medical care for their patients if they do not have an idea of their patients' preferences in advance. Living wills, decisions about cardiopulmonary resuscitation, and the designation of a surrogate decision maker are being discussed routinely. We should also make the discussion of organ donation routine. Inquiries about a patient's willingness to donate organs should also become a routine part of every hospital admission.

Some might object that this subject is too macabre for an interview on admission to the hospital. It might even be seen as bad public relations, suggesting to a patient that death is a likely outcome of the encounter. But surely, sensitive questions are already asked in such sessions. Physicians ask about sexual histories; hospital admission interviews include questions about who will pay the bills. Skilled professionals learn how to pose these questions diplomatically. If these discussions occur as part of all routine physical examinations and admission interviews, both patients and clinicians will grow accustomed to them, and they will provide an occasion for reflection.

Perhaps equally promising would be opportunities for routine inquiry outside the context of health care. Routine inquiry should become a part of other social encounters, as in religious and fraternal groups. At a more formal, legal level, many states now ask people about organ donation when they renew their driver's licenses. It would be a small additional step to require that the question be answered. Of course, persons would not be required to answer in the affirmative. They could even be given an opportunity to answer "I don't know." In that case, the provisions in the Uniform Anatomical Gift Act for decisions by a surrogate would come into play. Some might see routine inquiry during license renewals as an offensive intrusion of the state into private matters, but it seems little to ask for what could be a lifesaving decision. All that would be asked is that one think enough about the lifesaving potential of a donation to make a decision, not that a particular decision be made. Our obligation to the community surely goes far enough to require that the question be addressed in order for a license application to be completed. That, after all, is what happens with other questions that must be answered, such as questions about insurance.

There are other nonmedical ways that routine inquiry could take place. One of the most practical would be to have a question about organ donation on the income-tax return. The form is completed by virtually all adults; it is updated yearly; and the data could easily be entered into a central computer. A tape of the responses to that question only could be sent to the United Network for Organ Sharing or some other central organ-procurement agency. As long as there were provisions for negative answers and for expressing uncertainty, such routine inquiries would seem to affirm the primacy of the individual and the model of donation. Other ways to connect routine inquiries about organ donation to existing computerized data banks might also be considered.

Routine Retrieval of Organs with Provisions for Refusal

Some may be convinced that none of the voluntarist approaches will be adequate, that we need something more communal in focus. In that case, it seems far better to go explicitly to a scheme based on routine retrieval of organs (perhaps with a provision for opting out), so that we admit we are simply subordinating the will of the individual to the needs of the society. That seems far more honest than pretending we can presume consent when we really cannot. The fact is that the organ-procurement agencies are in a delicate and precarious position. They need to build trust and confidence, not impose a false presumption of consent or an explicit policy of routine retrieval. Making sure that people understand that we will ask their permission rather than assume that we have it seems the wise and responsible policy.

REFERENCES

1. United Network for Organ Sharing. Number of patients on UNOS waiting lists by organ needed and ABO blood group. UNOS Update 1991;7(5):19.

2. Sadler AM Jr, Sadler BL, Stason EB. The uniform anatomical gift act: a model for reform. JAMA 1968;206:2505–6.

3. Dukeminier J Jr, Sanders D. Organ transplantation: a proposal for routine salvaging of cadaver organs. N Engl J Med 1968;279:413–9.

4. Stuart FP, Veith FJ, Cranford RE. Brain death laws and patterns of consent to remove organs for transplantation from cadavers in the United States and 28 other countries. Transplantation 1981;31:238–44.

5. Caplan AL. Organ transplants: the costs of success. Hastings Cent Rep 1983;13(6): 23–32.

6. Starzl TE. Implied consent for cadaveric organ donation. JAMA 1984;251:1592.

7. Matas AJ, Veith FJ. Presumed consent for organ retrieval. Theor Med 1984;5:155–66.

8. *Idem*. Presumed consent—a more humane approach to cadaver organ donation. In: Hardy MA, Appel GB, Kiernan JM, et al., eds. Positive approaches to living with end-stage renal disease: psychosocial and thanatological aspects. New York: Praeger, 1986: 37–51.

9. Spital A. The shortage of organs for transplantation—where do we go from here? N Engl J Med 1991;325:1243–6.

10. Randall T. Too few human organs for transplantation, too many in need . . . and the gap widens. JAMA 1991;265:1223–7.

11. Organ and tissue donation. In: Task Force on Organ Transplantation. Organ transplantation: issues and recommendations. Washington, D.C.: Department of Health and Human Services, 1986:30–1.

12. Gerson WN. Refining the law of organ donation: lessons from the French law of presumed consent. N Y Univ J Int Law Polit 1987;19:1013–32.

13. Veatch RM. Death, dying, and the biological revolution: our last quest for responsibility. Rev. ed. New Haven, Conn.: Yale University Press, 1989.

27 Organs for Sale? Propriety, Property, and the Price of Progress

LEON R. KASS, M.D.

Leon Kass, M.D. is the Henry Luce Professor of the Liberal Arts of Human Biology at the University of Chicago.

J ust in case anyone is expecting to read about new markets for Wurlitzers, let me set you straight. I mean to discuss organ transplantation and, especially, what to think about recent proposals to meet the need for transplantable human organs by permitting or even encouraging their sale and purchase. If the reader will pardon the impropriety, I will not beat around the bush: the subject is human flesh, the goal is the saving of life, the question is, "To market or not to market?"

Such blunt words drive home a certain impropriety not only in my topic but also in choosing to discuss it in public. But such is the curse of living in interesting times. All sorts of shameful practices, once held not to be spoken of in civil society, are now enacted with full publicity, often to applause, both in life and in art. Not the least price of such "progress" is that critics of any impropriety have no choice but to participate in it, risking further blunting of sensibilities by plain overt speech. It's an old story: opponents of unsavory practices are compelled to put them in the spotlight. Yet if we do not wish to remain in the dark, we must not avert our gaze, however unseemly the sights, especially if others who do not share our sensibilities continue to project them—as they most certainly will. Besides, in the present matter, there is more than impropriety before us—there is the very obvious and unquestionable benefit of saving human lives.

About two years ago I was asked by a journal to review a manuscript that advocated overturning existing prohibitions on the sale of human organs, in order to take advantage of market incentives to increase their

This article appeared in The Public Interest *107 (Spring 1992): 65–86.*

supply for transplantation. Repelled by the prospect, I declined to review the article, but was punished for my reluctance by finding it in print in the same journal. Reading the article made me wonder at my own attitude: What precisely was it that I found so offensive? Could it be the very idea of treating the human body as a heap of alienable spare parts? If so, is not the same idea implicit in organ *donation*? Why does payment make it seem worse? My perplexity was increased when a friend reminded me that, although we allow no commerce in organs, transplant surgeons and hospitals are making handsome profits from the organ-trading business, and even the not-for-profit transplant registries and procurement agencies glean for their employees a middleman's livelihood. Why, he asked, should everyone be making money from this business except the person whose organ makes it possible? Could it be that my real uneasiness lay with organ donation or with transplantation itself, for, if not, what would be objectionable about its turning a profit?

Profit from human tissue was centrally the issue in a related development two years ago, when the California Supreme Court ruled that a patient had no property rights in cells removed from his body during surgery, cells which, following commercial genetic manipulation, became a patented cell-line that now produces pharmaceutical products with a market potential estimated at several billion dollars, none of it going to the patient. Here we clearly allow commercial ownership of human tissue, but not to its original possessor. Is this fair and just? And quite apart from who reaps the profits, are we wise to allow patents for still-living human tissue? Is it really necessary, in order to encourage the beneficial exploitation of these precious resources, to allow the usual commercial and market arrangements to flourish?

With regard to obtaining organs for transplantation, voluntary donation rather than sale or routine salvage has been the norm until now, at least in the United States. The Uniform Anatomical Gift Act, passed in all fifty states some twenty years ago, altered common-law practices regarding treatment of dead bodies to allow any individual to donate all or any part of his body, the gift to take place upon his death. In 1984, Congress passed the National Organ Transplantation Act to encourage and facilitate organ donation and transplantation, by means of federal grants to organ-procurement agencies and by the creation of a national procurement and matching network; this same statute prohibited and criminalized the purchase or sale of all human organs for transplant (if the transfer affects interstate commerce). Yet in the past few years, a number of commentators have been arguing for change, largely because of the shortage in organs available through donation. Some have, once again, called for a system of routine salvage of cadaveric organs, with organs always removed unless there is prior objection from the deceased or, after death, from his family—this is the current practice in most European countries (but not in Britain). Others, believing that it is physician diffidence or neglect that is to blame for the low yield, are experimenting with a system of required request, in which physicians are legally obliged to ask next of kin for permission to donate. Still others, wishing not to intrude upon either individual rights or family feelings regarding the body of the deceased, argue instead for allowing financial incentives to induce donation, some by direct sale, others by more ingenious methods. For example, in a widely discussed article, Lloyd Cohen proposes and defends a futures market in organs, with individuals selling (say, to the government) future rights to their cadaveric organs for money that will accrue to their estate if an organ is taken upon their death and used for transplant.

In this business, America is not the leader of the free-market world. Elsewhere, there already exist markets in organs, indeed in live organs. In India, for example, there is widespread and open buying and selling of kidneys, skin, and even eyes from living donors—your kidney today would fetch about 25,000 rupees, or about $1,200, a lifetime savings among the Indian poor. Rich people come to India from all over the world to purchase. Last summer, the *New York Times* carried a front-page story reporting current Chinese marketing practices, inviting people from Hong Kong to come to China for fixed-price kidney-transplant surgery, organs—from donors unspecified—and air fare included in the price. A communist country, it seems, has finally found a commodity offering it a favorable balance of trade with the capitalist West.

What are we to think of all this? It is, for me, less simple than I first thought. For notwithstanding my evident revulsions and repugnances, I am prepared to believe that offering financial incentives to prospective donors could very well increase the supply—and perhaps even the quality—of organs. I cannot deny that the dead human body has become a valuable resource which, rationally regarded, is being allowed to go to waste—in burial or cremation. Because of our scruples against sales, potential beneficiaries of transplantation are probably dying; less troubling but also true, their benefactors, actual and potential—unlike the transplant surgeons—are not permitted to reap tangible rewards for their acts of service. Finally, and most troublesome to me, I suspect that regardless of all my arguments to the contrary, I would probably make every effort and spare no expense to obtain a suitable life-saving kidney for my own child—if my own were unusable. And though I favor the pre-modern principle, "One man, one liver," and am otherwise disinclined to be an organ donor, and though I can barely imagine it, I think I would readily sell one of my own kidneys, were the practice legal, if it were the only way to pay for a life-saving operation for my children or my wife. These powerful feelings of love for one's own are certainly widely shared; though it is far from clear that they should be universalized to dictate mores or policy in this matter, they cannot be left out of any honest consideration.

The question "Organs for sale?" is compelling and confusing also for philosophical reasons. For it joins together some of the most powerful ideas and principles that govern and enrich life in modern, liberal Western society: devotion to scientific and medical progress for the relief of man's estate; private property, commerce, and free enterprise; and the primacy of personal autonomy and choice, including freedom of contract. And yet, seen in the mirror of the present question, these principles seem to reach their natural limit or at least lose some of their momentum. For they painfully collide here with certain other notions of decency and propriety, pre-modern and quasi-religious, such as the sanctity of man's bodily integrity and respect owed to his mortal remains. Can a balance be struck? If not, which side should give ground? The stakes would seem to be high—not only in terms of lives saved or lost but also in terms of how we think about and try to live the lives we save and have.

How to proceed? Alas, this, too, poses an interesting challenge—for in whose court should one conduct the inquiry? Shall we adopt the viewpoint of the economist or the transplant facilitator or the policy analyst, each playing largely by rational rules under some version of the utilitarian ethic: find the most efficient and economical way to save lives? Or shall we adopt the viewpoint of the strict libertarian, and place the burden of proof on those who would set limits to our autonomy to buy and sell or to treat our bodies in any way we wish? Or shall we adopt a moralist's position and defend the vulnerable, to argue that a great harm—say, the exploitation or degradation of even one person—cannot be overridden by providing greater goods to others, perhaps not even if the vulnerable person gives his less-than-fully-free consent?

Further, whichever outlook we choose, from which side shall we think about restrictions on buying and selling—what the experts call "inalienability"? Do we begin by assuming markets, and force opponents to defend non-sale as the exception? Or do we begin with some conception of human decency and human flourishing, and decide how best to pursue it, electing market mechanisms only where they are appropriate to enhancing human freedom and welfare, but remaining careful not to reduce the worth of everything to its market price? Or do we finesse such questions of principle altogether and try to muddle through, as we so often do, refining our policies on an *ad hoc* basis, in light of successes, costs, and public pressures? Whose principles and procedures shall we accept? And on whom shall we place the burden of what sort of proof?

Because of the special nature of this topic, I will not begin with markets and not even with rational calculations of benefits and harms. Indeed, I want to step back from policy questions altogether and consider more philosophically some aspects of the *meaning* of the idea of "organs for sale." I am especially eager to understand how this idea reflects and bears on our cultural and moral attitudes and sensibilities about our own humanity and, also, to discover the light it sheds on the principles of property, free contract, and medical progress. I wish, by this means, also to confront rational expertise and policy analysis with some notions outside of expertise, notions that are expressed and imbedded in our untutored repugnance at the thought of markets in human flesh. One would like to think that a proper understanding of these sentiments and notions—not readily rationalizable or measurable but not for that reason unreasonable or irrational—might even make a difference to policy.

I. Propriety

The non-expert approaching the topic of organ transplantation will begin with questions of propriety, for it is through the trappings of propriety that we normally approach the human body; indeed, many of our evolved conventions of propriety—of manners and civility—are a response to the fact and problem of human embodiment. What, then, is the fitting or suitable or seemly or decent or proper way to think about and treat the human body, living and dead? This is, indeed, a vast topic, yet absolutely central to our present concern; for what is permissible to do to and with the body is partly determined by what we take the human body to be and how it is related to our own being.

I have explored these questions at some length elsewhere, in an essay entitled "Thinking About the Body,"† from which I transplant some conclusions without the argument. Against our dominant philosophical outlooks of reductive corporealism (that knows not the soul) and person-body dualism (that deprecates the body), I advance the position of psychophysical unity, a position that holds that a human being is largely, if not wholly, self-identical with his enlivened body. Looking up to the body and meditating on its upright posture and on the human arm and hand, face and mouth, and the direction of our motion (with the help of Erwin Straus's famous essay on "The Upright Posture"), I argue for the body's intrinsic dignity:

---

† Leon R. Kass, M.D., *Toward a More Natural Science: Biology and Human Affairs* (New York: The Free Press, 1985).

The dumb human body, rightly attended to, shows all the marks of, and creates all the conditions for, our rationality and our special way of being-in-the-world. Our bodies demonstrate, albeit silently, that we are more than just a complex version of our animal ancestors, and, conversely, that we are also more than an enlarged brain, a consciousness somehow grafted onto or trapped within a blind mechanism that knows only survival. The body-form *as a whole* impresses on us its inner powers of thought and action. Mind and hand, gait and gaze, breath and tongue, foot and mouth—all are part of a single package, suffused with the presence of intelligence. We are *rational* (i.e., *thinking*) animals, down to and up from the very tips of our toes. No wonder, then, that even a corpse still shows the marks of our humanity.

And, of course, it shows too the marks of our particular incarnation of humanity, with our individual and unique identity.

Yet this is only part of the story. We are *thinking* animals, to be sure, but we are simultaneously also and merely thinking *animals.* Looking down on the body, and meditating on the meaning of its nakedness (with the help of the story of man and woman in the Garden of Eden), we learn of human weakness and vulnerability, and especially of the incompleteness, insufficiency, needy dependence, perishability, self-division, and lack of self-command implicit in our sexuality. Yet while perhaps an affront to our personal dignity, these bodily marks of human abjection point also to special interpersonal relationships, which are as crucial to our humanity as is our rationality.

For in the navel are one's forebears, in the genitalia our descendants. These reminders of perishability are also reminders of perpetuation; if we understand their meaning, we are even able to transform the necessary and shameful into the free and noble. . . . [The body, rightly considered,] reminds us of our debt and our duties to those who have gone before, [teaches us] that we are not our own source, neither in body nor in mind. Our dignity [finally] consists not in denying but in thoughtfully acknowledging and elevating the necessity of our embodiment, rightly regarding it as a gift to be cherished and respected. Through ceremonious treatment of mortal remains and through respectful attention to our living body and its inherent worth, we stand rightly when we stand reverently before the body, both living and dead.

This account of the meaning of the human body helps to make sense of numerous customs and taboos, some of them nearly universal. Cannibalism—the eating of human flesh, living and dead—is the pre-eminent defilement of the body; its humanity denied, the human body is treated as mere meat. Mutilation and dismemberment of corpses offend against bodily integrity; even surgery involves overcoming repugnance at violating wholeness and taboos against submitting to self-mutilation, overridden here only in order to defend the imperiled body against still greater threats to its integrity. Voyeurism, that cannibalism of the eyes, and other offenses against sexual privacy invade another's bodily life, objectifying and publicizing what is, in truth, immediate and intimate, meaningful only within and through shared experience. Decent burial— or other ceremonial treatment—of the mortal remains of ancestors and kin pays honor to both personal identity and generational indebtedness, written, as it were, into the body itself. How these matters are carried out will vary from culture to culture, but no culture ignores them—and some cultures are more self-consciously sensitive to these things than others.

Culture and the Body

The Homeric Greeks, who took embodiment especially to heart, regarded failure to obtain proper burial as perhaps the greatest affront to human dignity. The opposite of winning great glory is not cowardice or defeat, but becoming an unburied corpse. In his invocation to the Muse at the start of the *Iliad,* Homer deplores how the wrath of Achilles not only caused strong souls of heroes to be sent to Hades, but that *they themselves* were left to be the delicate feastings of birds and dogs; and the *Iliad* ends with the funeral of Hector, who is thus restored to his full humanity (above the animals) after Achilles's shameful treatment of his corpse: "So they buried Hector, breaker of horses." A similarly high re-gard for bodily integrity comes down to us through traditional Judaism and Christianity. Indeed, the Biblical tradition extends respect for bodily wholeness even to animals: while sanctioning the eating of meat, the Noachide code—widely regarded as enunciating natural rather than divine law—prohibits tearing a limb from a living animal.

Most of our attitudes regarding invasions of the body and treatment of corpses are carried less by maxims and arguments, more by senti-ments and repugnances. They are transmitted inadvertently and indi-rectly, rarely through formal instruction. For this reason, they are held by some to be suspect, mere sentiments, atavisms tied to superstitions of a bygone age. Some even argue that these repugnances are based mainly on strangeness and unfamiliarity: the strange repels *because* it is unfamil-iar. On this view, our squeamishness about dismemberment of corpses is akin to our horror at eating brains or mice. Time and exposure will cure us of these revulsions, especially when there are—as with organ transplantation—such enormous benefits to be won.

These views are, I believe, mistaken. To be sure, as an empirical matter, we can probably get used to many things that once repelled us—organ swapping among them. As Raskolnikov put it, and he should know, "Man gets used to everything—the beast." But I am certain that the repugnances that protect the dignity and integrity of the body are not based solely on strangeness. And they are certainly not irrational. On the contrary, they may just be—like the human body they seek to protect—the very embodiment of reason. Such was the view of Kant, whose title to rationality is second to none, writing in *The Metaphysical Principles of Virtue:*

> To deprive oneself of an integral part or organ (to mutilate oneself), e.g., to *give away* or *sell* a tooth so that it can be planted in the jawbone of another person, or to submit oneself to castration in order to gain an easier livelihood as a singer, and so on, belongs to partial self-murder. But this is not the case with the amputation of a dead organ, or one on the verge of mortification and thus harmful to life. Also, it cannot be reckoned a crime against one's own person to cut off something which is, to be sure, a part, but not an organ of the body, e.g., the hair, although selling one's hair for gain is not entirely free from blame.

Kant, rationalist though he was, understood the rational man's duty to himself as an animal body, precisely because this special animal body was the incarnation of reason:

> [T]o dispose of oneself as a mere means to some end of one's own liking is to degrade the humanity in one's person (*homo noumenon*), which, after all, was entrusted to man (*homo phenomenon*) to preserve.

Man contradicts his rational being by treating his body as a mere means.

Respect for the Living and the Dead

Beginning with notions of propriety, rooted in the meaning of our precarious yet dignified embodiment, we start with a series of presumptions and repugnances *against* treating the human body in the ways that are required for organ transplantation, which really is—once we strip away the trappings of the sterile operating rooms and their astonishing technologies—simply a noble form of cannibalism. Let me summarize these *prima facie* points of departure.

(1) Regarding *living donors,* there is a presumption against self-mutilation, even when good can come of it, a presumption, by the way, widely endorsed in the practice of medicine: Following venerable principles of medical ethics, surgeons are loath to cut into a healthy body not for its own benefit. As a result, most of them will not perform transplants using kidneys or livers from unrelated living donors.

(2) Regarding *cadaver donation,* there is a *beginning* presumption that mutilating a corpse defiles its integrity, that utilization of its parts violates its dignity, that ceremonial disposition of the total remains is the fitting way to honor and respect the life that once this body lived. Further, because of our body's inherent connection with the embodied lives of parents, spouses, and children, the common law properly mandates the body of the deceased to next of kin, in order to perform last rites, to mourn together in the presence of the remains, to say ceremonial farewell, and to mark simultaneously the connection to and the final separation from familial flesh. The deep wisdom of these sentiments and ways explains why it is a strange and indeed upsetting departure to allow the will of the deceased to determine the disposition of his remains and to direct the donation of his organs after death: for these very bodily remains are proof of the limits of his will and the fragility of his life, after which they "belong" properly to the family for the reasons and purposes just indicated. These reflections also explain why doctors—who know better than philosophers and economists the embodied nature of all personal life—are, despite their interest in organ transplantation, so reluctant to press the next of kin for permission to remove organs. This, and not fear of lawsuit, is the reason why doctors will not harvest organs without the family's consent, even in cases in which the deceased was a known, card-carrying organ donor.

(3) Regarding the *recipients of transplantation,* there is some primordial revulsion over confusion of personal identity, implicit in the thought of walking around with someone else's liver or heart. To be sure, for most recipients, life with mixed identity is vastly preferable to the alternative, and the trade is easily accepted. Also, the alien additions are tucked safely inside, hidden from sight. Yet transplantation as such—especially of vital organs—troubles the easygoing presumption of self-in-body, and ceases to do so only if one comes to accept a strict person-body dualism or adopts, against the testimony of one's own lived experience, the proposition that a person is or lives only in his brain-and-or-mind. Even the silent body speaks up to oppose transplantation, in the name of integrity, selfhood, and identity: its immune system,

which protects the body against all foreign intruders, naturally rejects tissues and organs transplanted from another body.

(4) Finally, regarding *privacy and publicity,* though we may celebrate the life-saving potential of transplantation or even ordinary surgery, we are rightly repelled by the voyeurism of the media, and the ceaseless chatter about this person's donation and that person's new heart. We have good reason to deplore the coarsening of sensibilities that a generation ago thought it crude of Lyndon Johnson to show off his surgical scar, but that now is quite comfortable with television in the operating suite, requests for organ donation in the newspaper, talk-show confessions of conceiving children to donate bone marrow, and the generalized talk of spare parts and pressed flesh.

I have, I am aware, laid it on thick. But I believe it is necessary to do so. For we cannot begin in the middle, taking organ transplantation simply for granted. We must see that, from the point of view of decency and seemliness and propriety, there are scruples to be overcome and that organ transplantation must bear the burden of proof. I confess that, on balance, I believe the burden can be easily shouldered, for the saving of life is indeed a great good, acknowledged by all. Desiring the end, we will the means, and reason thus helps us overcome our repugnances— and, unfortunately, leads us to forget what this costs us, in coin of shame and propriety. We are able to overcome the restraints against violating the integrity of dead bodies; less easily, but easily enough for kin, we overcome our scruple against self-mutilation in allowing and endorsing living donation—though here we remain especially sensitive to the dangers of coercion and manipulation of family ties.

How have we been able to do so? Primarily by insisting on the principle not only of voluntary consent but also of *free donation.* We have avoided the simple utilitarian calculation and not pursued the policy that would get us the most organs. We have, in short, acknowledged the weight of the non-utilitarian considerations, of the concerns of propriety. Indeed, to legitimate the separation of organs from bodies, we have insisted on a principle which obscures or even, in a sense, denies the fact of ultimate separation. For in a *gift* of an organ—by its living "owner"—as with any gift, what is given is not merely the physical entity. Like any gift, a *donated* organ carries with it the donor's generous good will. It is accompanied, so to speak, by the generosity of soul of the donor. Symbolically, the "aliveness" of the organ requisite for successful transplant bespeaks also the expansive liveliness of the donor—even, or especially, after his death. Thus, organ removal, the partial alienation-of-self-from-body, turns out to be, in this curious way, a *reaffirmation* of the self's embodiment, thanks to the generous act of donation.

We are now ready to think about buying and selling, and questions regarding the body as property.

II. Property

The most common objections to permitting the sale of body parts, especially from live donors, have to do with matters of equity, exploitation of the poor and the unemployed, and the dangers of abuse—not excluding theft and even murder to obtain valuable commodities. People deplore the degrading sale, a sale made in desperation, especially when the seller is selling something so precious as a part of his own body. Others deplore the rich man's purchase, and would group life-giving organs with other most basic goods that should not be available to the rich when the poor can't afford them (like allowing people to purchase substitutes for themselves in the military draft). Lloyd Cohen's proposal for a futures market in organs was precisely intended to avoid these evils: through it he addresses only increasing the supply without embracing a market for allocation—thus avoiding special privileges for the rich; and by buying early from the living but harvesting only from the dead he believes—I think mistakenly—that we escape the danger of exploiting the poor. (This and other half-market proposals seeking to protect the poor from exploitation would in fact cheat them out of what their organs would fetch, were the rich compelled to bid and buy in a truly open market.)

I certainly sympathize with these objections and concerns. As I read about the young healthy Indian men and women selling their kidneys to wealthy Saudis and Kuwaitis, I can only deplore the socioeconomic system that reduces people to such a level of desperation. And yet, at the same time, when I read the personal accounts of some who have sold, I am hard-pressed simply to condemn these individuals for electing apparently the only non-criminal way open to them to provide for a decent life for their families. As several commentators have noted, the sale of organs—like prostitution or surrogate motherhood or baby-selling—provides a double-bind for the poor. Proscription keeps them out of the economic mainstream, whereas permission threatens to accentuate their social alienation through the disapproval usually connected with trafficking in these matters.

Torn between sympathy and disgust, some observers would have it both ways: they would permit sale, but ban advertising and criminalize brokering (i.e., legalize prostitutes, prosecute pimps), presumably to eliminate coercive pressure from unscrupulous middlemen. But none of these analysts, it seems to me, has faced the question squarely. For if there were nothing fundamentally wrong with trading organs in the first place, why should it bother us that some people will make their living at it? The objection in the name of exploitation and inequity—however important for determining policy—seems to betray deeper objections, unacknowledged, to the thing itself—objections of the sort I dealt with in the discussion of propriety. For it is difficult to understand why someone who sees absolutely no difficulty at all with transplantation and donation should have such trouble sanctioning sale.

True, some things freely giveable ought not to be marketed because they cannot be sold: love and friendship are prime examples. So, too, are acts of generosity: it is one thing for me to offer in kindness to take the ugly duckling to the dance, it is quite another for her father to pay me to do so. But part of the reason love and generous deeds cannot be sold is that, strictly speaking, they cannot even be *given*—or, rather, they cannot be given *away*. One "gives" one's love to another or even one's body to one's beloved, one does not donate it; and when friendship is "given" it is still retained by its "owner." But the case with organs seems to be different: obviously material, they are freely alienable, they can be given and given away, and, therefore, they can be sold, and without diminishing the unquestioned good their transfer does for the recipient— why, then, should they not be for sale, of course, only by their proper "owner"? Why should not the owner-donor get something for his organs? We come at last to the question of the body as property.

Whose Body?

Even outside of law and economics, there are perhaps some common-sense reasons for regarding the body as property. For one thing, there is the curious usage of the possessive pronoun to identify my body. Often I do indeed regard my body a tool (literally, an organ or instrument) of my soul or will. My organism is organized for whose use?—why, for my own. My rake is mine, so is the arm with which I rake. The "my-ness" of my body also acknowledges the privacy and unsharability of my body. More importantly, it means also to assert possession against threats of unwelcome invasion, as in the song "My Body's Nobody's Body But Mine," which reaches for metaphysics in order to teach children to resist potential molesters. My body may or may not be mine or God's, but as between you and me, it is clearly mine.

And yet, I wonder. What kind of *property* is my body? Is it mine or is it me? Can it—or much of it—be alienated, like my other property, like my car or even my dog? And on what basis do I claim property *rights* in my body? Is it really "my own"? Have I labored to produce it? Less than did my mother, and yet it is not hers. Do I claim it on merit? Doubtful: I had it even before I could be said to be deserving. Do I hold it as a gift— whether or not there be a giver? How does one possess and use a gift? Are there limits on my right to dispose of it as I wish—especially if I do not know the answer to these questions? Can one sell—or even give away—that which is not clearly one's own?

The word property comes originally from the Latin adjective *proprius* (the root also of "proper"—fit or apt or suitable—and, thus, also of "propriety"), *proprius* meaning "one's own, special, particular, peculiar." Property is both that which is one's own, and also the right—indeed, the exclusive right—to its possession, use, or disposal. And while there might seem to be nothing that is more "my own" than my own body, common sense finally rejects the view that my body is, strictly speaking, my property. For we do and should distinguish among that which is *me*, that which is *mine*, and that which is mine as *my property*. My body is me; my daughters are mine (and so are my opinions, deeds, and speeches); my car is my property. Only the last can clearly be alienated and sold at will.

Philosophical reflection, deepening common sense, would seem to support this view, yet not without introducing new perplexities. If we turn to John Locke, the great teacher on property, the right of property traces home in fact to the body:

> Though the earth and all creatures be common to all men, yet every man has a property in his own person; this nobody has a right to but himself. The labour of his body and the work of his hands we may say are properly his.

The right to the fruits of one's labor seems, for Locke, to follow from the property each man has in his own person. But unlike the rights in the fruits of his labor, the rights in one's person are for Locke surely inalienable (like one's inalienable right to liberty, which also cannot be transferred to another, say, by selling oneself into slavery). The property in my own person seems to function rather to limit intrusions and claims possibly made upon me by others; it functions to exclude me—and every other human being—from the commons available to all men for appropriation and use. Thus, though the right to property stems from the my-own-ness (rather than the in-commons-ness) of my body and its labor, the body itself cannot be, for Locke, property like any other. It is, like property, exclusively mine to use; but it is, unlike property, not mine to dispose of. (The philosophical and moral weakness in the very idea of property is now exposed to view: Property rights stem from the my-own-ness of my labor, which in turn is rooted in the my-own-ness of my body; but this turns out to be only relatively and politically my own.)

Yet here we are in trouble. The living body as a whole is surely not alienable, but parts of it definitely are. I may give blood, bone marrow, skin, a kidney, parts of my liver, and other organs without ceasing to be me, as the by-and-large self-same embodied being I am. It matters not to my totality or identity if the kidney I surrendered was taken because it was diseased or because I gave it for donation. And, coming forward to my cadaver, however much it may be me rather than you, however much it will be *my* mortal remains, it will not be me; my corpse and I will have gotten divorced, and, for that reason, I can contemplate donating from it without any personal diminution. How much and what parts of the bodily me are, finally, not indispensably me but merely mine? Do they thus become mine as my property? Why or why not?

The analysis of the notion of the body as property produces only confusion—one suspects because there is confusion in the heart of the idea of property itself, as well as deep mystery in the nature of personal identity. Most of the discussion would seem to support the common-sense and common-law teaching that *there is no property in a body*—not in my own body, not in my own corpse, and surely not in the corpse of my deceased ancestor. (Regarding the latter, the common-law courts had granted to next of kin a quasi-property right in the dead body, purely a custodial right for the limited purpose of burial, a right which also obliged the family to protect the person's right to a decent burial against creditors and other claimants. It was this wise teaching that was set aside by the Uniform Anatomical Gift Act.) Yet if my body is not my property, if I have no property right in my body—and here, philosophically and morally, the matter is surely dubious at best—by what *right* do I give parts of it away? And, if it be by right of property, how can one then object—in principle—to sale?

Liberty and Its Limits

Let us try a related but somewhat different angle. Connected to the notion of private property is the notion of free contract, the permission to transfer our entitlements at will to other private owners. Let us shift our attention from the vexed question of ownership to the principle of freedom. It was, you will recall, something like the principle of freedom—voluntary and freely given donation—that was used to justify the gift of organs, overcoming the presumption against mutilation. In contrast to certain European countries, where the dead body now becomes the property of the state, under principles of escheatage or condemnation, we have chosen to stay with individual rights. But why have we done so? Is it because we want to have the social benefits of organ transplantation without compromising respectful burial, and believe that leaving matters to individual choice is the best way to obtain these benefits? Or is the crucial fact our liberal (or even libertarian) belief in the goodness of autonomy and individual choice *per se*? Put another way, is it the dire need for organs that justifies opening a freedom of contract to dispose of organs, as the best—or least bad—instrument for doing so? Or is the freedom of contract paramount, and we see here a way to take social advantage of the right people have to use their bodies however they wish? The difference seems to me crucial. For the principle of autonomy, separated from specific need, would liberate us for all sorts of subsequent uses of the human body, especially should they become profitable.

Our society has perceived a social need for organs. We have chosen to meet that need not by direct social decision and appropriation, but, indirectly, through permitting and encouraging voluntary giving. It is, as I have argued, generosity—that is, more the "giving" than the "voluntariness"—that provides the moral ground; yet being liberals and not totalitarians, we put the legal weight on freedom—and hope people will use it generously. As a result, it looks as if, to facilitate and to justify the practice of organ donation, we have enshrined something like the notions of property rights and free contract in the body, notions that usually include the possibility of buying and selling. This is slippery business. Once the principle of private right and autonomy is taken as the standard, it will prove difficult—if not impossible—to hold the line between donation and sale. (It will even prove impossible, philosophically, to argue against voluntary servitude, bestiality, and other abominations.) Moreover, the burden of proof will fall squarely on those who want to set limits on what people may freely do with their bodies or for what purposes they may buy and sell body parts. It will, in short, be hard to prevent buying and selling human flesh not only for transplantation, but for, say, use in luxury nouvelle cuisine, once we allow markets for transplantation on libertarian grounds. We see here, in the prism of this case, the limits and, hence, the ultimate insufficiency of rights and the liberal principle.

Astute students of liberalism have long observed that our system of ordered liberties presupposes a certain kind of society—of at least minimal decency, and with strong enough familial and religious institutions to cultivate the sorts of men and women who can live civilly and responsibly with one another, while enjoying their private rights. We wonder whether freedom of contract regarding the body, leading to its being bought and sold, will continue to make corrosive inroads upon the kind of people we want to be and need to be if the uses of our freedom are not to lead to our willing dehumanization. We have, over the years, moved the care for life and death from the churches to the hospitals, and the disposition of mortal remains from the clergy to the family and now to the individual himself—and perhaps, in the markets of the future, to the insurance companies or the state or to enterprising brokers who will give new meaning to insider trading. No matter how many lives are saved, is this good for how we are to live?

Let us put aside questions about property and free contract, and think only about buying and selling. Never mind our rights, what would it mean to fully commercialize the human body even, say under state monopoly? What, regardless of political system, is the moral and philosophical difference between giving an organ and selling it, or between receiving it as a gift and buying it?

Commodification

The idea of commodification of human flesh repels us, quite properly I would say, because we sense that the human body especially belongs in that category of things that defy or resist commensuration—like love or friendship or life itself. To claim that these things are "priceless" is not to insist that they are of infinite worth or that one cannot calculate (albeit very roughly, and then only with aid of very crude simplifying assumptions) how much it costs to sustain or support them. Rather it is to claim that the bulk of their meaning and their human worth do not lend themselves to quantitative measures; for this reason, we hold them to be incommensurable, not only morally but factually.

Against this view, it can surely be argued that the entire system of market exchange rests on our arbitrary but successful attempts to commensurate the (factually) incommensurable. The genius of money is precisely that it solves by convention the problem of natural incommensurability, say between oranges and widgets, or between manual labor and the thinking time of economists. The possibility of civilization altogether rests on this conventional means of exchange, as the ancient Greeks noted by deriving the name for money, *nomisma*, from the root *nomos*, meaning "convention"—that which has been settled by human agreement—and showing how this fundamental convention made possible commerce, leisure, and the establishment of gentler views of justice.

Yet the purpose of instituting such a conventional measure was to facilitate the satisfaction of *natural* human needs and the desires for well-being and, eventually, to encourage the full flowering of human possibility. Some notion of need or perceived human good provided always the latent non-conventional standard behind the nomismatic convention—tacitly, to be sure. And there's the rub: In due course, the standard behind money, being hidden, eventually becomes forgotten, and the counters of worth become taken for worth itself.

Truth to tell, commodification by conventional commensuration always risks the homogenization of worth, and even the homogenization of things, all under the aspect of quantity. In many transactions, we do not mind or suffer or even notice. Yet the human soul finally rebels against the principle, whenever it strikes closest to home. Consider, for example, why there is such widespread dislike of the pawnbroker. It is not only that he profits from our misfortunes and sees the shame of our having to part with heirlooms and other items said (inadequately) to have "sentimental value." It is especially because he will not and cannot appreciate their human and personal worth and pays us only their market price. How much more will we object to those who would commodify our very being?

We surpass all defensible limits of such conventional commodification when we contemplate making the convention-maker—the human being—just another one of the commensurables. The end comes to be treated as mere means. Selling our bodies, we come perilously close to selling out our souls. There is even a danger in contemplating such a prospect—for if we come to think about ourselves like pork bellies, pork bellies we will become.

We have, with some reluctance, overcome our repugnance at the exploitative manipulation of one human body to serve the life and health of another. We have managed to justify our present arrangements not only on grounds of utility or freedom but also and especially on the basis of generosity, in which the generous deed of the giver is inseparable from the organ given. To allow the commodification of these exchanges is to forget altogether the impropriety overcome in allowing donation and transplantation in the first place. And it is to turn generosity into trade, gratitude into compensation. It is to treat the most delicate of human affairs as if everything is reducible to its price.

There is a euphemism making the rounds in these discussions that makes my point. Eager to encourage more donation, but loath to condone or to speak about buying and selling organs, some have called for the practice of "rewarded gifting"—in which the donor is rewarded for his generosity, not paid for his organ. Some will smile at what looks like double-talk or hypocrisy, but even if it is hypocrisy, it is thereby a tribute paid to virtue. Rewards are given for good deeds, whereas fees are charged for services, and prices are paid merely for goods. If we must continue to practice organ transplantation, let us do so on good behavior.

Anticipating the problem we now face, Paul Ramsey twenty years ago proposed that we copy for organ donation a practice sometimes used in obtaining blood: those who freely give can, when in need, freely receive. "Families that shared in premortem giving of organs could share in freely receiving if one of them needs transplant therapy. This would be—if workable—a civilizing exchange of benefit that is not the same as commerce in organs." Ramsey saw in this possibility of organized generosity a way to promote civilized community and to make virtue grow out of dire necessity. These, too, are precious "commodities," and provide an additional reason for believing that the human body and the extraordinary generosity in the gift of its parts are altogether too precious to be commodified.

III. The Price of Progress

The arguments I have offered are not easy to make. I am all too well aware that they can be countered, that their appeal is largely to certain hard-to-articulate intuitions and sensibilities that I at least believe belong intimately to the human experience of our own humanity. Precious though they might be, they do not exhaust the human picture, far from it. And perhaps, in the present case, they should give way to rational calculation, market mechanisms, and even naked commodification of human flesh—all in the service of saving life at lowest cost (though, parenthetically, it would be worth a whole separate discussion to consider whether, in the longer view, there are not cheaper, more effective, and less indecent means to save lives, say, through preventive measures that forestall end-stage renal disease now requiring transplantation: the definitions of both need and efficiency are highly contingent, and we should beware of allowing them to be defined for us by those technologists—like transplant surgeons—wedded to present practice). Perhaps this is not the right place to draw a line or to make a stand.

Consider, then, a slightly more progressive and enterprising proposal, one anticipated by my colleague, Willard Gaylin, in an essay, "Harvesting the Dead," written in 1974. Mindful of all the possible uses of newly dead—or perhaps not-quite-dead—bodies, kept in their borderline condition by continuous artificial respiration and assisted circulation, intact, warm, pink, recognizably you or me, but brain dead, Gaylin imagines the multiple medically beneficial uses to which the bioemporium of such "neomorts" could be put: the neomorts could, for example, allow physicians-in-training to practice pelvic examinations and tracheal intubations without shame or fear of doing damage; they could serve as unharmable subjects for medical experimentation and drug testing, provide indefinite supplies of blood, marrow, and skin, serve as factories to manufacture hormones and antibodies, or, eventually, be dismembered for transplantable spare parts. Since the newly dead body really is such a precious resource, why not really put it to full and limitless use?

Gaylin's scenario is not so far-fetched. Proposals to undertake precisely such body-farming have been seriously discussed among medical scientists in private. The technology for maintaining neomorts is already available. Indeed, in the past few years, a publicly traded corporation has opened a national chain of large, specialized nursing homes—or should we rather call them nurseries?—for the care and feeding solely of persons in persistent vegetative state or ventilator-dependent irreversible coma. Roughly ten establishments, each housing several hundred of such beings, already exist. All that would be required to turn them into Gaylin's bioemporia would be a slight revision in the definition of death (already proposed for other reasons)—to shift from death of the whole brain to death of the cortex and the higher centers—plus the will not to let these valuable resources go to waste. (The company's stock, by the way, has more than quadrupled in the last year alone; perhaps someone is already preparing plans for mergers and manufacture.) Repulsive? You bet. Useful? Without doubt. Shall we go forward into this brave new world?

Forward we are going, without anyone even asking the question. In the twenty-five years since I began thinking about these matters, our society has overcome longstanding taboos and repugnances to accept test-tube fertilization, commercial sperm-banking, surrogate motherhood, abortion on demand, exploitation of fetal tissue, patenting of living human tissue, gender-change surgery, liposuction and body shops, the widespread shuttling of human parts, assisted-suicide practiced by doctors, and the deliberate generation of human beings to serve as transplant donors—not to speak about massive changes in the culture regarding shame, privacy, and exposure. Perhaps more worrisome than the changes themselves is the coarsening of sensibilities and attitudes, and the irreversible effects on our imaginations and the way we come to conceive of ourselves. For there is a sad irony in our biomedical project, accurately anticipated in Aldous Huxley's *Brave New World:* We expend enormous energy and vast sums of money to preserve and prolong bodily life, but in the process our embodied life is stripped of its gravity and much of its dignity. This is, in a word, progress as tragedy.

In the transplanting of human organs, we have made a start on a road that leads imperceptibly but surely toward a destination that none of us wants to reach. A divination of this fact produced reluctance at the start. Yet the first step, overcoming reluctance, was defensible on benevolent and rational grounds: save life using organs no longer useful to their owners and otherwise lost to worms.

Now, embarked on the journey, we cannot go back. Yet we are increasingly troubled by the growing awareness that there is neither a natural nor a rational place to stop. Precedent justifies extension, so does rational calculation: We are in a warm bath that warms up so imperceptibly that we don't know when to scream.

And this is perhaps the most interesting and the most tragic element of my dilemma—and it is not my dilemma alone. I don't want to encourage; yet I cannot simply condemn. I refuse to approve; yet I cannot moralize. How, in this matter of organs for sale, as in so much of modern life, is one to conduct one's thoughts if one wishes neither to be a crank nor to yield what is best in human life to rational analysis and the triumph of technique? Is poor reason impotent to do anything more than to recognize and state this tragic dilemma?

28 Which Ills To Bear?: Reevaluating the "Threat" of Modern Genetics

ALEXANDER MORGAN CAPRON

Alexander Morgan Capron is Professor of Law and Medicine at the University of Southern California.

For more than a century, archaeologists, anthropologists, and biologists have been digging through layers of dirt and rock, sieving fossils and artifacts, in an attempt to figure out when, where, and how human beings differentiated from other primates to become a unique species. . . .

The development of molecular genetic techniques for analyzing DNA offers a new source of evidence in the ongoing debate about human origins. Techniques for mapping and sequencing DNA allow researchers to compare different species and different individuals from the same species at the most basic level.

—*Office of Technology Assessment*[1]

I don't think these scientists are thinking about mankind at all. I think that they're getting the thrills and the excitement and the passion to dig in and keep digging to see what the hell they can do.

—*Alfred E. Vellucci*
Mayor of Cambridge, Massachusetts[2]

This article first appeared in Emory Law Review *39 (Summer 1990): 665–696.*

The synthetic chemistry and molecular biology of yesterday
are curing disease today, just as the theoretical physics of yesterday provides the nuclear power of today. Only twenty years
ago heredity was hidden in abstract genetic language; today it
has found explicit chemical terms to work with in ameliorating
human faults and constructing better bodies. . . . Great expectation, great hopes, push us on. . . . It is no longer possible to
entertain a self-image as complacent as the one we used to have
because we assumed we were fixed in whatever shape we were
given by nature.

—*Joseph Fletcher*[3]

[W]ho would fardels bear,
To grunt and sweat under a weary life,
But that the dread of something after death,
The undiscover'd country, from whose bourn
No traveller returns, puzzles the will,
And makes us rather bear those ills we have
Than fly to others that we know not of?

—*William Shakespeare,* Hamlet[4]

INTRODUCTION

That molecular genetics is the quintessential life science of the twen-
tieth century—as nuclear physics is the quintessential physical science—
is obvious. Still to be determined is whether genetics will also spawn the
most important medical advances, thus rivaling antibiotics and vaccines
(fields that rely heavily on the tools of molecular biology).

Less in doubt is that—at a rate that is disproportionate to its manifest consequences—the field of genetics has provoked public excitement
and terror, which in turn have engendered statutes, regulations, and
court rulings. Ever since the rediscovery of Mendel's experimental findings at the beginning of this century, genetic theories and tools have
been employed in framing public policy. Likewise, government involvement with genetics has also been a source of major criticism and concern, from the revulsion at the misuse of genetics by Nazi eugenicists to
latter day alarm over genetic engineering.[5]

Categorizing developments in genetics is no easy task. Though
Mendel is the "father" of genetics, his now famous paper of 1865[6] never
used the term "genes." Similarly, a century later Rollin Hotchkiss coined
the term "genetic engineering" before the tools that made genetic engineering feasible had even been detected.[7] For purposes of this paper,
I will refer to the period prior to the early 1970s, when restriction

enzymes were discovered and first used to create "recombinant molecules," as the period of "classical genetics," and the period since then as
that of "modern genetics." (This description is quite arbitrary; many
people would date modern genetics to the discovery of the structure
of DNA [deoxyribonucleic acid] by James Watson and Francis Crick
in 1953, but as I am more concerned with the uses of genetics than
with theoretic discoveries, the development of the means to manipulate
genes seems a more important dividing point.)

As enthusiastic as biologists—to say nothing of physicians and drug
companies—have been about modern genetic developments, the field
has repeatedly been perceived as a "threat" by some members of the
public and public officials. My thesis is that, for the most part, the public
has gotten the "threat" wrong. Genetics does hold peril as well as promise, but the perils that ought most to concern us have gotten considerably
less attention than those that have been most loudly trumpeted.

To the extent that society has responded to concerns voiced about
genetics, those responses have not been notably productive. There are
several possible explanations for this failure. One could be that the concerns raised have related to things which turned out not to involve the
harm alleged, hence obviating the need for the proposed response. Second, some of the attempts to respond have gotten tangled up in related
subjects (particularly the abortion controversy), thus impeding the ability of anyone to take effective action on the specifically genetic issues.
Third, the concerns may have been about things that amount to wrongs,
rather than harms; as to the former, the law does not offer adequate
means of control and its usually most potent tool—tort law—fits poorly
with those wrongs that do occur, as it tends to compensate for wrongs
(often labelled "dignitary harms") only if they are intentionally imposed
on their victims.

A fourth explanation is that the real "threat" posed by modern genetics is to the collectivity, by the changes that genetics can bring about
in values and the alterations it generates in our perception and understanding of the world, not merely because of its *discoveries* (as was true of
Copernicus and Darwin) but also because of its *ability to modify* living
things, including human beings. The legal mechanisms of a liberal society—much less the rudimentary means for collective action available
to the world at large—are ill-suited for responding to such conceptual
challenges, not the least because, as Joshua Lederberg has observed,
"[t]he suppression of knowledge appears . . . unthinkable, not only on
ideological, but merely on logical grounds. How can the ignorant know
what they should not know?"[8]

By both misstating and exaggerating the hazards posed by developments in genetic knowledge and practical capabilities, past responses

have risked erecting unnecessary barriers to beneficial uses, thus leaving persons with genetic diseases to bear their ills so that the rest of us can avoid purely hypothetical risks.[9] Perhaps if we refocused on those "threats" to human beings that are more concrete and comprehensible—and, one might argue, more probable—we could develop responses that would actually be effective in directing the powers of genetics into their most beneficial uses. Identifying genetic screening as one such area of inquiry, this article suggests some appropriate responses in that area and addresses concerns raised by the more controversial fields of genetic engineering and gene mapping at a more conceptual level, drawing (loosely) on critical theory.

I. THE GREATEST THREAT: GENETIC ENGINEERING?

Human beings have a long history of interfering with living things, themselves included. The cultivation of food plants and the domestication of animals are older than recorded history; the remarkable accomplishments of botanists and plant breeders like Luther Burbank and George Washington Carver are more than familiar schoolbook tales, for they also led to the adoption of statutes to create a protectable interest for the "inventors" of novel plant varieties. To the opposite effect, medical interventions, by saving lives that would otherwise be lost to disease, have subtly increased the frequency of certain deleterious (even lethal) genes in the population.

A. The Perception of a "Fundamental Danger"

For some people, this history of human intervention—even, in the "remaking" of human beings themselves—is merely a reflection of what makes us human, that is, our ability to plan, to organize, to act, and to remember. In Judeo-Christian terms, man, created in the image of God, was given dominion over the earth and the power (and responsibility) to act as a co-creator. Yet, for other people, this history provides no sanction for the use of modern genetics techniques to intervene more directly and in a more directed fashion with living things. In reviewing the first application for a patent on an "engineered" microorganism, Chief Justice Burger noted the objections that had been raised to research of the type that underlay that patent:

> Scientists, among them Nobel laureates, are quoted suggesting that genetic research may pose a serious threat to the human race, or, at the very least, that dangers are far too substantial to permit such research to proceed apace at this time. We are told that genetic research and related technological developments may spread pollution and disease, that it may result in a loss of

genetic diversity, and that its practice may tend to depreciate the value of human life.[10]

Rather than become enmeshed in this debate, the Supreme Court concluded that it was "the business of elected representatives," not judges, to decide whether genetic engineering was a "serious threat" or presented "fantasies generated by fear of the unknown."[11] Shortly thereafter, the General Secretaries of the National Council of Churches, the Synagogue Council of America, and the United States Catholic Conference requested that President Carter remedy the lack of "adequate oversight or control" concerning especially the issues relating to the uses on human beings of the genetic technology. They declared:

> We are rapidly moving into a new era of fundamental danger triggered by the rapid growth of genetic engineering. Albeit, there may be opportunity for doing good; the very term suggests the danger.[12]

1. Protecting Against Biohazards

For the clerics, the "danger" may have been apparent in the term "genetic engineering" itself. Yet the initial concerns about this technology—raised by researchers themselves,[13] and culminating in an unprecedented moratorium in 1974 to 1975 on certain types of experiments using the newly discovered restriction enzymes[14]—were much more practical and resided not in the fact of the technology but in particular uses of it. Those concerns centered on the creation of novel pathogenic microorganisms, and they were met by the development of what are known as the "NIH Guidelines for Research Involving Recombinant DNA Molecules."[15]

Although the impetus for, and initial formulation of, the guidelines had come from the researchers involved, the process under which they are now applied rests with a committee known as the RAC (for Recombinant DNA Advisory Committee) which includes social scientists, ethicists, lawyers, and other nonscientists, serving as advisors to the Director of the National Institutes of Health, the agency responsible for providing most of the federal support for genetic engineering studies. Crudely described, the NIH Guidelines simply impose on institutions where research using recombinant techniques is performed requirements for the use of methods of physical and biological containment that are comparable to (or somewhat in excess of) the standards that microbiologists dealing with virulent organisms apply in their work (but which seem to have been unfamiliar to molecular biologists when they first began using the recombinant DNA techniques to manipulate bacteria and viruses).

The involvement of nonscientists in the process, and the high degree of public scrutiny that it has received for the past fifteen years, seems more an historical artifact than an accurate reflection of any unusual "threat" in the gene splicing research now being carried out in laboratories. (Indeed, many requirements of the original guidelines have been relaxed, as the RAC found them to be unduly restrictive or demanding in light of actual risks.) Ironically, the areas that might well generate the most concern—release of altered organisms into the environment (for agricultural or industrial purposes) and the large-scale manufacturing of altered organisms (for pharmaceutical or industrial purposes)—have received less rigorous and less publicly visible scrutiny, although these large projects and field tests continue to be the source of occasional objection from private parties.[16] Again, whatever the risks of such activities, it seems dubious in many cases that they are any greater than comparable activities that use methodologies other than genetic engineering.[17] The net result has been that genetic engineering research has probably been subjected to a more stringent process of prior review, in which the weighing of risks against benefits incorporates the views of the nonscientific "public," than any other area of science.

2. Human Gene Therapy—Means and Ends

This extraordinary degree of public scrutiny did not, however, alter the sense of some people—like the clerical leaders, in their 1980 letter to the President—that once genetic engineering is employed to alter human beings a "fundamental danger" will be posed, beyond that which the RAC was capable of addressing. The reassertion of concern over inadequate oversight was doubtless largely a result of a certain basic horror at the notion of direct intervention in human life (which manifested itself from the first genetic engineering controversies in the frequency with which analogies were drawn to Dr. Frankenstein);[18] perhaps it also resulted from a sense that the RAC had never addressed such questions as whether different burdens of proof might be appropriate in judging the risks of means, especially physical risks (standard fare for the RAC), as compared with the risks of ends, particularly social risks.[19]

The examination of the clerics' concerns that the President's Commission for the Study of Ethical Problems in Medicine and Biomedical and Behavioral Research undertook at the request of President Carter's Science Advisor relied upon the distinction between means and ends. As to the former, the commissioners found nothing inherently unethical or socially unacceptable in attempts to place functional genes in patients who suffer from a genetic disorder. The alarm over scientists "who would play God" (in the words of the clerics) served at best as a reminder of the need for caution when human beings exercise greater powers, but the religious scholars who examined the "playing God" objection at the request of the President's Commission rejected the notion that medical interventions to save lives and relieve suffering violate divinely pre-scribed laws. Indeed, changes in genetic material of the type that would be involved in "gene therapy" occur in nature all the time, in human beings as in other living things; medicine, in harnessing these same techniques, merely aims to provide an intentional benefit rather than the random harm that nature often dispenses.

B. Evaluating Consequences

1. For Individuals—Like Any Innovative Therapy

Turning to the consequences of using genetic engineering on hu-man beings, the Commission first addressed the consequences for in-dividuals who undergo such interventions. The Commission found that for these individuals, the issues are the same as for any other patient-subjects and revolve around a balancing of the risks and benefits of using an experimental means of therapy, especially when conventional means are nonexistent or only partially effective. This balancing is ultimately performed by the patient-subject in conjunction with the physician-investigator, but before such individual "informed consent" can be ob-tained, the design of the research and the content of the consent form are typically subject to review by others, such as both the institutional re-view board (IRB) and the institutional biosafety committee at the hospi-tal or university where the physician works, by the peer review process of the National Institutes of Health, and by the Food and Drug Adminis-tration. Under a process adopted as a consequence of recommendations of the President's Commission, a group—now known as the Human Gene Therapy Subcommittee (HGTS)—was created to provide the NIH with additional, specialized review of all research in which recombinant DNA would be used to insert a "foreign" gene into a human being.

The HGTS has spent most of its six years of existence developing and refining a set of "Points to Consider in the Design and Submission of Protocols for the Transfer of Recombinant DNA into the Genome of Human Subjects," in which it sets forth the issues that will guide its deliberations on research proposals, rather than providing a statement of the requirements for approval.[20] In 1989, the HGTS and the RAC recommended, and the Director of NIH approved, the first officially sanctioned use of recombinant DNA technology in the treatment of human beings, although the research—in which the gene coding for neomycin-resistance was inserted into tumor-infiltrating lymphocytes used in immunotherapy for advanced melanoma—involved transfer of a gene as a marker rather than as an active factor in bringing about the therapeutic goal of the intervention.

In March 1990, nearly ten years after the church leaders warned of the need for an urgent response to a rapidly developing danger, the RAC and HGTS had before them the first proposal for a therapeutic use of a "foreign" gene in a human being.[21] Though this protocol is a landmark in modern genetics, it involves the insertion of the gene into lymphocytes rather than into bone marrow stem cells, so that the new genetic information—intended to supply the genetic message for adenosine deaminase (ADA) that is missing in some people who suffer severe combined immunodeficiency disease—is expected to persist only as long as the lymphocytes remain in a patient's bloodstream.

At this writing, the HGTS and the RAC appear to be on the brink of approving the protocol.[22] Not surprisingly, in light of the panels' past discussions and the suggestions implicit in the "Points to Consider," the review process at NIH has focused on practical issues that—rather than being unique to human gene therapy—are merely magnified beyond the extent they would occur in any novel treatment program. Among these will be such issues as: (i) the comparative risk-benefit ratios for gene therapy versus existing modes of treatment for the disease (such as enzyme replacement therapy that is being tested for ADA); (ii) the safety (for treatment personnel and other parties as well as for the patient) in using a disabled retrovirus to transfer the relevant gene into the lymphocytes; (iii) the adequacy of *in vitro* and animal studies to establish both the probable efficacy and absence of side effects expectable in human use of the technique; (iv) the acceptability of surrogate decisionmaking on behalf of the patient-subjects (who, by the nature of the disease, will be minors); and (v) the ability of the researchers to protect the privacy of the patient-subjects, in light of the media's likely interest in the first approved trials of genetic engineering in human beings.

2. For Future Generations—Germ-Line Experiments

Given that the President's Commission concluded that somatic cell gene therapy is comparable to any other medical treatment, it is hardly surprising that the NIH advisory committees charged with reviewing the protocols should function more or less like super-specialized IRBs. A distinction drawn by the Commission[23] and followed by the HGTS, however, would limit the introduction of genes to body cells only and would not allow alteration of the germ-line cells, which determine the genetic information passed on to offspring. Thus, in addition to requesting information from which one can estimate the risk of a transferred gene infecting third parties, the "Points to Consider" requests comparable information about "the possibility that the proposed experiment will inadvertently affect reproductive cells."[24] In a burst of subtlety that will probably be lost on most designers of gene therapy experiments, the "Points" proclaims, "The RAC and its Subcommittee will not at present entertain proposals for germ-line alterations but will consider for approval protocols involving somatic cell gene therapy."[25] Apparently, researchers may submit protocols that involve intentional or unintentional germ-line genetic alterations, but the HGTS and RAC will not yet "entertain" them "for approval," although if preparatory research has progressed to the point where human germ-line alterations are a real possibility, the review groups at the NIH want to be made cognizant of that fact.

The major reasons for drawing a line between somatic-cell and germ-line interventions—beyond the greater risk of harm in the latter to the individuals directly affected and doubts that there are many situations in which alternative, simpler means would not be available[26]—are that germ-line changes not only run the risk of perpetuating any errors made into future generations of nonconsenting "subjects" but also go beyond ordinary medicine and interfere with human evolution. Again, it must be admitted that all of medicine obstructs evolution. But that is inadvertent, whereas with human germ-line genetic engineering, the interference is intentional. Still, the results produced by evolution at any point in time are hardly sacrosanct; indeed, genetic diseases are a reminder that evolution can fail to be either "wise" or "kind" where individuals are concerned. Thus, the fact that germ-line genetic engineering would produce intentional changes in humankind's genetic inheritance is not a sufficient reason to foreswear the technique forever,[27] though it is reason enough to distinguish it from somatic-cell interventions.

3. For Society in General

Given the level of anxiety that surfaced in many public discussions of human genetic engineering a decade ago—and that may well still exist, just waiting for the provocation of sufficient growth in the field to make the threat seem real again—it is noteworthy how little progress has been made in grappling with the wider implications of human genetic alteration. The President's Commission surveyed a range of possible consequences at the level of concepts and attitudes that might be transformed by the availability of germ-line genetic engineering. Among these were alterations in parental rights and responsibilities,[28] in societal obligations regarding care,[29] and in society's commitment to equality of opportunity.[30] Even more fundamentally, were genetic engineering capable of altering important human traits (such as intelligence, dexterity, or personality) rather than simply overcoming single-gene metabolic defects and the like, it could transform what it means to be human and our sense of personal identity. As one geneticist boldly declared two decades ago, genetic engineering would provide a simple means to convert "all the unfit to the highest genetic level," for today "[w]e seek not in the stars but in our genes for the herald of our fate."[31] Finally, the techniques of genetic engineering might be used not merely to bring all people up to a "normal" level but actually to "enhance" human capabilities by providing genes not usually found in a particular form in humans.

Further examination is plainly needed of such questions as: what is "human nature" from a genetic vantagepoint, and where ought limits be drawn on its alteration? Or, alternatively, when if ever would genetic alterations render the ensuing being not human? The Biomedical Ethics Advisory Committee (BEAC), the successor to the President's Commission, was expected to deal with issues of this sort, but abortion politics have deadlocked the Congressional Biomedical Ethics Board to which the Committee reports, resulting in the BEAC being placed like a frozen embryo into the equivalent of bureaucratic liquid nitrogen. The HGTS once seemed intent on taking on the fundamental issues implicated in human genetic engineering but was deterred from this undertaking by its role in the grant-approval process at the NIH because it seemed unfair to condition approval of any particular genetics researcher's project on his or her developing and justifying a theory about the relationship of that project (much less the entire field of gene therapy) to the larger, long-term issues.[32] Instead, the Subcommittee now states that "[i]n recognition of the social concern that surrounds the subject of gene transfer," it will cooperate with other groups in assessing "the possible long-term consequences" of the field,[33] but the latest revision of the "Points" dropped the specification of the effects the HGTS and RAC would be examining, as had been spelled out in the 1985 version.[34]

II. The Current Threat: The Human Genome Project

Surprisingly, despite the lack of genuine societal or global risk in *current* avenues of gene therapy, anxiety on the subject continues to bubble up. For example, at the Fifth Summit Conference on Bioethics, hosted by the Italian government in Rome in April 1988 on behalf of the "Group of Seven," for the purpose of discussing the ethical issues in mapping and sequencing the human genome, French delegate Jean Dausset urged that a formal moratorium be imposed on genetic engineering of human germ-line cells. The other delegates rejected this step as unduly confining. Instead, they "agreed that there are neither medical indications nor ethical justification for intentional genetic manipulation of human germ-line cells at this time."[35] Six months later, Professor Dausset, invoking the image of the Nazi horrors, nearly persuaded the delegates to a workshop in Valencia on international cooperation on the human genome to adopt a germ-line moratorium, a move which failed when Norton Zinder, the chair of the NIH advisory committee on the Human Genome Project, argued that the workshop had no means to enforce such a moratorium.[36]

What is remarkable is less Dausset's anxieties over germ-line interventions than the settings in which they were manifested: meetings supposedly concerned with human genome mapping. My personal sense is that persons assigned to examine the ethics of genome mapping quickly find themselves discussing related subjects, because the topic-in-chief is regarded as pretty thin gruel.

A. The Articulated (Albeit Inchoate) Concerns

The human genome—that is, the complement of 50,000 to 150,000 genes estimated as the molecular basis for human life—is now the object of concerted scrutiny by thousands of biological cartographers around the world. The largest effort is underway in the United States (with principal sponsorship coming from a new "center" at the National Institutes of Health headed by James Watson and from a special program in the Department of Energy), but many other countries are linked together in a cooperative/competitive arrangement coordinated by the international Human Genome Organization (HUGO).

The objective is first to produce a list of DNA "markers," sequences of DNA, with or without known biological effect, which are polymorphic, that is, which vary slightly, making it possible to differentiate their location. The list must be large enough so that every gene could be located on a chromosome between two markers with a high degree of accuracy (say, 90% or higher).[37] Developing and using markers requires painstaking study of large pedigrees (the patterns of inheritance over several generations in families with many living relatives). Different restriction enzymes cause the genetic material drawn from these families to be cut at different sites, which produce different markers, referred to as RFLPs (restriction fragment length polymorphisms). Several different sets of markers have been produced by different research teams. When the information is combined, chromosome by chromosome, the result should be genetic linkage maps.[38]

In addition to these genetic maps, physical maps are also being constructed. These also rely on cutting up pieces of DNA with restriction enzymes and cloning the resulting fragments; the DNA sequences of the clones are then analyzed to see where they overlap, thus allowing the order of the clones to be determined. The result is a "contig map," the detail of which is determined by the amount of DNA being studied and the number of fragments produced.

The final stage in mapping will be to produce a listing of the sequence of DNA base-pairs for the entire human genome, approximately 2,800,000,000 base-pairs in all. This is plainly a time-consuming process. To be completed in full, it will require further advances in the automated techniques for reading the DNA sequences.

The large appropriations being requested from (and largely supplied by) Congress for this process of mapping and sequencing the human genome give it the aura of a massive project, the sort of "big science" associated with high energy physics and moon rocket launches. While the wisdom of making the Genome Project a scientific priority at this time has been sharply debated by scientists over the past several years, it is generally recognized that the "big science" image is somewhat misleading. Even granted that a good deal of the research is being carried out at the "national laboratories" affiliated with the Department of Energy, which have previously carried on physics studies requiring a major concentration of resources and personnel, most of the work is decentralized and a good deal of it derives from studies being carried out for other purposes besides mapping the human genome.[39]

Thus far, conflicts over the appropriate strategy to follow in mapping and sequencing the human genome (e.g., how much to spend, how fast, and in what fashion)[40] have overshadowed the ethical controversy. The project is regarded rather banefully by some lawyers and ethicists, who seem to think that any major undertaking involving genetics must be loaded with ethical issues.[41] Yet only one novel ethical-legal topic has emerged from the Genome Initiative, the issue of ownership and control of use over the information generated.[42]

This is not to say that the conventional issues do not take on a novel twist in the context of the Genome Project. As mentioned, large pedigrees are a requisite of map-building; through them, researchers can study patterns of inheritance by determining how frequently particular DNA sequences, located within certain distances of each other, are inherited together. The most obvious concern is that a great deal of information about the people who participate in genetic registries—including "information" in the form of genetic material—must be collected, stored, and then sent out to researchers. Care must be taken that the confidentiality of registry participants is ensured.[43] As with all records in an era of computerization, such assurances are difficult to fulfill.

A more subtle issue is the risk that the decision of any particular person to participate in a family linkage registry may not be truly voluntary. If the success of the registry is dependent upon a high degree of cooperation of families that are included in the registry, the risk is that any particular individual's reluctance will be overcome by pressure from others in the family or by researchers themselves, particularly when the initial involvement of the family with a genetics center arose because of the occurrence of a genetic disease in the family. In such a situation, failure to allow oneself to be studied might either seem a form of ingratitude or, worse, an impediment to the development of a medical response to the disease that burdens the family (even if the likelihood that the genetic mapping project will provide anything of direct value to understanding, much less correcting, the familial genetic disease is extremely remote).

B. Deconstructing the Human Genome

Although I do not believe that the Human Genome Initiative *in and of itself* poses any major ethical problems, some of the uses of the knowledge gained through mapping the genome may raise significant issues. Before turning to those issues in the context in which I think they will have their major effect in the immediate future (genetic screening), I also want to say a few words about the conceptual significance of the initiative to map and sequence the human genome. As one way into this undertaking, it is interesting to attempt to apply the philosophical practices associated with Jacques Derrida and his colleagues regarding the interpretation of texts. It seems to me that the enterprise of mapping and sequencing the human genome might benefit from some deconstructionist consciousness.

Deconstruction is associated with several practices that may prove illuminating for us. First, at the heart of the activity is understanding the connection between what we say and how we say it or, conversely, the gap between that which represents and that which is represented. Deconstructive practice applied to the Human Genome Initiative might treat the genome itself as a text and a genetic map or a physical map as attempts to "read" it. What is one saying when one expresses the human genome in terms of a sequence of nucleotides? What gap may exist when it is said of a compact disc with the full transcription of base pairs, "Here I have a human being"? Ecce homo? Similarly, when looking at DNA sequences, what is involved in our reading them as "genes," as Mendel's units of inheritance?

Second, deconstruction also involves what Derrida calls the "metaphysics of presence,"[44] that is the privilege given to that which is most apparent to our consciousness over that which is absent. This has several implications for our topic. First, it makes us aware of the paradigm shift as we move from manifestations of disease to their chromosomal location, their genetic linkage, or even their point-mutational location. Second, rather than give preference to the "normal," Derrida argues that we should invert the hierarchy: do not think of the "normal" as the rule and the "abnormal" as the exception.[45] After all, the normal depends for its existence (as a concept) on the abnormal, and we could just as well define the normal in terms of the abnormal instead of the other way around. I find this particularly intriguing because, while Derrida's point may be novel in literary interpretation, what he describes is actually reflected in the work of biomedical scientists. The understanding of *normal* metabolic functioning has, on many occasions, proceeded from observations about *abnormal* functioning. Thus, while *descriptively* the normal has preference, *scientifically* the abnormal has precedence.

The presence/absence notion also has a further implication, which is to challenge the very concept of a genetic disease. To speak of a genetic disease presupposes the category of nongenetic diseases. But genes do not have diseases, only organisms do.

And the human organism always exists in an environment. In a different environment, that which is manifested as a "genetic disease" would be no disease at all. On the other hand, some aspects of our normal environment such as the usual array of microorganisms—are not lethal for most people but are fatal for a person with ADA-deficiency, which is thus labelled a genetic disease. For David, "the boy in the bubble" in Houston, however, perhaps one should term ADA-deficiency an environmental disease, because it was only when David wanted greater interaction with the world outside the bubble that he perished. Conversely, some aspects of our environment—like an automobile accident—are so abnormal that they have disastrous effects even in the absence of what we term "genetic disease." Yet, a particular trauma will not have identical consequences for all who experience it, because of differences in strength and susceptibility in bones and muscles that are themselves the results of genetic-environmental interactions. Thus, all diseases are multifactorial.

Finally, the "extentionalist" slogan of Alfred Korzybski, "a map is not the territory,"[46] is plainly provocative for gene-mappers. In one sense, this statement seems correct. There is, most of us believe, some underlying reality as to which a representation, a map for example, is merely an approximation. It is not the same thing as that which it represents. But there is another way in which the map *is* the territory, because the map—and how we set out to draw it—determines what we will find and what we will think the territory is. Columbus sailed west to find the Indies and, blocked by North America, he found some Caribbean Islands, which thus became known as the West Indies and their residents as Indians. Likewise, in some fundamental way, what scientists *think* the territory of the human genome is, *is* (that is, becomes) what it is, because it exists only in our mind, only in our textual representation of it. For what do geneticists look on their maps? For genes? Do they look for diseases? For abnormalities? For a genetic or a physical description of the territory? For a nucleic record of human history, to links with other species, to humankind's burden of viral infections?

The applications of the deconstructionist dictum *il n'y a pas de hors-texte* to the "text" of the human genome may seem perverse because Derrida had in mind the *constructed* text as opposed to "the absolute present, Nature" which "ha[s] never existed." Yet without this text, we would not exist—though human beings have long existed with no glimmer of this text in their conscious minds and with very different explanations for their existence. Let us say, then, that in decoding the human genome we are engaged in the process of simultaneously deconstructing *and* constructing our text.

III. The Real Threat: Genetic Screening

I have suggested throughout this article that the real "threat" of modern genetics has been misperceived, first and rather dramatically, as coming from genetic engineering, particularly human gene therapy, and second and somewhat inchoately, as flowing from the Human Genome Initiative. While attention has focused on these highly technical areas, the less flashy field of genetic screening actually poses more significant issues. Perhaps, however, with the long-awaited ability close at hand to screen for carrier status (i.e., heterozygotes) for cystic fibrosis, the most common fatal autosomal recessive disease in the American population, the ethical and legal issues in genetic screening will begin to receive renewed attention.

The past lack of attention may have originated in the belief that all issues in genetic screening were well disposed of by that familiar bioethical triumvirate, the principles of autonomy, beneficence, and justice. From the principle of autonomy, for example, are derived rules about informed consent to testing; the right to refuse to be informed about test results; and rights of privacy and confidentiality regarding dissemination of test results. But none of these are absolutes. Just as consent and confidentiality are particularly important in this context because one is dealing with *genetic* information which is, after all, *inherent in*—and, indeed, one might say, *constitutive of*—an individual and thus is a matter of unusual sensitivity for many people, so too one must recognize that the genetic nature of the data may place limits on the usual rules. For example, might individuals have a moral (even if not usually a legal) obligation of beneficence to cooperate in a family linkage study—even at the risk of learning unwanted information—if the individual's tissue sample is necessary to establish the pattern of inheritance that other family members need to know so that they can safeguard their health or that of potential offspring?[47]

Putting flesh on the bones of the principles of beneficence and justice is of particular importance. Specifically, what is the definition of "doing good" in the area of genetic mapping or genetic therapy? And how is justice manifested when one is dealing with rare diseases that in an earlier era might have been explained as manifestations of fate or of God's judgment? How do we behave justly in selecting patients to treat or diseases to study, or indeed, in allocating resources to this exciting and challenging field of biomedicine that may some day have great benefit for future sufferers, when the alternative is to spend these funds to address the unmet needs of present sufferers?

A. Four Varieties of Genetic Screening

The fact that these topics elicit more questions than well-defined public policy answers probably reflects the relatively low level of visibility that genetic screening has had until late.[48] Indeed, one might even say that the most prominent instances of genetic screening were not really conceived or described by those who promoted them as instances of genetic testing. Although genetic tests have gotten public attention in certain legal settings—such as the recent, and still controversial use of DNA analysis to create "genetic fingerprints" for forensic purposes, or the use of genetic tests to resolve paternity disputes—the more widespread use of genetic screening has gone largely unremarked and perhaps even unnoticed by millions of people who are subjected to it.

Genetic screening—that is, the search in an asymptomatic population for persons at elevated risk of genetic disease in themselves or their offspring—first came into general use in the early 1960s with the development of tests for several inborn errors of metabolism, particularly the Guthrie test of newborns for phenylketonuria (PKU), a condition that causes mental retardation unless the affected child is placed on a special diet that severely restricts intake of phenylalanine, a normal (indeed, essential) component of the human diet. These metabolic errors are rare (PKU occurs approximately once in every 14,000 births among Americans of European ancestry) and are typically autosomal recessive conditions, meaning that they arise when two people who carry the deviant gene mate; with each pregnancy, they have a one-in-four chance of producing a child who inherits the deviant gene from both of them and manifests the disease. In the case of PKU, Dr. Robert Guthrie developed a simple and inexpensive means of testing a small sample of blood from newborn children, taken at several days of age from a heel prick and sent on filter paper to the laboratory for automated testing.

In order to ensure that the test would be performed on all babies, most states—beginning with Massachusetts in 1963—adopted mandatory screening laws.[49] Although in some ways this was a "genetic" test, it was not generally so perceived. The statutes were championed by the state chapters of the Association for Retarded Persons as a means of preventing mental retardation, not by medical geneticists; furthermore, the true genetic nature of the condition, including its variations, was not well understood at the time, which led to a number of problems in screening and diagnosing some cases. Finally, because they were not thinking in genetic terms, the potential effects of the disease on the offspring of the children treated were neglected; only in recent years has it become apparent that girls who suffer from PKU should be urged to go back on the special low-phenylalanine diet (which the children ordinarily stop following by adolescence) before becoming pregnant, lest their metabolic problem damage the brain of their developing fetus.

From a legal vantagepoint, the major issue in newborn screening has been that the PKU statutes—and those adopted in some states that encompass a wider range of inborn metabolic problems—make screening mandatory, with some legal sanction. Even when these statutes provide that parents may exercise a religious or conscientious objection to testing, the right to do so is often not conveyed in a timely fashion.[50] Yet mandatory laws seem difficult to justify, both in light of the principle of autonomy and because a voluntary program, with good information and education of parents and health care providers, produces as high a rate of screening as mandatory programs.[51] Furthermore, screening by itself offers no benefit to children affected with PKU: first, a positive screening result must be confirmed through diagnostic testing, and then, affected children must receive the special diet. Yet neither of these additional steps is either required or guaranteed by legislation in most states.

Although screening of newborns in order to determine which ones may need treatment is the most common form of genetic testing today, two other types of screening related to reproduction are likely to become more prevalent in the near future, testing for carrier-status and prenatal tests. The best examples of such screening now are testing for Tay-Sachs disease among Ashkenazi Jews and for sickle-cell disease among African-Americans. The tests for the genetic defects that cause cystic fibrosis, while still not ready for use in screening the general population,[52] may soon generate screening programs with orders of magnitude larger than any heretofore.

Tay-Sachs disease causes progressive neurological deterioration and early death in affected children. About one Jew in thirty of East

European extraction is a carrier of the gene (four times the rate of PKU carriers); for two decades, screening programs that employ a relatively simple blood test have been carried out in Jewish communities in the United States, initially with sponsorship by local Jewish organizations and today usually through ordinary medical channels. Since the condition is recessive, "carrier couples" face a one-in-four chance of producing an affected child with each pregnancy, but prenatal screening permits diagnosis of affected fetuses (usually before the end of the second trimester). One of the issues that arose in the initial screening programs was whether testing should be limited to couples of reproductive age (excluding not merely older persons but younger ones as well and persons who were not yet married), to avoid the risk that anyone would become the victim of discrimination or rejection.

Also beginning two decades ago, sickle-cell testing was widely promoted in the black community (where one-in-twelve Americans of African extraction carries the gene). It did not, however, achieve comparable acceptance to Tay-Sachs screening, in part because prenatal diagnosis was not then feasible, so that a person found to be a carrier faced the choice either to attempt to marry a non-carrier, not to have children if married to another carrier of the gene, or to risk giving birth to a child with the disease. Today, molecular medicine makes prenatal diagnosis possible, which in turn increases people's interest in learning whether they carry the gene and ought to consider prenatal testing. Another reason why sickle-cell testing has met with resistance is that, especially in its early years, some employers (including the United States Armed Services) and others (such as schools) excluded or placed restrictions on persons found to be carriers, despite the lack of evidence that being heterozygous for the sickle-cell gene elevated the risk of health problems. Since few employers or others ran their own screening programs,[53] the best way to avoid suffering this discrimination was thus not to have oneself tested.

A fourth type of screening now coming into prominence is susceptibility testing. In effect, a good deal of medical monitoring could be described as testing for genetic susceptibilities—for example, screening for serum lipid levels, as a means to predict atherosclerosis and other risks. Yet, despite the fact that some physicians may point to the relationship between test results and familial patterns of heart disease and stroke, this testing is not typically described as "genetic screening." The development of the genome map and other tools from genetic engineering will greatly increase the number of tests available to reveal one's personal risk of experiencing particular diseases and disabilities, ranging from small percentage risks to virtual certainty of certain late-onset conditions (such as Huntington's disease) that are inherited in a dominant fashion.

B. Screening, Insurability, and Employability

Newborn screening aimed at detecting who is in need of protective interventions (e.g., PKU screening) is relevant to present discussions mostly as an historical precedent for the ease with which genetic testing became a part of common practice and accepted public policy with little thought having been given to the implications. Turning now to screening relevant to reproduction (i.e., carrier screening and prenatal testing) and to personal susceptibility, this earlier history suggests several concerns that deserve careful attention before these other types of screening move from their present place within medical practice into more widespread use by public and private authorities and institutions. Of particular interest are the issues of insurability and employability that may arise more often as accurate and inexpensive means are developed for a larger number of genetic conditions.

What makes this field complicated is that there are strong reasons that a person would want the information that can be gained from both reproductive and susceptibility-type screening, while at the same time the results of such screening will also be of interest to others with whom the person has voluntary relationships (such as employment) and who might wish to take actions that would be harmful to the person (such as denial of insurance). Several tensions are thus created: between the rights or interests of the individual screened and the rights or interests of others, and between failing to obtain or ignoring potentially useful information and having that information become the only factor guiding important decisions.

These tensions are exacerbated by another, inescapable reality, namely that discoveries and developments do not occur evenly across the whole of genetics nor do they necessarily touch first on those genetic conditions that are most common in the population. Instead, both the potential benefits and possible risks of genetic screening and diagnosis will attach very unevenly across the population. Although all of us carry five to seven lethal recessive genes as well as a still undetermined number of genes that make us susceptible to developing diseases based on interactions with the environment (e.g., through work, diet, etc.), persons who carry those particular genes for which screening first becomes available are in greater danger of suffering discrimination because of their apparent singularity. Once the widespread and basically random nature of genetic risks becomes more apparent, the need for concern about stigma—and specifically about loss of insurability and employability—may be lessened, even though it will never be the case that all people face identical genetic risks (defined in terms of the probability and severity of ourselves or our children suffering a disease of genetic origin).

Thus, the central question in my view involves the degree to which inborn differences should be regarded as ethically and legally relevant. To ignore them totally would not only be foolhardy but would also amount to a radical departure from our traditions—after all, the measurements of "merit" on which many decisions in our society rest do not equate merit with effort alone (indeed, they often separate aptitude from achievement). On the other hand, permitting inborn differences to play a decisive role in allocating a variety of benefits, such as access to employment and insurance, risks blaming the victim. Furthermore, to the extent that genetic screening is either inaccurate or partial (in the sense of uncovering some but not all genetic risks), too heavy a reliance on this one method in framing policy will lead to nonoptimal outcomes.

The tensions that need to be addressed can be seen in the relationship between reproductive screening and insurance and between susceptibility screening and employment. Regarding the former, suppose that tests are developed that can identify persons who carry a rare gene that causes a severe, crippling illness when inherited from both parents; further suppose that besides carrier testing, prenatal diagnosis can also be performed for the disease during the first trimester of pregnancy. If the carrier test is inexpensive enough and the costs of treating the illness are heavy enough, it may well be financially advisable for health insurance companies to provide the test. Focusing for the moment solely on persons who are already enrolled in a particular health insurance plan and who agree to undergo carrier screening voluntarily, what should be the insurance company's response when an identified "carrier couple" declines to undergo prenatal diagnosis? Under many indemnity insurance plans, coverage is not provided for "preexisting conditions." Could treatment of the genetic disease in an affected child be excluded on this ground? Alternatively, could the plan's exclusion from coverage for "self-inflicted" conditions be invoked? Though both of these limitations have themselves been criticized, both can also be defended on moral as well as prudential grounds. And both have at least some applicability to the hypothetical case, since insurance is meant to spread the risk of unexpected and inescapable harms, and the birth of an affected child is both foreseeable to, and avoidable by, the insured couple. Yet requiring prenatal diagnosis and abortion would deeply intrude into a protected realm of personal, private decisionmaking. Furthermore, if generalized, it would amount to a eugenics program by the insurance company, as it decided which children it thought fit enough to allow to be born.

Thus far, insurers have, to the best of my knowledge, not yet adopted such draconian measures. Indeed, it is unlikely for competitive reasons that a single company would dare to act alone toward a mandatory approach. But, by being willing to pay for genetic testing and by encouraging its use in appropriate cases, companies are able to achieve many of the results that they would want, even though there is no legal compulsion on prospective parents to use such tests, much less to act on their results.[54] As genetic tests become more widespread, it does not exceed the bounds of credibility to suppose that insurers will insist that their enrollees at least avail themselves of the tests, even if acting on the results is left up to them.

For most people, the door to health insurance is found in the workplace; thus, the question of insurability is in part a question of employability. Moreover, since they bear a portion of the cost of their employees' health care (which looms as an ever increasing portion of the cost of doing business), employers have the same interest as insurance carriers in excluding high-cost patients or at least in avoiding having to pay certain costs such patients generate.

Besides the interest they have in the risk that their employees and prospective employees will produce children burdened with genetic disorders, employers have an additional concern with their workers' own susceptibility to illness and injury. First, an employee who is prone to get sick will generate expenses: medical treatment costs, sick days, and potentially even disability benefits. Second, if the problem might be described as job-related, then the genetic condition could lead directly to workers compensation payments—for instance, a genetic predisposition to a bad back in an employee who has to do a lot of lifting. Finally, employers generally want to avoid hiring persons who are going to be sick a great deal because such persons cannot be relied upon to be present when needed and the expense of training them may thus be wasted if they become totally disabled.

Again, employers have yet to turn heavily to genetic testing, although some of the screening done in pre-employment physical exams is aimed at uncovering conditions in which genetics plays an important role. But as more genetic screens for disease susceptibility are perfected and made available at reasonable prices, it is likely that employers will be inclined to use them, especially if these tests identify employees who are at higher than average risk in particular work environments, from which they can therefore be excluded.[55]

IV. If We Were Clear on the Threat, What Should We Do?

I have argued in this essay that the "threat" of modern genetics has largely been misidentified with technologically glamorous developments such as human genetic engineering and the major effort to map and sequence the human genome, thereby overlooking the problems generated by genetic screening. The latter is the route through which the findings of the more glamorous areas of genetic engineering and genome mapping will probably first affect the lives of most Americans. In particular, I have suggested that a rapid increase in the number and technical capacity of screening methods for inherited conditions will affect two important relationships: between insured and insurer, and between employee and employer.

Plainly, some specific legal responses are possible, such as the passage of legislation to protect the confidentiality of genetic information and to prevent discrimination against those who have—or who are believed to be at high risk of developing—a genetic disability. Indeed, the report of the House-Senate conference committee on the recently adopted Americans With Disabilities Act makes clear that the scope of its protections encompasses genetic discrimination.[56]

Yet such responses, valuable as they may be, only address symptoms and do not respond to the underlying problems that the genetic techniques uncover. If we are to address the fundamental issues, we need to elevate them to a level of much greater public visibility. This is more than just the usual prescription for openness in a democracy, for it seems to me that if the deeper problems are going to be overcome some collective redefinitions of concepts and standards will be required.

Plainly, as the deconstructionist discussion suggested, some of that simply relates to reorienting how we think about normality and abnormality. Genetics, by illuminating the ways in which the line of difference between the two may be nothing more than the rearrangement of a single DNA base-pair (out of the billions in every cell), may make abnormalities less strange and "different." Some of the needed rethinking will have to extend to the concepts by which we describe our relationships and duties. For example, in light of the genetic connections that bind people to one another, in terms not only of inheritance but also of molecular diagnostics, what are the proper meanings of "autonomy" and "privacy"?

To be successful, what will be needed is a true social reexamination of the use that these concepts have in people's lives, not a mere "redefinition" by lawyers, who are capable of changing the meaning of any word, within the confines of a statute or contract. A further, more practical predicate is the kind of legal protection already mentioned: people will only be able to think about a less restrictive view of "privacy" if they are assured that they have been protected from any repercussions of sharing a genetic diagnosis.

A second task—somewhat more pragmatic but grounded also on principles—will be to reexamine our notions of insurance and employment. Especially in the field of health insurance, we have moved from a risk-sharing model to a group-narrowing model—in other words, from seeing ourselves as all being in roughly the same situation (thereby making it morally desirable to spread risks as broadly as possible) to seeking our individual advantage in placing ourselves in a group from which we have excluded people who are at higher risk than ourselves. When the exclusions are based on voluntarily acquired risks (such as from smoking), they do not seem very pernicious, so long as we apply a fairly relaxed understanding of the term "voluntary." But exclusions grounded in genetic differences are less benign. Nonetheless, the acceptability of one practice or the other depends not on abstract ethical principles but on our conception of the purpose of insurance. If the purpose is simply to spread out the costs of paying for illness across a lifetime, then narrow groupings of people at comparable risk make sense; if, on the other hand, the purpose is to manifest solidarity in the face of misfortunes (which do not strike all people equally) then narrowing of insurance pools based on ever-finer genetic differentiations would be unacceptable.

Another issue raised already by genetic screening that probably remains many years off in genetic engineering or genome mapping is the issue of mandatoriness. It strikes me as unlikely that laws will soon be passed requiring anyone to undergo gene therapy or to provide personally identifiable genetic material for purely scientific uses. Yet mandatory laws already exist in the area of genetic screening, and private parties (insurers and employers), who already border on compelling the use of such tests, are likely to move even further and faster in this direction.

We begin with a strong predisposition to protect free choice in private matters generally and in medical care in particular. Yet the consequences for other people in the choices we make cannot be totally ignored. If taking those consequences into account means putting the costs of the choices onto the shoulders of those who make the choices, then voluntariness has a very different meaning—closer, perhaps, to the sense in which one has the "choice" to violate a criminal statute, provided that one is willing to be penalized. Yet the alternative—totally insulating a person making a choice in the face of a known genetic risk from having to shoulder any of the consequences of that choice—seems equally undesirable.

Thus, more than a reexamination of voluntariness and mandatoriness will be needed: along the way, we will need to examine what we mean by such concepts as "responsible parenthood." Again, we have traditionally regarded reproductive decisions as appropriately made within the family; the state gets involved only when there is family breakdown (divorce), when children are at risk (child abuse and neglect), or when family status is rearranged (marriage, adoption). My personal preference is to preserve family choice as much as possible. In many ways, it seems a bedrock of diversity in other spheres in society because, by bolstering the integrity of the family unit, choice about reproduction supports an institution that is important for individual self-definition, for the fostering of varied cultural and religious viewpoints, and the like.

Yet individuals are also members of their society, and they depend on the larger community in many ways. For some individuals, the choices made by their families have disastrous consequences. Rather than being solely concerned with not having to bear the costs of correcting those consequences after-the-fact, might not the community assert an interest in avoiding them in the first place? Regarding some consequences, the answer adopted by society already is "yes"—for example, through removal of children from abusive or neglectful homes. The implications of genetic screening go much further, however, because it may provide information about the risk to certain children in even being conceived or born.

I have argued against the use of tort law to restrict the choices of parents about whether to reproduce in the face of genetic risks.[57] Yet it seems inevitable that such a position will need to be reexamined and redefended in the light both of increased medical capabilities and of other pressures in society.

That such reexamination of a wide range of practical issues and fundamental principles seems inevitable strikes me as a good rather than a bad thing. It is much more likely to occur if we reevaluate the "threat" of modern genetics and spend less time on distant prospects involving genome mapping and genetic engineering and more time thinking about genetic screening.

NOTES

1. Office of Technology Assessment, U.S. Congress, *Mapping Our Genes: The Genome Projects: How Big, How Fast?* 71 (1988).

2. President's Commission for the Study of Ethical Problems in Medicine and Biomedical and Behavioral Research, *Splicing Life: The Social and Ethical Issues of Genetic Engineering with Human Beings* 16 (1982) [hereinafter *Splicing Life*] (quoting Mayor Vellucci concerning Harvard University's plans for a laboratory to conduct recombinant DNA research).

3. J. Fletcher, *The Ethics of Genetic Control: Ending Reproductive Roulette* 188–89 (1974).

4. W. Shakespeare, *Hamlet* Act III, scene 1, lines 76–82 (Cambridge Univ. Press ed. 1934).

5. For an excellent history of "eugenics"—the term coined in 1883 by Charles Darwin's cousin, Francis Dalton—and its social impact, see D. Kevles, *In the Name of Eugenics: Genetics and the Uses of Human Heredity* (1985).

6. Mendel, "Experiments in Plant Hybridization", reprinted in *Classic Papers in Genetics* 1 (J. Peters ed. 1959).

7. Hotchkiss, "Portents for a Genetic Engineering", 56 *J. Heredity* 197 (1965).

8. Lederberg, "Orthobiosis: The Perfection of Man", in *The Place of Value in a World of Facts* 29, 54 (A. Tiselius & S. Nilsson eds. 1970). Another eminent biologist has taken the opposite viewpoint:

> Do we want to assume that basic responsibility for life on this planet—to develop new living forms for our own purposes? . . . Shall we take into our hands our own future evolution? . . . Perverse as it may, initially, seem to the scientist, we must face the fact that there can be unwanted knowledge.

Dixon, "Tinkering with Genes", 235 *Spectator*, Aug. 30, 1975, at 289 (quoting Robert L. Sinsheimer, then Chair of the Biology Department at the California Institute of Technology).

9. At an earlier (and more optimistic?) moment, Robert Sinsheimer (*supra* note 8) suggested that those who find the prospect of designed genetic change "repugnant—who fear, with reason, that we may unleash forces beyond human scale and who recoil from this responsibility"—are not seeing the situation from the vantagepoint of the "losers in that chromosomal lottery":

> We are among those who were favored in the chromosomal lottery and, in the nature of things, it will be our very conscious choice whether as a species we will continue to accept the innumerable, individual tragedies inherent in the outcome of this mindless, age-old throw of the dice, or instead will shoulder the responsibility for intelligent genetic intervention.

Sinsheimer, "The Prospect of Designed Genetic Change", 32 *Engineering & Science*, Apr. 1969, at 8, 13.

10. Diamond v. Chakrabarty, 447 U.S. 303, 316 (1980).

11. *Id.* at 317.

12. Letter of Dr. Claire Randall, Rabbi Bernard Mandelbaum & Bishop Thomas Kelly to President Jimmy Carter, June 20, 1980, reprinted in *Splicing Life, supra* note 2, at 95–96.

13. See, *e.g.*, Berg, Baltimore, Boyer, Cohen, *et al.*, Potential Biohazards of Recombinant DNA Molecules (Letter), 185 *Science* 303 (1974); Singer & Soll, Guidelines for DNA Hybrid Molecules (Letter), 181 *Science* 1114 (1973).

14. See M. Rogers, *Biohazard* 51–101 (1977); Swazey, Sorenson & Wong, "Risks and Benefits, Rights and Responsibilities: A History of the Recombinant DNA Research Controversy", 51 *So. Cal. L. Rev.* 1019 (1978).

15. The guidelines were first published at 41 Fed. Reg. 27,902 (1976). The basic current set of guidelines can be found at 51 Fed. Reg. 16,958 (1986), although the specific provisions are subject to minor modifications and amendments from time to time.

16. See, *e.g.*, Foundation on Economic Trends v. Heckler, 756 F.2d 143 (D.C. Cir. 1985) (upholding injunction against approval of a deliberate release experiment proposed by a scientist at the University of California because the NIH had failed to follow rules on environmental impact statements). Only after three years of further delay were the scientists able to conduct their field trials of a bacterium altered to lower the temperature at

which it triggered frost damage on plants. *L.A. Times,* June 9, 1987, pt. 1, at 3, col. 3. A private research firm, not wishing to become mired in the delays inherent in NIH-approval during the period of the injunction, applied to and received approval in 1985 from the Environmental Protection Agency for a comparable field trial.

17. See, *e.g.,* Brill, "Safety Concerns and Genetic Engineering in Agriculture", 227 *Science* 381 (1985) (quoting the scientist whose work was delayed by the case cited *supra* note 16, who argued that genetically engineered bacteria are probably safer because the alternations are limited in a known fashion to the frost-genes, while chemically muted bacteria—which can be tested without going through as rigorous a governmental approval process—may incorporate genetic changes that are more pathological).

18. See generally *Splicing Life, supra* note 2, at 13–17.

19. See Capron, "Prologue: Why Recombinant DNA?", 51 *S. Cal. L. Rev.* 973, 977 (1978).

20. The latest version appears at 55 Fed. Reg. 7438, 7444–48 (1990). Although the "Points to Consider" in effect provide "questions" rather than "answers," one may safely assume that the criteria for beginning trials of human gene therapy stated in articles such as Anderson & Fletcher, "Gene Therapy in Human Beings: When is it Ethical to Begin?", 303 *New Eng. J. Med.* 1293 (1980), would be regarded as applicable by the HGTS and the RAC: (1) the new gene should be put into target cells and remain in them, (2) the new gene should be regulated appropriately, and (3) the presence of the new gene should not harm the cell.

21. See 55 Fed. Reg. 6954 (1990). (The author is a member of the Human Gene Therapy Subcommittee.)

22. See 55 Fed. Reg. at 26,349 (1990). [On July 30 and 31, 1990 the HGTS and RAC, respectively, approved both the ADA-deficiency protocol and one to use gene transfer techniques to enable tumor infiltrating lymphocytes to make multiple copies of tumor necrosis factor as a therapy for melanoma. Angier, "Gene Treatment for Human Illness May Be Tried Soon", *N.Y. Times,* Aug. 1, 1990, at 1, col. 1.—EDS.]

23. Therefore, the technical uncertainties, the ethical implications, and the low probability of actually treating an affected person are strong contraindications against therapy of fertilized eggs or embryos becoming a useful clinical option in the near future. *Splicing Life, supra* note 2, at 48.

24. 55 Fed. Reg. at 7445.

25. *Id.* at 7444.

26. Germ-line therapy would probably have to be done at an early (two- to four-cell) stage of an *in vitro* zygote; it would only make sense to do it once it had been determined that a particular zygote carried the "abnormal" gene; and it is likely that most prospective parents would be equally willing at that point simply to limit embryo-insertion and attempted pregnancy to zygotes found to be free of the abnormal gene.

27. Quite the contrary, the ability to manipulate inheritable genes may actually come to be an aid to the very same "end" that evolution has: species survival. One might extend to human beings a point philosopher Stephen Stitch has made about crops:
> There may . . . come a time when, because of natural or man-induced climactic change, the capacity to alter quickly the genetic constitution of agricultural plants will be necessary to forestall catastrophic famine.

Stitch, "The Recombinant DNA Debate", 7 *Phil. & Pub. Affs.* 187, 191 (1978).

28. For example, the ability to treat genetic disease prenatally would alter what it means to be a "good parent" and what is meant by "defective" and "normal," as well as altering our sense of familial continuity. *Splicing Life, supra* note 2, at 64–66.

29. For example, whether to provide somatic treatment for conditions that could have been avoided through genetic alteration. *Id.* at 66.

30. For example, deciding what would be a fair system for distributing the benefits of the new technology. *Id.* at 66–68.

31. Sinsheimer, *supra* note 9.

32. The first version of the "Points to Consider" asked a researcher submitting a protocol to answer a series of questions, including: "3. Is it likely that somatic-cell therapy for human genetic disease will lead to: (a) germ-line gene therapy, (b) the enhancement of human capabilities through genetic means, or (c) eugenic programs encouraged or even mandated by governments?" 50 Fed. Reg. 2940, 2944 (1985).

33. 55 Fed. Reg. 7445 (1990).

34. In explaining the need to assess long-term consequences, the HGTS also stated its sense that such consequences should not stand in the way of appropriate somatic-cell therapy: "While research in molecular biology could lead to the development of techniques for germ-line intervention or for the use of genetic means to enhance human capabilities rather than to correct defects in patients, the [Subcommittee] does not believe that these effects will follow immediately or inevitably from experiments with somatic-cell gene therapy." 8 *Recomb. DNA Tech. Bull.* 181. 183 (1985).

35. *Analisi del Genoma Umano* (G. Tocchini-Valentini ed. 1989).

36. Roberts, "Carving Up the Human Genome", 246 *Science* 1244 (1989). Professor George Annas has suggested that enacting Dausset's ban would have signalled "that the scientists [at the Valencia meeting] could handle the ethical issues alone, and could monitor their own work." Annas, "Who's Afraid of the Human Genome?", 19 *Hastings Center Rep.*, July/Aug. 1989, at 19, 21.

37. An excellent introduction to the technologies for mapping the genome is provided by Chapter Two of the Office of Technology Assessment report, *Mapping Our Genes, supra* note 1, at 19–51.

38. See Roberts, "The Genetic Map is Back on Track After Delays", 249 *Science* 805 (1990).

39. See, *e.g.,* the description of the project, originated by Sydney Brenner of Cambridge University in 1963, "to learn everything there is to know about the nematode *Caenorhabditis elegans*"—a project that is now culminating in an effort "to decipher its complete genetic instructions." Roberts, "The Worm Project", 248 *Science* 1310, 1310 (1990).

40. See, *e.g.,* Roberts, "Genome Backlash Going Full Force", 248 *Science* 804 (1990).

41. See, *e.g.,* Annas, *supra* note 36. The sense that important ethical problems are at hand is probably magnified by the unprecedented plan of NIH's National Center for Human Genome Research to allocate from one to three percent of its funds for ethical analysis; perhaps this is nothing more than the formula under which one percent of the construction costs of new buildings is set aside in some cities to purchase works of art—it does not guarantee more aesthetic buildings, but it does ensure that artists will be kept busy producing ornaments for what gets built.

42. See, *e.g.*, Eisenberg, "Patenting the Human Genome", 39 *Emory L. J.* 721 (1990).

43. From a scientific standpoint, researchers do not need to know the personal identity of the people from whom DNA samples come. In generating their maps, the genetic cartographers will use samples from many people; while each person's DNA differs slightly from other people's, any two people share about 99% of their genetic makeup.
> Referring to the donor of the X-chromosome region [David] Schlessinger's group [at the Center for Genetics in Medicine at Washington University in St. Louis] is studying, he states, "The identity of the donor is locked away. . . . [T]hat individual is the genetic equivalent of the unknown soldier."

Fink, "Whose Genome Is It, Anyway?", 2 *Human Genome News,* July 1990, at 5.

44. J. Derrida, *Of Grammatology* 49 (G. Spivak trans. 1976).

45. See J. Derrida, *Writing and Difference* 278–79 (A. Bass trans. 1978).

46. A. Korzybski, *Science and Sanity* 58 (1958).

47. Cf. President's Commission for the Study of Ethical Problems in Medicine and Biomedical and Behavioral Research, *Screening and Counseling for Genetic Conditions* 44 (1983) (discussing circumstances in which professional's ethical duty of confidentiality may be overridden by the need to prevent harm to relative of person who has undergone genetic testing).

48. After an initial flurry of ethical and legal analysis nearly two decades ago, the subject receded to a less prominent status. See, *e.g.*, National Research Council, Committee for the Study of Inborn Errors of Metabolism, *Genetic Screening: Programs, Principles, and Research* (1975) [hereinafter *Genetic Screening*]; *Genetic Counseling: Facts, Values, and Norms* (A. Capron, M. Lappé, R. Murray, T. Powledge, S. Twiss & D. Bergsma eds. 1979); Research Group on Ethical, Social and Legal Issues in Genetic Counseling and Genetic Engineering of the Institute of Society, "Ethical and Social Issues in Screening for Genetic Disease", 286 *New Eng. J. Med.* 1129 (1972). One report by the President's Commission (*supra* note 47), and an OTA report, Office of Technology Assessment, U.S. Congress, *The Role of Genetic Testing in the Prevention of Occupational Disease* (1983) [hereinafter *Role of Genetic Testing*], both in 1983, stimulated some interest, but only recently has genetic screening again begun to receive concerted analysis. See, *e.g.*, N. Holtzman, *Proceed with Caution* (1989); Netherlands Scientific Council for Government Policy, *The Social Consequences of Genetic Testing, Preliminary and Background Studies* 64 (1990).

49. See generally *Genetic Screening, supra* note 48, at 44–87.

50. *Id.*

51. See Faden, Chalow, Holtzman & Horn, "A Survey to Evaluate Parental Consent As Public Policy for Neonatal Screening", 72 *Am. J. Pub. Health* 1347 (1982).

52. "Statement from the National Institutes of Health Workshop on Population Screening for the Cystic Fibrosis Gene", 323 *New Eng. J. Med.* 70 (1990).

53. See *Role of Genetic Testing, supra* note 48, at 34. The OTA found that, despite a good deal of hype on the subject, few employers were actually using genetic tests to screen workers, but the perception that technical improvements have lately increased employers' interest in using genetic screening has recently led the OTA to update its survey of practices.

54. Some courts have recognized an obligation in medical professionals to offer appropriate genetic tests, the breach of which obligation can result in civil liability under the

confusing labels of "wrongful birth" and "wrongful life," but no court has yet held parents liable to an affected child for failing to take steps to prevent the child's birth. See Capron, "Wrongful Life: Will Common Sense Prevail?", 3 *Bioethics Rptr.*, Commentary 23–27 (1985).

55. Employers have already been permitted to take one comparable factor (namely, the risk to fetuses of women workers exposed to lead) into account in excluding certain employees from certain types of work. The Supreme Court is now reviewing a Seventh Circuit ruling under Title VII of the Civil Rights Act of 1964 (which forbids discrimination on gender grounds) upholding an automobile battery manufacturer's policy that bars women from certain positions unless they can provide evidence of infertility. The circuit court found the policy "well reasoned and scientifically documented" and thus justified either as a "bona fide occupational qualification" or as a "business necessity." International Union, UAW v. Johnson Controls, Inc., 886 F.2d 871 (7th Cir. 1989), *cert. granted*, 58 U.S.L.W. 3609 (U.S. Mar. 27, 1990) (No. 89-1215).

56. See "Conference Report on S.393, Americans With Disabilities Act of 1990," 136 *Cong. Rec.* H4614, H4627 (1990).

57. See, *e.g.*, Capron, "Informed Decisionmaking in Genetic Counseling: A Dissent to the 'Wrongful Life' Debate", 48 *Ind. L. J.* 581 (1973); Capron, "Tort Liability in Genetic Counseling", 79 *Colum. L. Rev.* 618 (1979).

29 Public Health Policy and the AIDS Epidemic: An End to HIV Exceptionalism?

Ronald Bayer, Ph.D.

Professor Ronald Bayer teaches at Columbia University, New York.

I n the early and mid-1980s, when democratic nations were forced to confront the public health challenge posed by the epidemic of the acquired immunodeficiency syndrome (AIDS), it was necessary to face a set of fundamental questions: Did the history of responses to lethal infectious diseases provide lessons about how best to contain the spread of human immunodeficiency virus (HIV) infection? Should the policies developed to control sexually transmitted diseases or other communicable conditions be applied to AIDS? If AIDS were not to be so treated, what would justify such differential policies?

To understand the importance of these questions, it is necessary to recall that conventional approaches to public health threats were typically codified in the latter part of the 19th or the early part of the 20th century. Even when public health laws were revised in subsequent decades, they tended to reflect the imprint of their genesis. They provided a warrant for mandating compulsory examination and screening, breaching the confidentiality of the clinical relationship by reporting to public health registries the names of those with diagnoses of "dangerous diseases," imposing treatment, and in the most extreme cases, confining persons through the power of quarantine.

As the century progressed, the most coercive elements of this tradition were rarely brought to bear, because of changing patterns of

This article first appeared in The New England Journal of Medicine *324 (23 May 1991): 1500–1504.*

morbidity and mortality and the development of effective clinical alternatives. Nevertheless, it was the specter of these elements that most concerned proponents of civil liberties and advocates of gay rights as they considered the potential direction of public health policy in the presence of AIDS.[1] Would there be widespread compulsory testing? Would the names of the infected be recorded in central registries? Would such registries be used to restrict those with HIV infection? Would the power of quarantine be used, if not against all infected persons, then at least against those whose behavior could result in the further transmission of infection?

Although there were public health traditionalists in the United States and abroad who pressed to have AIDS and HIV infection brought under the broad statutory provisions established to control the spread of sexually transmitted and other communicable diseases, they were in the distinct minority. Typically, it was those identified with conservative political parties or movements who endorsed such efforts—e.g., the Christian Social Union of Bavaria—although not all conservatives pursued such a course.[2] Liberals and those identified with the democratic left tended to oppose such efforts. There were striking exceptions, such as the Swedish Social Democrats,[3] but in the end it was those who called for "HIV exceptionalism" who came to dominate public discourse.

In the first decade of the AIDS epidemic, an alliance of gay leaders, civil libertarians, physicians, and public health officials began to shape a policy for dealing with AIDS that reflected the exceptionalist perspective. As the second decade of the epidemic begins, it is clear that the potency of this alliance has begun to wane. The evidence of this change with regard to HIV testing, reporting, partner notification, and even quarantine is most visible in the United States, but it may begin to appear in other democratic nations as well. What follows is drawn from the American experience, but it most certainly has parallels in other countries.

TESTING AND SCREENING

The HIV-antibody test, first made widely available in 1985, was the subject of great controversy from the outset. Out of the confrontations emerged a broad consensus that, except in a few well-defined circumstances, people should be tested only with their informed voluntary and specific consent. When the clinical importance of identifying those with asymptomatic HIV infection became clear in mid-1989, the political context of the debate over testing underwent a fundamental change. Gay organizations began to urge homosexual and bisexual men to have their antibody status determined under confidential or anonymous conditions. Physicians pressed for AIDS to be returned to the medical mainstream and for the HIV-antibody test to be treated like other blood tests—that is, given with the presumed consent of the patient.

Thus, four clinical societies in New York State, including the New York Medical Society, unsuccessfully sued the commissioner of health in 1989 to compel him to define AIDS and HIV infection as sexually transmitted and communicable diseases.[4] Among the goals of the suit was the liberalization of the stringent consent requirements for HIV testing. In December 1990 the House of Delegates of the American Medical Association called for HIV infection to be classified as a sexually transmitted disease. Although the delegates chose not to act on a resolution that would have permitted testing without consent, their decision on classification had clear implications for a more routine approach to HIV screening, one in which the standard of specific informed consent would no longer prevail.[5]

The movement toward routine or mandatory testing has been especially marked in the case of pregnant women and newborns. Pregnant women are already tested in this way for syphilis and hepatitis B. The screening of newborns for phenylketonuria and other congenital conditions is standard. Although as of this writing a deeply divided AIDS task force of the American Academy of Pediatrics had not recommended mandatory HIV screening of newborns, that decision was a function of the lack of specificity of the test and the lack of a definitive clinical regimen for seropositive newborns. The publication in the *Morbidity and Mortality Weekly Report* on March 15, 1991,[6] of recommendations for the prophylaxis of *Pneumocystis carinii* pneumonia in newborns will undoubtedly affect future discussion of the importance of identifying infants born to mothers with HIV infection.

REPORTING OF NAMES

Clinical AIDS has been a reportable condition in every state since 1983. But since the inception of HIV testing, there has been a sharp debate about whether the names of all infected persons should be reported to confidential registries of public health departments. Gay groups and their allies have opposed HIV reporting because of concern about privacy and confidentiality. Many public health officials opposed such a move because of the potential effect on the willingness of people to seek HIV testing and counseling voluntarily. By 1991 only a few states, typically those with relatively few AIDS cases, had required such reporting.[7]

Divisions have begun to appear in the alliance against the reporting of names in states where the prevalence of HIV infection is high and where gay communities are well organized. In New York State, as noted above, four medical societies have demanded that HIV infection be made a reportable condition.[4] In 1989, Stephen Joseph, then commissioner of health in New York City, stated that the prospects of early clinical intervention warranted "a shift toward a disease-control approach to HIV infection along the lines of classic tuberculosis practices," including the "reporting of seropositives."[8] Although political factors thwarted the commissioner, it is clear that his call represented part of a national trend.

At the end of November 1990, the Centers for Disease Control declared its support for reporting. In a carefully crafted editorial note in the *Morbidity and Mortality Weekly Report,* the agency stated that

> by using measures to maintain confidentiality, the implementation of a standardized system for HIV reporting to state health departments can enhance the ability of local, state, and national agencies to project the levels of required resources . . . [and aid] in the establishment of a framework for providing partner notification and treatment services. . . .[9]

Within a week, the House of Delegates of the American Medical Association endorsed the reporting of names as well.

Notification of Partners

Most important in the move toward the reporting of names has been the belief on the part of public health officials that effective programs of partner notification require reporting the names of persons with HIV infection as well as the names of those with a diagnosis of AIDS. Despite its long-established, though recently contested, role in the control of other venereal diseases, notification of the sexual and needle-sharing partners of patients with HIV infection or AIDS has been the exception rather than the rule. Opponents of such notification or contact tracing have denounced it as a coercive measure, even though it has always depended on cooperation with the index patient and protection of that patient's anonymity.

The early opposition to partner notification by gay and civil-liberties groups has begun to yield, as a better understanding of the practice has developed. Since 1988 the Centers for Disease Control has made the existence of partner-notification programs in states a condition for the granting of funds from its HIV-prevention program.[10] Such programs have also been endorsed by the Institute of Medicine, the National

Academy of Sciences,[11] the Presidential Commission on the HIV Epidemic,[12] the American Bar Association,[13] and the American Medical Association.[14]

Many of the early strict-confidentiality statutes relating to HIV infection and AIDS appeared to prevent physicians from acting when confronted with infected patients who indicated that they would neither inform their partners nor alter their sexual practices. More recent acknowledgment of clinicians' ethical responsibilities under such circumstances has led to modifications of the stringent prohibitions on breaches of confidentiality. Both the American Medical Association[15] and the Association of State and Territorial Health Officials[16] have endorsed legislative provisions that would permit disclosure to people placed at risk by the HIV infection of a partner.

As of 1990, only two states had imposed on physicians a legal duty to warn spouses that they were at risk for HIV infection. Approximately a dozen states had passed legislation granting physicians a "privilege to warn or inform" sexual and needle-sharing partners, thus freeing clinicians from liability whether or not they issued such warnings.[17] In a remarkable acknowledgment of the extreme sensitivity of the issues involved, some of the legislation stipulated that the warnings could not involve revealing the identity of the source of the threat to the person being warned.[18]

QUARANTINE AND CRIMINALIZATION

On epidemiologic, pragmatic, and ethical grounds, there has been virtually no support for extending the power to quarantine to apply to all HIV-infected persons. There has, however, been periodic discussion of whether the tradition of restricting liberty in the name of the public health should be invoked when a person's behavior poses a risk of HIV transmission.[1] Although bitter opposition has greeted all attempts to bring such behavior within the scope of existing quarantine statutes, more than a dozen states did so from 1987 through 1990. When such measures have been enacted, they have generally provided an occasion to revise state disease-control laws to reflect contemporary constitutional standards of due process (Intergovernmental Health Policy Project: unpublished data). There have been a few well-reported instances of efforts to impose control over recalcitrant persons for reasons of public health. Almost always, states have used the existence of the authority to quarantine to warn those who persist in unsafe sexual practices and to counsel them aggressively about the need for a change in behavior.

More common, though still relatively rare, has been the use of the criminal law under such circumstances. From 1987 through 1989, 20 states enacted statutes permitting the prosecution of persons whose behavior posed a risk of HIV transmission (Intergovernmental Health Policy Project: unpublished data), a move broadly endorsed by the Presidential Commission on the HIV Epidemic.[19] The 1990 Ryan White Comprehensive AIDS Resources Emergency (CARE) Act requires that all states receiving funds have the statutory capacity to prosecute those who engage in behavior linked to the transmission of HIV infection to unknowing partners. Perhaps more crucial, aggressive local prosecutors have relied on the general criminal law to bring indictments against some people for HIV-related behavior, even in the absence of statutes specifically defining such behavior as criminal.

In the vast majority of instances, such prosecutions have resulted either in acquittal or in a decision to drop the case. When there have been guilty verdicts, the penalties have at times been unusually harsh.[20]

The Roots of the Challenge to HIV Exceptionalism

What accounts for the pattern of changes described above? When the communal welfare is threatened, public health policy always requires more than the application of a repertoire of standard professional practices. Inevitably, public health officials must contend with a range of extraprofessional considerations, including the prevailing political climate and the unique social forces brought into play by a particular public health challenge. In the first years of the AIDS epidemic, U.S. officials had no alternative but to negotiate the course of AIDS policy with representatives of a well-organized gay community and their allies in the medical and political establishments. In this process, many of the traditional practices of public health that might have been brought to bear were dismissed as inappropriate. As the first decade of the epidemic came to an end, public health officials began to reassert their professional dominance over the policy-making process and in so doing began to rediscover the relevance of their own professional traditions to the control of AIDS.

This process has been fostered by changing perceptions of the dimensions of the threat posed by AIDS. Early fears that HIV infection might spread broadly in the population have proved unfounded. The epidemic has been largely confined to the groups first identified as being at increased risk. As the focus of public health concern has shifted from homosexual men, among whom the incidence of HIV infection has remained low for the past several years, to poor black and Hispanic drug users and their sexual partners, the influence of those who have spoken on behalf of the gay community has begun to wane. Not only do black and Hispanic drug users lack the capacity to influence policy in the way that homosexual men have done, but also those who speak on their behalf often lack the singular commitment to privacy and consent that so characterized the posture of gay organizations. Furthermore, policy directed toward the poor is often characterized by authoritarian tendencies. It is precisely such authoritarianism that evokes the traditions of public health. Finally, in the United States as in virtually every Western democracy, the estimates of the level of infection put forth several years ago have proved to be too high.[21] As AIDS has become less threatening, the claims of those who argued that the exceptional threat would require exceptional policies have begun to lose their force.

The most important factor in accounting for the changing contours of public health policy, however, has been the notable advances in therapeutic prospects. The possibility of managing HIV-related opportunistic infections better and the hopes of slowing the course of HIV progression itself have increased the importance of early identification of those with HIV infection. That, in turn, has produced a willingness to consider traditional public health approaches to screening, reporting, and partner notification.

CONCLUSIONS

As of the end of 1990, 11 states had classified AIDS and HIV infection as sexually transmitted or venereal diseases. Twenty-two states had classified them as communicable diseases, infectious diseases, or both. Strikingly absent from this group are New York, California, and New Jersey, the three states that have borne the heaviest burdens during the epidemic (Intergovernmental Health Policy Project: unpublished data). Whether they and other states will follow will depend on epidemiologic and clinical developments. But more important will be the balance of political forces.

The pattern that has begun to emerge so clearly in the United States may not be replicated in every respect in other democratic nations where HIV exceptionalism has held sway in the first years of the epidemic. Much will depend on the tradition of public health practice with regard to sexually transmitted and communicable diseases and on the relative strength and viability of the alliances forged in the phase of the epidemic marked by therapeutic impotence. But what is clear is that the effort to sustain a set of policies treating HIV infection as fundamentally different from all other public health threats will be increasingly difficult. Inevitably, HIV exceptionalism will be viewed as a relic of the epidemic's first years.

Finally, the broad political context within which decisions will be made about the availability of resources for prevention, research, and the provision of care will be affected by the changing perspective on AIDS. The availability of such resources has always been the outcome of a competitive process, however implicit. In the beginning, the desperate effort to wrest needed resources from an unresponsive political system in the context of a health care system that failed to provide universal protection against the cost of illness compelled AIDS activists and their allies to argue that AIDS was different and required funding commitments of a special kind. However late these funds were in coming, and however grudgingly they were provided, it was inevitable that in a resource-constrained climate there would be challenges to the allocations that were made. Thus, in 1990 the Office of Technology Assessment was compelled to address the question of whether the resources made available for AIDS research had distorted the funding allocated for other medical conditions.[22] Winkenwerder et al. argued in 1989 that further increases in federal expenditures for AIDS would be disproportionate to the burden of disease in the population.[23] Such concern has begun to find expression in the popular media as well.[24] The erosion of the exceptionalist perspective on HIV infection will inevitably foster the further expression of such doubt, precisely when greater resources are required to treat those with HIV disease.

That the difference between the public health response to the HIV epidemic and the response to other conditions has been eroding does not necessarily mean that public health traditionalists will inevitably win out over those who have argued for a new public health practice. In Denmark, for example, the experience with AIDS has led to a reconsideration of the traditional approach to venereal disease.[25] Indeed, there are many reasons, both pragmatic and ethical, that some of the practices that have emerged over the past decade in response to AIDS should inform the practice of public health more generally. There are good reasons, for example, to argue that the principle of requiring informed consent for HIV testing ought to apply to all clinical tests to which competent adults may be subject. Furthermore, the lessons learned—about mobilizing an effective campaign of public health education, about the central importance of involving in the process of fashioning such efforts those who speak on behalf of those most at risk, and about the very limited and potentially counterproductive consequences of recourse to coercion in seeking to effect a radical modification of private behavior—could be applied profitably to the patterns of morbidity and mortality that represent so much of the contemporary threat to the public health.

Were the end of HIV exceptionalism to mean a reflexive return to the practices of the past, it would represent the loss of a great opportunity to revitalize the tradition of public health so that it might best be adapted to face the inevitable challenges posed not only by the continuing threat of AIDS but also by threats to the communal health that will inevitably present themselves in the future.

REFERENCES

1. Bayer R. Private acts, social consequences: AIDS and the politics of public health. New Brunswick, N.J.: Rutgers University Press, 1991.

2. Frankenberg G. In the beginning all the world there was America: AIDS policy in West Germany. In: Bayer R, Kirp D, eds. Passions, politics and policy: AIDS in eleven democratic nations. New Brunswick, N.J.: Rutgers University Press (in press).

3. Henriksson B, Ytterberg H. Swedish AIDS policy: a question of contradictions. In: Bayer R, Kirp D, eds. Passions, politics and policy: AIDS in eleven democratic nations. New Brunswick, N.J.: Rutgers University Press (in press).

4. New York State Society of Surgeons et al. v. Axelrod, 1989.

5. Jones L. HIV infection labeled as STD; board to clarify testing policy. American Medical News. December 14, 1990:3, 28.

6. Working Group on PCP Prophylaxis in Children. Guidelines for prophylaxis against *Pneumocystis carinii* pneumonia for children infected with human immunodeficiency virus. MMWR 1991;40(RR-2):1–13.

7. Intergovernmental Health Policy Project. HIV reporting in the states. Intergovernmental AIDS Reports. November–December 1989:1–3.

8. Joseph SC. Remarks at the Fifth International Conference on AIDS, Montreal, June 4–9, 1989.

9. Update: public health surveillance for HIV infection—United States, 1989 and 1990. MMWR 1990;39:861.

10. Fed Regist 1988;53:3554.

11. Altering the course of the epidemic. In: Institute of Medicine, National Academy of Sciences. Confronting AIDS: update 1988. Washington, D.C.: National Academy Press, 1988:82.

12. Report of the Presidential Commission on the Human Immunodeficiency Virus Epidemic: submitted to the President of the United States. Washington, D.C.: Presidential Commission on the Human Immunodeficiency Virus Epidemic, 1988:76.

13. American Bar Association, House of Delegates. Report from the House of Delegates, August 1989: annual meeting. Chicago: American Bar Association, 1989:23–5.

14. Abraham L. AIDS contact tracing, prison test stir debate. American Medical News. July 8–15, 1988:4.

15. American Medical Association Board of Trustees. Report X: AMA HIV policy update. In: AMA Proceedings of the House of Delegates, December 3–6, 1989, 43rd interim meeting. Chicago: American Medical Association, 1989:76–95.

16. Association of State and Territorial Health Officials, National Association of County Health Officials, Conference of Local Health Officers. Guide to public health practice: HIV partner notification strategies. Washington, D.C.: Public Health Foundation, 1988.

17. Intergovernmental Health Policy Project. 1989 legislative overview. Intergovernmental AIDS Reports. January 1990:3.

18. New York State Public Health Law, Article 27-F.

19. Report of the Presidential Commission on the Human Immunodeficiency Virus Epidemic: submitted to the President of the United States. Washington, D.C.: Presidential Commission on the Human Immunodeficiency Virus Epidemic, 1988:130–1.

20. Gostin LO. The AIDS litigation project: a national review of court and human rights commission decisions, part 1: the social impact of AIDS. JAMA 1990;263:1961–70.

21. Estimates of HIV prevalence and projected AIDS cases: summary of a workshop, October 31–November 1, 1989. MMWR 1990;39:110–9.

22. Office of Technology Assessment. How has federal research on AIDS/HIV disease contributed to other fields? Washington, D.C.: Government Printing Office, 1990.

23. Winkenwerder W, Kessler AR, Stolec RM. Federal spending for illness caused by the human immunodeficiency virus. N Engl J Med 1989;320:1598–603.

24. Krauthammer C. AIDS getting more than its share? Time. June 25, 1990:80.

25. Alback E. AIDS: the evolution of a non-controversial issue in Denmark. In: Bayer R, Kirp D, eds. Passions, politics and policy: AIDS in eleven democratic nations. New Brunswick, N.J.: Rutgers University Press (in press).

30 *An Ethical Framework for Rationing Health Care*

NANCY S. JECKER, PH.D. AND
ROBERT A. PEARLMAN, M.D., M.P.H.

Nancy S. Jecker, Ph.D., teaches in the Department of History and Ethics, School of Medicine, University of Washington, Seattle. Robert A. Pearlman, M.D., M.P.H., serves in the Department of Medicine, School of Medicine, University of Washington, Seattle.

Recently we have witnessed the emergence of various proposals for rationing health care. One increasingly popular approach calls for rationing certain forms of medical care by age (Callahan, 1987). Elsewhere (Jecker *et al.*, 1989; Jecker, 1988, 1989), we argue that age does not constitute an ethically sound basis for limiting care. Yet rejecting an age criterion leads us to ask, What alternative rationing criteria are ethically defensible? This paper critically evaluates several alternatives for rationing publicly-financed health care. Part one proposes a framework that classifies these criteria according to their ethical basis and examines the ethical arguments supporting each. Part two summarizes these findings and sets forth an ethical framework for rationing publicly supported health care.

PART I: ALTERNATIVE CRITERIA FOR RATIONING HEALTH CARE

Rationing takes place whenever health care resources are insufficient to make them available to all who could benefit. Despite continued debate about the just distribution of health care, there appears to be no general terms to indicate the *ethical basis* for rationing choices. We propose grouping different ethical criteria under two broad categories. The first we shall call resource-centered rationing. Resource-centered criteria treat specific aspects of health care resources as ethically important, such as the price resources command, the newness or technological sophistication resources display, or the rehabilitative, curative, palliative or

---

This article appeared in The Journal of Medicine and Philosophy 17 *(February 1992): 79–96.*

preventive function resources serve. Resource-centered criteria ignore differences between persons and instead rest rationing decisions on features of health services themselves. In general, appeals to resource-centered criteria occur between different health care categories. For instance, it might be argued that Medicaid dollars should be invested in basic or preventive health care, rather than costly acute care services. The individuals authorized to make resource-centered rationing decisions typically include policy makers, legislators, hospital administrators, and state and federal governments. One appeal of resource-centered rationing is that it offers a way of avoiding controversial comparisons between persons. Of course, this aspect of resource-centered rationing cuts both ways: to the extent that morally relevant differences exist between individuals, resource-based rationing can be faulted for ignoring these.

A second ethical basis for rationing is patient-centered. Patient-centered rationing claims to identify morally relevant qualities of individuals and make these the determining ground of individuals' entitlement to health care. A person's age, ability to pay, place of residence, life expectancy, needs, past or future contributions, and lifestyle choices are examples of patient-centered standards. In general, appeals to patient-centered criteria occur within health care categories. For example, a particular person may be denied a liver-transplant because that person has a history of alcohol abuse. Persons directly involved with patient care and management are most likely to assume responsibility for patient-centered rationing decisions. The challenge of patient-centered rationing is to guard against a tendency to denigrate the worth of individuals or groups and to avoid resting rationing on differences between persons that are arbitrary from a moral point of view.

In this section we critique four rationing criteria. Two criteria are resource-centered: rationing high technology services and rationing non-basic services. Two are patient-centered: rationing services to patients that receive the least medical benefit and rationing services that are not equally available to all patients. Throughout the paper we will be considering the use of these criteria only in the context of government funded care, and many of our arguments will not apply to privately purchased health care. It should be noted at the outset that the brief arguments we offer in support of some national plan for basic health care do not purport to settle the issue, but only to make the idea plausible enough for the reader to entertain our central arguments, which concern rationing within the context of some form of publicly financed care. Even in the absence of a national plan, however, our arguments are relevant to the way health care dollars are spent. After all, even under the present piecemeal approach public financing of health care is significant. It includes not only programs such as Medicare and Medicaid, but also the enormous public subsidy that goes into the training of doctors, the support of medical research, and the tax subsidy for employer-sponsored health insurance. Understood in this light, the rationing of publicly-financed care will affect many of us if it is done even-handedly.

1. Resource-Centered Criteria

a. Rationing High Technology Services

One form of resource-centered rationing holds the success of recent medical technology chiefly responsible for problems of distributive justice in health care. For example: diagnostic technologies, such as magnetic resonance imaging; curative procedures, such as organ transplantation; and therapies, such as total parenteral nutrition raise rationing problems that did not exist previously. This approach regards rationing publicly-financed high technology as a natural antidote to our present health care crisis. "High technology" usually refers in this context to apparatus and procedures based on modern sciences, as opposed to the simpler healing arts (McGregor, 1989). High technology also connotes: new, as opposed to long accepted; scientifically complex, as distinct from common sense; costly, rather than inexpensive; and limited, rather than widespread, expertise in using a particular technique.

Advocates of rationing publicly-financed high technology medicine defend their view by pointing, first, to a growing consensus among intellectual leaders in the health care field that much technically curative medicine costs a great deal in comparison to alternative uses of the money for other health purposes (Price, 1978; Wennberg, 1984; Abel-Smith, 1978). Subjective factors, such as practice-style or the prestige associated with new technologies, have been suggested as influencing clinical treatment much more than scientific evidence. As Abel-Smith (1978, p. 17) writes,

> If a physician wants to order diagnostic tests or use surgery . . . he expects the sky to be the limit. But if he were to decide to prescribe . . . just a concrete ramp to enable a wheel chair patient to get in and out of his home the physician's expectations and the public's suddenly become circumscribed.

In the academic setting especially, centers of excellence depend upon enterprising groups of individuals becoming experts and specialists in the latest technologies. Critics charge that high technologies are sought primarily to advance professional careers, rather than to provide medical benefits to patients. Strategies for controlling runaway technology include adjusting the way physicians are reimbursed to reduce the incentive to use expensive technologies (Hsiao *et al.,* 1988a,b); improving technology assessment and eliminating non-beneficial or only marginally beneficial technologies; preventing physicians from profiting from referrals to high technology service centers (Hyman *et al.,* 1989; Morreim, 1989; Todd *et al.,* 1989; Stark, 1989; Relman, 1987); educating clinicians to be more prudent in judging the costs and benefits of new technologies (Soumerai *et al.,* 1990); and curbing citizens demands for high technologies (Brett *et al.,* 1986; Callahan, 1990). In general, these authors maintain that the burden of proof in high technology medicine should be shifted to those who urge proceeding with new technologies full speed ahead.

Further support for rationing medical technology is based on the belief that no one has a right to receive the latest medical technologies in the first place. Such a stance is consistent with beliefs we hold in other areas. For example, in the area of education, we do not think that students' rights are infringed because public schools do not provide them with ergonomic chairs or the latest computer software. Likewise, in the area of health care, denying public support for the leading edge does not imply that our health care system treats patients unjustly.

Despite its appeal, the proposal to ration publicly-supported high technology can be faulted on several grounds. First, although certain forms of health care are above and beyond what society is morally obligated to provide, the practical difficulty is to identify forms of care that fall under this heading. Technological sophistication alone is not an adequate gauge. Especially where technology is defined broadly, to include technical complexity, newness, costliness, and related features, such as scarcity and professional expertise, it is not a sensitive tool.

Second, much of the criticism directed against public support for high technology medicine speaks to the unwarranted *use* of medical technologies in clinical practice (Jennett, 1986). These objections do not establish that *technology per se* should be rationed. The soundness of limiting the use of technologies will depend upon the extent of medical benefits those technologies afford in specific, clinical applications and whether they qualify as basic or non-basic forms of medical care. We discuss these criteria in more detail below.

Finally, a major drawback of rationing publicly-financed high technology is that today's high technologies are tomorrow's low technologies. Developing new technologies is important as a pathway to improving the overall level of health care in society. For example, if Congress had failed to extend Medicare to cover the cost of hemodialysis, then many patients who can now live happy and productive lives would have died prematurely. We regard this objection as important and decisive.

b. Rationing Non-basic Services

A second form of resource-centered rationing advocates rationing non-basic services that exceed a basic floor (Schelling, 1978). On this model, those whose primary concern is obtaining a basic floor depend on the imposition of a ceiling for the resources they need.

The floor is elaborated in a variety of ways. Some elaborate the floor in terms of the government's minimum obligation defined as the least health services the public feels compelled to provide individuals, merely because they need help (Rosenthal, 1978). Others identify the floor as including those services most people use most of the time. Still others judge that the basic floor should encompass primary care generally, and include such items as immunizations, basic health education, inexpensive curative therapies, relief for chronic conditions, emergency care and palliative care (Churchill, 1987). Finally, some associate basic care with less technologically sophisticated services.

We submit that basic health care refers to health services that prevent, cure or compensate for deficiencies in the normal opportunities persons enjoy at each stage of life (Daniels, 1985). We define the normal range both *biologically,* in terms of typical species functioning, and *socially,* in terms of the level of health care resources available in society-at-large. For example, in old age, disabilities in activities of daily living can restrict normal opportunities; home health care is a form of basic care that can compensate for these restrictions. Yet basic care does not include the most advanced form of computer-assisted rehabilitative care. Although the most advanced form of computer-assisted rehabilitative care may compensate for opportunities that are normal for a typical member of the species, such care does not restore opportunities that are normal within the context of our society, i.e., given our present level of technological development and the amount of money we devote to health care.

In contrast to basic care, non-basic care either aims to improve conditions unrelated to normal opportunities *or* it aims to correct or compensate for deficiencies in normal opportunities but is ineffective in doing so. Efforts to improve conditions unrelated to normal opportunity include face lifts, breast augmentation or genetic engineering designed to enhance athletic skill or physical beauty beyond some average base line. By contrast, using penicillin to treat a viral infection is an example of an ineffective effort to improve a condition (viral infection) that has the potential to impair normal opportunities. Another example of an ineffective effort is maintaining a patient who is in a permanently vegetative state on a respirator. So long as normal opportunities remain forever beyond the patient's reach, treatment merely continues the patient's unconscious existence.

Proposals to ration non-basic health care are justified, first, by establishing that government is responsible to provide basic health care; and second, by arguing that society must ration publicly-financed non-basic care in order to prevent the cost of basic health care for all citizens from becoming prohibitive. In support of the first claim, it has been argued that society should provide a decent standard of health care because failing to do so works against the interests of all of us. For example, persons who lack adequate health care are less able to make productive contributions to the economy and community.

A principle of enforced benevolence lends further support to the claim that the public should shoulder a responsibility to ensure that citizens' basic health care needs are met (Buchanan, 1983). On this view, there exists a moral obligation of charity or beneficence to help those in need, including providing the needy with certain forms of health care. However, private acts of charity are rarely adequate to provide many important forms of health care, such as technologies that require coordination of diverse groups or large scale interdisciplinary programs. The conclusion of this argument is that government mechanisms to ensure that sufficient contributions and coordination take place are justified.

Third, it has been claimed that basic health care is a societal obligation for the reason that individuals have a right to basic health care. A right to basic care may be held to follow from the fact that considerable public dollars are spent on health care. Although some have argued that physicians own the medical services they sell (Sade, 1971), it can be argued to the contrary that public dollars underwrite a significant share of the cost of medical education and medical research and the demand for medical services. Public institutions also afford the environment in which and the structure through which much medical activity occurs. A right to basic health care also might be thought to follow from a more general property right to natural resources (Brody, 1981). This argument begins with the claim that all members of society own natural resources, such as viruses, molds, minerals, and plants. It proceeds with the observation that many basic health care resources are produced from these resources. According to one estimate, one in four prescription drugs in the United States comes from natural resources (Altman, 1989). This implies that the public partly owns many health care resources, although those who invest the labor needed to create usable products out of national resources also own a share of these resources. The conclusion of this argument states that people possess rights to basic health care and a government that fails to ensure access to basic health care violates these rights.

A fourth and final argument supporting the idea that the responsibility for basic health care should be shouldered by the public is that the alternative of letting basic care be bought and sold on a free market is unacceptable. In the first place, distributing health care on a free market runs afoul of long standing ethical traditions in medicine. In its very first Code of Medical Ethics, the American Medical Association called upon physicians to offer care to individuals in indigent circumstances in a free and cheerful manner (American Medical Association, 1985). More recently, a 1987 American Medical Association House of Delegates affirmed this tradition by approving a policy which urged all physicians to share in the care of indigent patients (Lundberg et al., 1988). Furthermore, if all citizens partly own health care goods, then the sale of health services on a free market violates the rights of all citizens who do not share in the profits of free exchange.

If we accept the claim that there is a social obligation to provide basic health care, the corresponding claim that rationing non-basic care is essential to make basic health care affordable gains support on several grounds. First, if health care is to occupy a responsible place in our common life, we must not allocate so much of our national wealth to health that we impoverish support of other social goods, such as education and the environment. This argument continues that a government that chooses to pay the cost of non-basic, as well as basic, care, will be forced to shirk its responsibilities in other areas. The remedy is for government to limit its sights to basic health care and broaden its perspective to include the full range of social goods.

Another way of mounting an argument for rationing non-basic health care appeals to the idea that persons have no right to receive extravagant health services in the first place; hence, rationing publicly-funded non-basic care to make more basic care affordable is consistent with justice. For example, no one has a right to receive luxurious treatments, such as liposuction or a face lift at the public's expense. Therefore, denying public support for such care violates no one's rights. Presumably, persons also have no right that society pay for other kinds of medical services that do not fall under the heading of basic care. For example, a patient with irreversible respiratory disease who is in the intensive care unit in a severely obtunded state, who cannot be weaned from the ventilator despite repeated efforts, and who will never recover to survive outside an intensive care setting, has no right to receive continued care at the public's expense. Under the circumstances, continued treatment does not represent a form of basic health care that the patient can claim as a matter of right.

2. Patient-Centered Criteria

a. Rationing Services to Patients Who Receive the Least Medical Benefit

Once public policies governing resource-centered rationing are enacted, persons who interface more directly with patients may employ patient-centered standards to distribute health care within specific categories. Patient-centered criteria highlight specific characteristics of individuals and regard these as the ultimate support for rationing policies. Under this heading fall rationing policies that seek to provide scarce services to individuals likely to receive the greatest medical benefit while denying them to patients likely to gain the least.

A medical benefit standard should be distinguished from a standard, such as Oregon's, that rations medical care for different illness categories based on whether that care, on average, offers greater improvements in health and quality of life per dollar spent. Under Oregon's plan, conditions falling under the same disease category are considered homogeneous, even though these conditions may have diverse etiologies and treatments may offer dissimilar medical benefits. For example, Aaron and Schwartz (1990) make the point that under Oregon's proposal, all stages of esophageal stricture are placed in one category in order to determine whether the state should pay for them. Yet degree of stricture of the esophagus can vary widely and require widely different interventions that have diverse benefits and costs. Similarly, Oregon lumps together all patients with renal failure, while ignoring a wide range of factors that affect outcome and benefits. Although some generalizing will of course be needed to put a medical benefit standard into practice, under a true medical benefit standard it will be medical benefit, not disease category, that is the basis for generalizing.

A foreseeable consequence of rationing by medical benefit is that certain visible groups may be denied specific treatments because these treatments can be more beneficial, on average, to other patient groups. For example, rationing intensive care unit services according to medical benefit may result in denial of these services to elderly persons in chronically poor health and with poor short-term survival rates (Knaus et al., 1983). However, a medical benefit approach is not the same as utilitarian approaches that incorporate social worth criteria. Whereas utilitarian approaches ask which use of resources produces the greatest benefit to *society at large,* a medical benefit approach is patient-centered, and asks which use of resources produces the greatest benefit to *particular patients or patient groups.*

Several arguments can be put forward in favor of rationing according to medical benefit. First, confining selection criteria to medical benefit avoids making comparisons between persons in terms of social worth. Second, not excluding outright any group from medical consideration also avoids invidious discrimination against particular groups. Finally, rationing on the basis of medical benefit builds on the idea that physicians' obligation to offer care strengthens as the quality and likelihood of benefits increase, yet no physician is obligated to offer futile treatment.[1] Futile treatment does not refer only to situations where the physician literally cannot do anything that will have any effect at all. It also includes cases in which medical benefits are highly improbable and situations where although the likelihood of some benefit may be good, the quality of benefit is extremely poor. For example, we agree with those who argue that medical treatment is futile where there is a negligible chance that a patient will wake up from a coma or where the best that can be hoped for is survival that requires the patient's entire preoccupation with intensive medical treatment (Schneiderman *et al.* 1990).

One objection to rationing based on medical benefit invokes the substantial difficulty of designing accurate and feasible tools for assessing benefit. Efforts to do so are often exceedingly cumbersome and difficult to implement. For example, Engelhardt and Rie (1986) developed an apparently simple equation for measuring societal obligation to pay for a patient's treatment in an ICU: societal obligation = PQL/C. In this equation, P refers to probability of successful outcome, Q to quality of success, L to length of life and C to cost required to achieve therapeutic success. However, the difficulty in measuring likelihood of success, quality of success, and length of survival is formidable. Rather than viewing this problem as decisive, however, we believe it points to a need to target research to developing accurate methods for assessing medical benefit.

A second objection to rationing by medical benefit insists that persons who knowingly choose to engage in unhealthy behaviors, such as excessive drinking or smoking, are less deserving of the medical benefits health services provide (Loewy, 1980; Knowles, 1990; Blank, 1988). Yet this objection is uncompelling. Much illness occurs at random and much is genetic (Price, 1978). Also, an individual's ability to consider the effects of decisions is itself an acquired skill that lower socioeconomic and educational groups are at a disadvantage to acquire. Thus, focusing on individual responsibility for health is likely to mask deeper social ills, such as poverty and lack of education, that influence the choice of risky lifestyles (Crawford, 1990). In addition, we are far from being able to tell accurately whether particular patients' health problems are caused by prior behaviors or would have occurred in the absence of these behaviors. More importantly, refusing health services to persons who live unhealthy lifestyles is at odds with our considered judgements about ethical medical practice. We would not accept the practice of physicians routinely refusing therapy to consumers of cholesterol, persons with venereal disease, those who choose to live in polluted urban areas, or the sedentary portion of the population (Atterbury, 1986). Our society's emphasis on liberty of the individual also places limits on any far reaching effort to compel or pressure people to lead healthy lives.

A final objection to rationing by medical benefit is that this approach does not incorporate the perspective of patients. According to this objection, medical benefit can be distinguished from *patient* benefit. Medical benefit refers to success in achieving significant goals of medicine, such as weaning a patient from a respirator or improving the patient's overall physiological condition. Determining whether or not a particular intervention will yield medical benefits requires the exercise of medical judgment and expertise, plus familiarity with medical facts and research findings. By contrast, patient benefit refers to success in achieving the goals of a particular patient.

The difficulty with this objection lies in the sharp distinction it tries to draw between patient and medical benefit. Properly understood, a medical benefit standard takes into account the values and goals a patient holds, as well as the physiological effects treatment will have for a particular patient. Thus, medical benefit does not mean the same thing as medical effect, nor is it merely equivalent to what the patient wishes. A broader interpretation of medical benefit is not vulnerable to the objection that the patient's perspective is not taken sufficiently into account.

b. Rationing Services That Are Not Equally Available

Unlike the patient-centered proposals glimpsed thus far, a principle of equality focuses on similarities, rather than differences, between persons. The guiding idea of this approach is that all individuals possess an equal worth and dignity. Thus, differences in persons' income, social productivity or wisdom do not imply that individuals are more or less worthy. In the area of health care, such a perspective lends support to the view that persons are equally entitled to receive health services. According to one interpretation, equal entitlement implies a principle of equal access. This principle states that whenever a health service is available to any individual, it should be effectively available to any other person who has similar medical needs (Gutmann, 1983). A second interpretation of equal entitlement allows some inequalities in health care, but seeks to eliminate differences in non-basic care. This approach either categorically restricts high levels of health care consumption, or requires that consumption at high levels benefit those who are least advantaged. For example, according to the latter approach if artificial hearts were likely to become available to the least advantaged in the future, then funding their selective use now can be ethically justified.

Both forms of an equality argument have merit. The first form resembles a medical benefit criterion in several key respects. Just as medical benefit implies that persons who will *benefit equally* from a particular treatment have an equal claim to receive it, a principle of equal access specifies that persons with *equal needs* for health care are equally entitled to that care. Both standards allow rationing health care to persons who would benefit less. Thus, much of the assessment given in connection with medical benefit applies to equal access as well. The alternative interpretation of equality, which favors imposing a ceiling on health care consumption, is made convincing by considering that our hesitancy to restrict access to high levels of health care may simply reflect the fact that we envision the possibility of ourselves being in a position to need and receive such care. Allowing or even applauding high levels of consumption keeps alive for us the idea of some day having access to high levels of consumption ourselves. If correct, this explanation bolsters the equality argument which calls for placing a ceiling on health care consumption. It reveals that our tolerance of inequalities is based more on the prospect of personal advantage than ethical considerations of justice and fairness.

Part II: Summary and Proposal

We have framed a variety of proposals concerning the just management of scarce health care resources in terms of resource- and patient-centered rationing. We now are prepared to evaluate this framework and weigh the strength and weakness of different rationing proposals. It is our hope that the framework we have identified affords clearer direction to present rationing debates and that the proposals we support furnish an ethically viable alternative to the age rationing proposals that are currently championed.

Our framework aims to achieve two central goals. First, it intends to clarify the context in which different rationing criteria apply. Proposals to ration high technology or ration non-basic care generally apply to legislators, hospital administrators, and governmental bodies who make choices about the distribution of scarce dollars between different health care categories. Proposals to ration based on medical benefit or the equality of persons generally apply to settings in which persons more directly involved with patient care and management distribute scarce health care resources between patients. A second goal of this framework is to highlight the ethical bases for different rationing choices. Arguments for rationing may point to ethically relevant features of resources themselves or to ethically important differences between persons.

Although the framework we have proposed marks progress toward achieving these goals, it is incomplete. Several features of it require further development. First, the categories of resource- and patient-centered rationing should be supplemented to accommodate rationing criteria that do not fit well into either category. For example, society-centered rationing may be added to accommodate criteria such as rationing based on social value. This criterion would deny scarce health care resources to individuals who have relatively less social value, where social value is measured by factors such as income, community service, occupation, or other standards. In addition to locating a fuller range of ethical reasons for rationing, a more complete approach should: consider a large number of rationing criteria; further clarify the ideas of high technology, basic care, and medical benefit; and place rationing within the broader context of the allocation of resources between health care and other social goods.

We now turn to the specific rationing criteria explored throughout the paper. These include rationing high technology services, rationing non-basic services, rationing services to patients who receive the least medical benefit, and rationing services that are not equally available. In light of the arguments discussed above, we submit the following four point proposal.

(1) First, we reject resource-centered rationing that calls for limiting the development of publicly-financed high technology medicine. As noted above, the critical flaws with this method are that it is insensitive to medical benefit and slows, or even stops, medical progress. Such progress holds out the hope of raising the level of health care for all. Rationing the use of high technology may be ethically defensible, but should not be done in a categorical fashion or any other manner that ignores relevant patient-centered factors. Neither the development nor the use of medical services should be rationed on the ground that they are high technology services.

(2) Second, we endorse resource-centered policies that place limits on publicly-financed non-basic health services. The practical problem will be determining which services fall under basic and non-basic health care categories. Making this determination requires qualitative assessment in which specific health services are classified as basic or non-basic. The classification is not static, but is relative both to the amount of money available to spend on health care and the level of medical technology available in the society at large. Nonetheless, it is possible to put forward a general standard: "basic health" care prevents, cures or compensates

for deficiencies in the normal range of opportunities people enjoy at each stage of life.

(3) Third, we hold that a medical benefit standard should be used to distribute health care resources between persons. Successfully implementing a medical benefit standard requires improving technology assessment in order to better predict the likelihood, magnitude, and duration of medical benefits to particular patients and patient groups. Here the goal should be to reduce, rather than eliminate, uncertainty.

(4) Finally, we submit that equality be the goal in provision of basic health care. This means that departures from equal basic care will require a special justification. For example, a non-basic health service that is on the leading edge of medical knowledge may be a candidate for public support if it promises to eventually improve basic health care for all. Generally speaking, the justification for support of non-basic services must be linked to improvements in basic care.

Ability to pay is another patient-centered standard that we have discussed more briefly in the context of discussing other rationing criteria. It is our view that inability to pay should not be a basis for excluding patients from basic health care. Instead, basic health care should be guaranteed. However, ability to pay can be used as a means to distribute non-basic health services. As noted above, funding of non-basic care is more accurately thought of as an act of supererogation, rather than a requirement of justice. Although people may ideally like government to pay for all the health care they desire, rationing non-basic care to persons who cannot afford its costs does not violate persons' rights. It also seems unlikely that individuals would be willing to give up completely their present freedom to use their own resources to purchase medical services. Individual freedom is an important value, and a viable approach to rationing must balance ethical factors against pragmatic considerations.

In summary, the cornerstone of our proposal is a commitment to basic care and patient-centered standards. Although age-based proposals represent a patient-centered approach, our proposal improves on the shortcomings of age rationing in several key respects. First, by emphasizing medical benefit, rather than age, our proposal is sensitive to differences between patients at each stage of life. For example, *within* age groups patients may have widely different life prospects and health status. And *between* age groups, healthier older persons may stand to gain much more than younger, sicker patients. Second, our proposal underscores the idea of equality and the related idea that persons at all ages possess an incalculable worth and dignity. By contrast, discriminating on the basis of age may denigrate the value and worth of elderly persons. Or it may signal that older persons can be legitimately disenfranchised from goods other than health care. Finally, our proposal supports funding basic health services for all age groups. Our arguments cast doubt on the idea that public support of non-basic care for the young or the old is a requirement of justice. Although tentative in nature, we believe our proposal constitutes a first step toward fashioning an ethical approach to rationing health care.

NOTE

1. Although the training and culture of modern medicine may reinforce a tendency to provide futile treatment and to do "everything possible" for the patient, this approach runs contrary to the historical and ethical roots of medicine (see Jecker, 1991; Schneiderman, Jecker, and Jonsen, 1990). This approach also reinforces the false belief that physicians have nothing to offer patients when no medical cure is possible (see Jecker and Self, 1991).

REFERENCES

Abel-Smith, B.: 1978, "Minimum adequate levels of personal health care: History and justification", *Milbank Memorial Fund Quarterly* 57, 212–213.

Altman, L.L.: 1989, "Tracking a new drug from the soil in Japan to organ transplants", *New York Times*, 31 October, B6.

American Medical Association: 1985, "Code of medical ethics", in S.J. Reiser, A.J. Dych, and W.J. Curran (eds.), *Ethics in Medicine: Historical Perspectives and Contemporary Concerns*, MIT Press, Cambridge, Massachusetts, pp. 26–34.

Atterbury, C.E.: 1986, "The alcoholic in the lifeboat: Should drinkers be candidates for liver transplant?", *Journal of Gastroenterology* 8, 1–4.

Blank, R.: 1988, *Rationing Medicine*, Columbia University Press, New York.

Brett, A. and McCullough, L.B.: 1986, "When patients request specific interventions: Defining the limits of the physician's obligation", *New England Journal of Medicine* 315, 1347–1351.

Brody, B.A.: 1981, "Health care for the haves and have nots: Toward a just basis of distribution", in E.E. Shelp (ed.), *Justice and Health Care*, Reidel Publishing Company, Dordrecht, The Netherlands, pp. 151–160.

Buchanan, A.: 1983, "The right to a decent minimum of health care", in President's Commission for the Study of Ethical Problems in Medicine and Biomedical and Behavioral Research, *Securing Access to Health Care*, Vol. 2, Government Printing Office, Washington, D.C., pp. 207–238.

Callahan, D.: 1987, *Setting Limits: Medical Goals in an Aging Society*, Simon and Schuster, New York.

Callahan, D.: 1990, *What Kind of Life: The Limits of Medical Progress,* Simon and Schuster, New York.

Churchill, L.R.: 1987, *Rationing Health Care in America: Perceptions and Principles of Justice,* University of Notre Dame Press, Notre Dame.

Crawford, R.: 1990, "Individual responsibility and health politics", in P. Conrad and R. Kern (eds.) *The Sociology of Health and Illness,* 3rd ed., St. Martin's Press, New York, pp. 387–395.

Daniels, N.: 1985, *Just Health Care,* Cambridge University Press, New York.

Engelhardt, H.T. and Rie, M.A.: 1986, "Intensive care units, scarce resources, and conflicting principles of justice", *Journal of the American Medical Association* 255, 1159–1164.

Gutmann, A.: 1983, "For and against equal access to health care", in President's Commission for the Study of Ethical Problems in Medicine and Biomedical and Behavioral Research, *Securing Access to Health Care,* Vol. 2, Government Printing Office, Washington, D.C., pp. 51–66.

Hsiao, W., Braun, P., Dunn, D., *et al.*: 1988a, "Results and policy implications of the resource-based relative-value study", *New England Journal of Medicine* 319, 881–888.

Hsiao, W., Braun, P., Yntema, D., *et al.*: 1988b, "Estimating physicians work for a resource-based relative-value scale", *New England Journal of Medicine* 319, 835–841.

Hyman, D.A. and Williamson, J.V.: 1989, "Fraud and abuse: Setting the limits on physicians' entrepreneurship", *New England Journal of Medicine* 320, 1275–1278.

Jecker, N.S.: 1988, "Disenfranchising the elderly from life-extending medical care", *Public Affairs Quarterly* 2, 51–68.

Jecker, N.S.: 1989, "Towards a theory of age group justice", *Journal of Medicine and Philosophy* 14, 655–676.

Jecker, N.S.: 1991, "Knowing when to stop: The limits of Medicine", *Hastings Center Report* 21, 5–8.

Jecker, N.S. and Pearlman, R.A.: 1989, "Ethical constraints on rationing medical care by age", *Journal of the American Geriatrics Society* 37,1067–1075.

Jecker, N.S. and Self, D.J.: 1991, "Separating care and cure: Historical and contemporary images of nursing and medicine", *Journal of Medicine and Philosophy* 16, 285–306.

Jennett, B.: 1986, *High Technology Medicine: Benefits and Burdens,* Oxford University Press, New York.

Knaus, W.A., Draper, E.A. and Wagner, D.P.: 1983, "The use of intensive care: New research initiatives and their implications for national health policy", *Milbank Memorial Fund Quarterly* 61, 561–583.

Knowles, J.H.: 1990, "The responsibility of the individual", in P. Conrad and R. Kern (eds.), *The Sociology of Health and Illness,* 3rd ed., St. Martin's Press, New York, pp. 376–386.

Loewy, E.: 1980, "Letter to the Editor", *New England Journal of Medicine* 302, 697.

Lundberg, G.D. and Bodine, L.: 1988, "Fifty houses for the poor", *Journal of the American Medical Association* 260, 3178.

McGregor, M.: 1989, "Technology and the allocation of resources", *New England Journal of Medicine* 320, 118–120.

Morreim, E.H.: 1989, "Conflicts of interest: Profits and problems in physician referrals", *Journal of the American Medical Association* 262, 390–394.

Price, D.: 1978, "Planning and administrative perspectives on adequate minimum personal health services", *Milbank Memorial Fund Quarterly* 56, 22–50.

Relman, A.: 1987, "Practicing medicine in the new business climate", *New England Journal of Medicine* 316, 1150–1151.

Rosenthal, G. and Fox, D.M.: 1978, "A right to what: Toward adequate minimum standards for personal health services", *Milbank Memorial Fund Quarterly* 56, 1–6.

Sade, R.: 1971, "Medical care as a right: A refutation", *New England Journal of Medicine* 285, 1288–1292.

Schelling, T.C.: 1978, "Standards for adequate minimum personal health services", *Milbank Memorial Fund Quarterly* 57, 212–213.

Schneiderman, L.J., Jecker, N.S. and Jonsen, A.R.: 1990, "Medical futility: Its meaning and ethical implications", *Annals of Internal Medicine* 112, 949–954.

Schwartz, W.B. and Aaron, H.J.: 1990, "The Achilles heel of health care rationing", *New York Times,* 9 July.

Soumerai, S.B. and Avron, J.: 1990, "Principles of educational outreach ('academic detailing') to improve clinical decision making", *Journal of the American Medical Association* 263, 549–556.

Stark, F.H.: 1989, "Physicians' conflicts in patient referrals", *Journal of the American Medical Association* 262, 397.

Todd, J.S. and Horan, J.K.: 1989, "Physician referral: The AMA view", *Journal of the American Medical Association* 262, 395–396.

Wennberg, J.E.: 1984, "Dealing with medical practice variations: A proposal for action", *Health Affairs* 3, 6–32.